Abnormal Hemoglobins in Human Populations

Abnormal Hemoglobins in Human Populations

Frank B. Livingstone

With a new introduction by Jonathan Marks

ALDINETRANSACTION
A Division of Transaction Publishers
New Brunswick (U.S.A.) and London (U.K.)

First paperback edition 2009
 All inquiries should be addressed to AldineTransaction, A Division of Transaction Publishers, Rutgers—The State University of New Jersey, 35 Berrue Circle, Piscataway, New Jersey 08854-8042. www.transactionpub.com

This book is printed on acid-free paper that meets the American National Standard for Permanence of Paper for Printed Library Materials.

Library of Congress Catalog Number: 2009008713
ISBN: 978-0-202-36264-9
Printed in the United States of America

Library of Congress Cataloging-in-Publication Data

Livingstone, Frank B.
Abnormal hemoglobins in human populations / Frank B. Livingstone.
p. ; cm.
Originally published: Chicago : Aldine, c1967, in series: Perspectives on the biology of man. With new introd.
Includes bibliographical references and index.
ISBN 978-0-202-36264-9 (alk. paper)
1. Hemoglobinopathy--Genetic aspects. I. Title.
[DNLM: 1. Hemoglobins, Abnormal. WH 190 L788ab 1967a]

RC641.7.H35L5 2009
362.196'157--dc22

2009008713

CONTENTS

List of Illustrations

List of Tables

Introduction to the AldineTransaction Edition

Frank Livingstone's career lay at the crossroads of anthropology and genetics, an intersection that has lately become heavily trafficked.

In the 1950s and 1960s, however, it was a very rare specialty. This was partly for historical, and partly for epistemic, reasons. Genetics and anthropology had converged twice before, in major scientific research programs, and they seemed to be fundamentally at odds with one another. In the first decades of the twentieth century, the eugenics movement, led by the geneticist Charles B. Davenport, framed itself specifically in opposition to the cultural-historical anthropology of Franz Boas. It visualized economic and social hierarchies as being rooted in underlying genetic hierarchies, and set out to sterilize the poor and to restrict immigration in the name of the American gene pool. The eugenics movement, however, lost much of its credibility with the stock market crash (reshuffling the economic hierarchy) and the accession of the Nazis (taking eugenics to its logical extreme).[1] The movement was nevertheless sufficiently mainstream in American science that when Charles Davenport died in 1944, he was the sitting President of the American Association of Physical Anthropologists.

The other intersection between anthropology and genetics spanned roughly the 1920s through the 1950s, and was known as racial serology. The problem of racial serology was not so much an embarrassing political history, but the difficulty in making any reasonable sense of its data. In an age when the classification and proper placement of human populations were the paramount questions in physical anthropology, what might it mean if, for example, the detectable ABO blood group allele frequencies were the same for Poles and Chinese? According to the geneticists, such as Laurence Snyder (1926), Alexander Weiner

(1946), and William Boyd (1950), it meant that the human groups identifiable to geneticists were more real than the groups identified by anthropologists. To the anthropologists, such as Earnest Hooton (1931), Ashley Montagu (1946), and T. Dale Stewart (1951), it meant that geneticists were simply doing something wrong, and were observing scientific artifacts that had no obvious connection to the major natural patterns of human variation.[2]

It is really only in the historical context of the antagonism between anthropology and human genetics—which itself has been replayed in various ways in recent generations—that Frank Livingstone's role in biological anthropology can be appreciated. While other biological anthropologists had collected genetic data, and had tried to integrate genetic data into their researches, Livingstone's work on the relationship between hemoglobins and malaria provided the first synthetic vision of human genetics and anthropology. He opened up anthropological genetics to anthropologists, and placed that specialization into the mainstream of anthropological research.

Abnormal Hemoglobins in Human Populations, first published in 1967, was the culmination of a decade of Livingstone's thought. Building on the work of geneticists and clinicians who postulated that certain hereditary blood diseases might be advantageous to unaffected carriers by protecting them against malaria, Livingstone tabulated the global frequencies of these hereditary diseases and explained them— perhaps a bit too deterministically!—in the context of local biological and cultural histories. While it probably doesn't matter whether any specific population has an allele frequency of 8% or 11%, given the vagaries of sampling error and human demography, certainly the demonstration that the allele frequencies (1) are clinal, (2) are correlated with malaria, and (3) involve multiple genetic loci and multiple alleles, permit as robustly as one could reasonably hope, the inference that natural selection is at work here. And perhaps the most interesting take-home lesson is that the human gene pools are co-evolving with human culture, as malaria itself as a major stressor on human populations is plausibly linked to the standing water brought by swidden agriculture in West Africa, and to domestic cattle as vectors in East Africa.

Certainly the most significant growth in our understanding of hemoglobin genetics since then has come at the molecular level. Sickle-cell is an allele of β (beta)–globin, located at the tip of human chromosome 11, and located alongside a specialized embryonic form of the gene (ε, epsilon), two fetal forms (γ, gamma), a non-functional copy or pseudogene (ψη, pseudo-eta), and a minor adult gene (δ, delta), which is transcribed at a very low rate compared with β-globin. The principal causes of β-thalassemia are point mutations in the regulatory signals, which compromise the activity of the gene. By contrast, the α-thalassemia genotype is primarily caused by deleting one of the tandemly duplicated α-globin genes, on chromosome 16. The α-globin cluster is composed of an embryonic gene (ζ, zeta), several pseudogenes, a gene whose function remains unknown

(θ, theta), and two α-globin genes. The wide range of expression of this disease results from five principal genotypes, which extend from having four functional α-globin genes to having none at all. Further, in East Asian populations α-thalassemia is now seen to play a genetic role analogous to that of sickle-cell.[3]

But perhaps even more interesting is the contemporary study of the hemoglobinopathies, and of human genetics in general, by social scientists, stimulated by the Human Genome Project's program called ELSI, or Ethical, Legal, and Social Implications. Anthropological interest in genetics has expanded to the extent that not only is significant work proceeding *qua* biological anthropology, but as well within the neighboring intellectual territory of medical anthropology.[4] It is in this context that we learn of sickle-cell not simply as an avatar of microevolution, but as a model of the general failure of a genetic screening program.[5] Moreover, we now encounter genetics as the basis for new forms of kinship relations, or biosociality—for example, in the bonds formed by otherwise unrelated bearers of disease genes, the formation of "mitochondrial clans," and the search for distant ancestral genetic ("real") roots.[6] Much of this takes place today in a privatized, free-market context, where results are bought and sold, analytic techniques are under patent and black-boxed, and the cultural meanings of genetic data are being actively transformed, largely disconnected from their scientific value.[7] Moreover, the collection and maintenance of genetic samples from indigenous peoples is being called into question from the perspective of property rights, and in the shadow of colonialism.[8] The intersection of anthropology and genetics is thus far more anthropological today, and in far more "holistic" senses, than was imaginable in 1967.[9]

Finally, we have the twin specters of race reification and scientific racism. Frank Livingstone will be remembered for his 1962 proclamation, "There are no races, there are only clines,"[10] which effectively summarized one aspect of the post-WWII synthesis known as "the new physical anthropology." In this view, the dynamic study of local populations under the sway of microevolutionary forces would replace the static classificatory practices which had dominated the scientific study of human diversity for two centuries.[11] Several decades later, however, some reactionary geneticists have begun to argue that the new physical anthropology got it all wrong—those macro-clusters of human populations that we thought were transient and ephemeral, the products of the classifying mind rather than the human gene pool, are really real, after all! Not coincidentally, this position is convergent with the attempt of pharmaceutical companies to develop racial niche markets for their products—the vanguard of which was BiDil, a specifically African-American heart medication.[12]

And this reification of race is complemented by more-or-less old-fashioned scientific racism, the kind that maintains large "natural" groups of people to be constitutionally deficient in one way or another. In political terms, this means that expenditures on social programs for disadvantaged minorities are doomed to failure, for the disadvantage is innate, and is thus not the result of injustice; the money could better be spent elsewhere.[13] In the 1960s, the issue was segregation, and its advocates numbered at least one prominent physical anthropologist among their numbers, Carleton S. Coon, who offered an idiosyncratic interpretation of the human fossil record and gene pool to support the cause.[14] Today *de jure* segregation is mercifully no longer an issue, but sadly, there is a new generation of scholars willing to abuse anthropological genetics similarly in support of reactionary social politics.[15] To them, Frank Livingstone's vision of an anthropological genetics will always be anathema; but to the rest of us, it remains a vigorous intellectual arena where the study of heredity and of culture converge and critically intersect one another, to their mutual benefit.

Jonathan Marks
University of North Carolina at Charlotte
September 2008

Notes

1. Davenport, C. B. (1911) *Heredity in Relation to Eugenics*. New York: Henry Holt. Boas, F. (1916) Eugenics. *Scientific Monthly*, 3:471-479. Allen, G. E. (1983) The Misuse of Biological Hierarchies: The American Eugenics Movement, 1900-1940. *History and Philosophy of the Life Sciences*, 5:105-128. Kevles, D. J. (1985) *In the Name of Eugenics*. Berkeley: University of California Press. Kühl, S. (1994) *The Nazi Connection*. New York: Oxford University Press.
2. Snyder, L. (1926) Human blood groups: Their inheritance and racial significance. *American Journal of Physical Anthropology*, 9: 233-263. Wiener, A. S. (1946) Blood Group Factors and Racial Relationships. *Science*, 103:147. Boyd, W. C. (1950) *Genetics and the Races of Man*. Boston: Little, Brown. Hooton, E. A. (1931) *Up from the Ape*. New York: Macmillan, p. 490. Montagu, M. F. A. (1946) Blood Group Factors and Ethnic Relationships. *Science*, 103:284. Rowe, C. (1950) Genetics vs. physical anthropology in determining racial types. *Southwestern Journal of Anthropology*, 6:197-211. Strandskov, H. H. and Washbum, S. L. (1951) Editorial: Genetics and Physical Anthropology. *American Journal of Physical Anthropology*, 9:261-263. Stewart, T. D. (1951) Objectivity in Racial Classifications. *American Journal of Physical Anthropology*, 9: 470-472. Birdsell, J. B. (1952) On Various Levels of Objectivity in Genetical Anthropology. *American Journal of Physical Anthropology*, 10: 355-362.
3. Marks, J. (1989) Human Micro- and Macro-Evolution in the Primate Alpha-Globin Gene Family. *American Journal of Human Biology*, 1:555-566.
4. Koenig, B., Lee, S., and Richardson, S. (2009) *Revisiting Race in a Genomic Age*, Piscataway, NJ: Rutgers University Press.
5. Duster, T. (1990) *Backdoor to Eugenics*. New York: Routledge. Wailoo, K. and Pemberton, S. (2006) *The Troubled Dream of Genetic Medicine: Disease and Ethnicity in Tay-Sachs, Cystic Fibrosis, and Sickle Cell Disease*. Baltimore, MD: Johns Hopkins University Press.
6. Sykes, B. (2001) *The Seven Daughters of Eve: The Science that Reveals our Genetic Ancestry*. New York: WW Norton. Rapp, R., Heath, D. and Taussig, K. (2001)

Genealogical Disease: Where Hereditary Abnormality, Biomedical Explanation, and Family Responsibility Meet. In: *Relative Values: Reconfiguring Kinship Studies*, ed. by Franklin, S. and McKinnon, S. Durham, NC: Duke University Press, pp. 384–412. Palmié, S. (2007) Genomics, Divination,"Racecraft." *American Ethnologist*, 34: 205-222. Bolnick, D. A., Fullwiley, D., Duster, T., Cooper, R. S., Fujimura, J., Kahn, J., Kaufman, J., Marks, J., Morning, A., Nelson, A., Ossorio, P., Reardon, J., Reverby, S., and Tallbear, K. (2007) The Science and Business of Genetic Ancestry Testing. *Science*, 318: 399-400.

7. Nelkin, D., and Lindee, M. Susan (1995) *The DNA Mystique: The Gene as Cultural Icon*. New York: Freeman.
8. Marks, J. and Harry, D. (2006) Counterpoint: Blood-Money. *Evolutionary Anthropology*, 15: 93-94.
9. Goodman, A., Heath, D. and Lindee, M., eds. (2003) *Genetic Nature/Culture: Anthropology and Science beyond the Two-Culture Divide*. Berkeley, CA: University of California Press.
10. Livingstone, F.B. (1962) On the Non-Existence of Human Races. *Current Anthropology*, 3: 279-281.
11. Washburn, S.L. (1951) The New Physical Anthropology. *Transactions of the New York Academy of Sciences, Series II*, 13:298-304. Washburn, S. L. (1963) The study of race. *American Anthropologist*, 65:521-531.
12. Kahn, J. (2004) How a Drug becomes 'Ethnic': Law, Commerce, and the Production of Racial Categories in Medicine. *Yale Journal of Health Policy, Law, and Politics*, 4:1-46. Duster, T. (2005) Race and Reification in Science. *Science*, 307: 1050-1051.
13. Herrnstein, R. and Murray, C. (1995) *The Bell Curve*. New York: Free Press.
14. Coon, C. S. (1962) *The Origin of Races*. New York: Knopf. Dobzhansky, T. (1968) More Bogus 'Science' of Race Prejudice. *Journal of Heredity*, 59:102-104. Jackson, J. P., Jr. (2001) "In Ways Unacademical": The Reception of Carleton S. Coon's *The Origin of Races*. *Journal of the History of Biology*, 34:247-285. Jackson, J. P., Jr. (2005) *Science for Segregation*. New York: NYU Press.
15. Sarich, V. and Miele, F. (2004) *Race: The Reality of Human Differences*. New York: Westview. Wade, N. (2006) *Before the Dawn: Recovering the Lost History of Our Ancestors*. New York: Penguin. Harpending, H. (2007) Anthropological Genetics: Present and Future. In: *Anthropological Genetics: Theory, Methods and Applications*, ed. by Crawford, M. H. New York: Cambridge University Press, pp. 456-466.

PREFACE

THIS STUDY is the outcome of my major scientific interest since graduate school, for which I have Dr. James V. Neel to thank, but the detailed compilation of the data was begun during a sabbatical leave from the University of Michigan, which I acknowledge with gratitude. Most of the data were collected at the University of Michigan Library, but the Harvard University Libraries and the National Library of Medicine were also visited and proved of great value. The assistance of all the librarians involved is acknowledged, and I especially want to thank Ruth L. Floyd of the University of Michigan Medical Library for tracking down and obtaining copies of all the obscure journal articles which I requested. In addition, several letters were written to colleagues whose permissions to use unpublished data are acknowledged. The graphs and maps were done by Leslie R. Thurston and the University of Michigan 7090 computer, both of whose assistance was invaluable. During the course of the study, conversations with Dr. Donald L. Rucknagel greatly assisted in the clarification of various points concerning the biochemical genetics of the hemoglobins, and Dr. George J. Brewer's assistance on the technical aspects of the glucose-6-phosphate dehydrogenase deficiency was of great value. However, neither is responsible for—nor even agrees with—the conclusions of the study. Dr. Gabriel W. Lasker also read much of the manuscript and his suggestions are gratefully acknowledged. This project has had no outside financial support, but the use of various budgets of the University of Michigan is acknowledged. Finally, I would like to thank Donna Proctor for typing the Appendix.

Frank B. Livingstone

ABNORMAL HEMOGLOBINS IN HUMAN POPULATIONS

I

INTRODUCTION

THIS BOOK is an attempt to compile the data on the frequencies of the abnormal hemoglobins, thalassemia, and the glucose-6-phosphate dehydrogenase deficiency in the world's populations. Since this is one of the most rapidly growing fields of scientific investigation, the book may become out of date even before it is published. This would seem to make it an exercise in futility. However, during the short span of the last ten years, when most of the data have been collected, we have come to know the world distributions of these traits in considerable detail, and the next few years will most likely only fill in the few existing gaps. Some surprising discoveries may still be made, but this seems an appropriate time to compile the data and attempt to interpret some of the features of these distributions.

That the growth in our knowledge of the abnormal hemoglobins, thalassemia, and the glucose-6-phosphate dehydrogenase deficiency has been explosive in the last ten years is aptly illustrated by the huge amount of data summarized in this book. Most of the studies cited appeared in medical journals, but many other sciences have contributed, especially anthropology, genetics, and biochemistry. This indicates that the data have interest for a diversity of scientific fields and is further justification for collecting the data in one place. The work on these traits has also been in the forefront of advances in these fields, and in the future it will probably continue to expand our genetic, anthropological, and medical horizons. Because we know so much about the chemistry and genetics of these traits, we can ask questions about their anthropological and populational significance that are unanswerable or even impossible to ask for most other inherited characteristics.

All the traits under consideration are inherited and for the most part due to the presence of a single gene. The basis of any interpretation of the differences among populations in these traits is, therefore, the genetic theory of evolution, which has been developed and refined over the past forty years. This theory is concerned with the forces or factors that can change the genetic characteristics of a population. There are three major forces: mutation, natural selection, and gene flow. Two other factors, random gene drift and the mating system of the population, can also influence the genetic characteristics or gene frequencies of a population. *Gene drift* is used here to include all random processes in the genetic reproduction of a finite population. The simpler deterministic models that we will consider are concerned with the effects of the first three major forces, but two computer simulations have been used to include the effects of random gene drift.

Gene flow or, in other words, migration and admixture, is the result of the exchange of individual organisms among populations. As an exchange of whole diploid sets of genes, the amount of gene flow between any two populations is the same for all individual genes or loci and hence is in no way a property of the individual gene. Similarly, random *gene drift*, which is simply the fluctuation in gene frequencies due to chance, is determined by the size of the population. The amount of gene drift that can occur varies inversely with the size of the population. It also is not a property of the individual gene in this sense. On the other hand, the remaining two forces of evolution, *mutation* and *natural selection*, can vary enormously from gene to gene. Because of this difference in the operation of the forces of evolution, when the variation in one genetic trait within the populations of a species is very different from the variation in another trait, it is difficult if not impossible to explain these differences without recourse to mutation or natural selection. Unfortunately we have very little knowledge of the effects of these two forces for most human genetic traits. The hemoglobin and glucose-6-phosphate dehydrogenase deficiency genes are two prominent exceptions to this generalization, particularly with regard to natural selection. The knowledge of the complete structure of the hemoglobin molecule has made it possible to determine the exact chemical change involved in mutation, and the anemias associated with homozygosity for many of these genes were a clear indication of the operation of natural selection. But the fact that there was so much selection against these genes implied that they must also have some selective advantage associated with them, which has since been found to be a relative resistance to malaria among the carriers for some of these traits.

Because we know so much more about the operation of the forces of evolution on the hemoglobin and glucose-6-phosphate dehydrogenase deficiency loci, we are able to use the genetic theory of evolution to interpret the distributions of these genes in much more detail than we can those of any other human genes. The major purpose of this book is to attempt such an interpretation. After a brief outline of the biochemistry and inheritance of the abnormal hemoglobins, thalassemia, and the glucose-6-phosphate dehydrogenase deficiency, the major part of the book will attempt to apply the general theorems of population genetics to the known distributions of these traits. Selection by malaria will be assumed to be the major factor causing high frequencies of these genes, so that much of this interpretation will be a correlation of the distribution of the genes with that of malaria. Most of the problems result from the absence of such a correlation in some populations.

The biochemical genetics of hemoglobin and glucose-6-phosphate dehydrogenase are the physical basis of their population genetics, but they are distinct spheres of knowledge in which I am no expert. The chapters on biochemistry have relied on the writings of specialists, in particular Ingram (339b) and the recent reviews of Braunitzer et al. (115), Huehns and Shooter(330), and Schroeder and Jones (612c).

II

THE ABNORMAL HEMOGLOBINS AND THALASSEMIA

THE ABNORMAL hemoglobins and thalassemia first came to our attention because of the anemia they can cause. In 1910 Herrick (318) first described sickle-cell anemia, and in 1925 Cooley and Lee (184) identified the thalassemia syndrome. These conditions seemed to cluster in certain families and "races," so that they were generally believed to be inherited, but it was not until the late 1940's that their inheritance was firmly established. During the intervening years the identification of these conditions was based on red blood cell morphology. For the detection of sickle cells, various kinds of sealed wet preparations were used; while for thalassemia, red cell size, shape, and resistance to lysis in hypotonic salt solution were used alone or in various combinations.

With the development and widespread use of filter paper electrophoresis in the early 1950's, knowledge of and work on the abnormal hemoglobins and thalassemia began to boom. This use of paper electrophoresis was the result of the discovery by Pauling and his associates (534a) that sickling was due to the presence of a different hemoglobin in the red cells of persons exhibiting this condition. This study also confirmed the hypothesis of Neel (506) and Beet (69) that the sickling phenomenon was due to the presence of a single gene that, when inherited from one parent, produced the benign sickle-cell trait, but when inherited from both parents resulted in sickle-cell anemia. Persons with the sickle cell trait, or heterozygotes for the sickle-cell gene, had two different kinds of hemoglobin, one like that of normal individuals and one like the hemoglobin found in persons with sickle-cell anemia, who were presumably homozygous for the sickle-cell gene.

The electrophoretic analysis of hemoglobin also resolved some of the questions raised by the hypothesis of the single gene inheritance for both the sickling phenomenon and thalassemia. It was found that some other abnormal hemoglobins when inherited in conjunction with a sickling gene would result in a clinical picture that resembled sickle-cell anemia but was not due to the simultaneous presence of two sickling genes. The reexamination of several "problem" familes, in which one parent did not sickle but one of the children had sickle-cell anemia, resulted in the discovery of new abnormal hemoglobins, which are now known as hemoglobins C and D.

In 1953 new hemoglobins began to be discovered in so many different areas of the world that an international conference was convened to set up a system to name these new discoveries (40a). At the conference it was decided to assign letters in alphabetic sequence to the new hemoglobins in the order of their discovery. Since the letter S had already been widely used for the hemoglobin causing the sickling phenomenon, it would continue to be used, although the letter B was also set aside for this hemoglobin. In addition, the letter F was reserved for fetal hemoglobin. This system proved rather unworkable because in several instances almost simultaneous publications used the same letter for different hemoglobins that they had discovered. But the system also became obsolete when techniques were developed that showed that hemoglobins assigned the same letter and thought to be identical were quite different in chemical structure.

Ingram's (339a) application of the technique of "fingerprinting" to hemoglobin was the innovation that necessitated changes in hemoglobin nomenclature. By digestion of the globin part of the hemoglobin molecule with trypsin, which broke it into several fragments or peptides, and then the successive use of electrophoresis in one direction and chromotography perpendicular to it, Ingram separated the molecule into these peptides. He first found the specific difference between normal adult hemoglobin and sickle-cell hemoglobin. That the sickling phenomenon was due to the presence of a single gene was further confirmed by Ingram's discovery that this hemoglobin differed by only one amino acid from normal hemoglobin. Hemoglobin C, which by family studies appeared to be an allele of the sickle-cell gene, also was found to differ by only one amino acid from normal hemoglobin; and in addition it differed at the same place as hemoglobin S. But when in the same laboratory different samples of hemoglobin D were examined, it was found that they were not the same, which resulted in their being labeled Dα, Dβ, and Dγ.

Although these discoveries may have rendered the letter nomenclature obsolete and have made changes in nomenclature necessary, they did not render the old nomenclature useless. Widespread and relatively frequent hemoglobins, such as S, C, and E, are still referred to only by letter because they seem to be the same hemoglobin wherever they are found. Of course, not many samples of these hemoglobins from geographically distant populations have been fingerprinted, so we do not really know whether or not the high frequencies of these hemoglobins in certain populations are due to the same identical mutation. This is only a supposition and will be more fully discussed when we consider the population genetics of the abnormal hemoglobins.

For other abnormal hemoglobins, a recent conference (41) has recommended that the place of discovery be included after the letter and, if the specific difference in amino acid structure from normal hemoglobin is known, then this be included. The letters have been retained to indicate the behavior of the hemoglobin on paper electrophoresis at pH 8.6. For adult hemoglobin variants we then have C and E in the slowest place; S, D, F, G, L, O, P, and Q in the next approximate position; A or normal hemoglobin in the next; and then the "fast" hemoglobins I, J, K, and N.

While the preceding discoveries as to the nature of adult hemoglobin were occurring, increasing knowledge of other kinds of human hemoglobin found at various stages in the life cycle was also accumulating. Since Korber in 1866 discovered that the hemoglobin of the fetus is more resistant to denaturation in alkaline solutions than is normal adult hemoglobin, we have known that different hemoglobins are synthesized at different times in the individual life cycle. More recently the hereditary persistance of fetal hemoglobin in both normal individuals and those with a serious anemia has been found in several human populations (247, 251, 348, 509). Thalassemia major is one of the most widespread anemias in which greatly increased amounts of fetal hemoglobin occur, but there are many cases of thalassemia which do not have this feature. Although the easiest method to detect fetal hemoglobin is still by its resistance to alkali denaturation, fetal hemoglobin does have a different electrophoretic mobility than normal hemoglobin at pH 8.6. The persistence of fetal hemoglobin in adults showed that an individual with only normal genes for adult hemoglobin could synthesize more than one hemoglobin at one time. Further, development of starch block and starch gel electrophoresis has shown that the normal individual synthesizes many different kinds of hemoglobin. In addition to small amounts of fetal hemoglobin, there have so far been discovered four hemoglobins that the normal individual synthesizes in varying quantities. These have been labeled A_1, which is the major component and had previously been known as hemoglobin A; A_2, which has the electrophoretic mobility of hemoglobins C and E; and A_3 and A_4, which are little known and about which there is some disagreement.

Although these discoveries of different types of hemoglobin, when coupled with the great variety of adult hemoglobin, seem to create a hodgepodge of miscellaneous information, the discovery of the complete chemical structures of the various types of hemoglobin has unified all these data and rendered them quite understandable. The human hemoglobin molecule has a molecular weight of about 67,000. It is composed of a heme group plus the protein globin, which is composed of two α- and two β- polypeptide chains.

TABLE 1
α-CHAIN VARIANTS OF HUMAN HEMOGLOBIN

Name(s)	Position	Substitution*	Reference(s)
J Toronto	5	ala → asp	190a
J Oxford, I Interlaken	15	gly → asp	425a, 462a
I, I Burlington	16	lys → asp	330, 519
J Medellín	22	gly → asp	330
G Honolulu, G Hongkong, G Singapore	30	glu → glm	330
D α Cyprus (Turkish)	αT-4		339b
L Ferrara, Umi, Kokura, Michigan-1, Tagawa II, Yukuhashi II	47	asp → gly	330, 304
Mexico, J Paris	54	glm → glu	362a
Shimonoseki, Hikoshima	54	glm → arg	304
Beilinson	αT-6		723
J Norfolk, Kagoshima, Nishiki I, Nishiki II, Nishiki III	57	gly → asp	330, 304
M Boston, M Leipzig-2, M Osaka, M Koln	58	his → tyr	330, 77, 304, 373
N Seattle	61	lys → glu	362a
G Philadelphia, G Bristol, G Azuokoli, D St. Louis, D Washington	68	asg → lys	330
M Iwate, M Kankakee, M Oldenberg	87	his → tyr	330
G Baltimore	αT-9	asp → his	573a
Q, G Paris, Ube-2, Matsue	αT-9		362a, 393a, 622
Tagawa I	αT-10		304
O Indonesia	116	glu → lys	330
Stanleyville II			303
L Bombay			656
Nicosia			244
Russ			331
K Madras, K Calcutta			407a
J India, J Malaya			407a
M Kiskunalas			323b
N α			636
Hopkins-2			612c
Karamojo			20
Columbia			499a

*Symbols used on tables and in text:

ala—alanine
arg—arginine
asg—asparagine
asp—aspartic acid
cys—cysteine
glm—glutamine
glu—glutamic acid
gly—glycine
his—histidine
ilu—isoleucine
leu—leucine
lys—lysine
met—methionine
phe—phenylalanine
pro—proline
ser—serine
thr—threonine
try—tryptophan
tyr—tyrosine
val—valine

TABLE 2
β-CHAIN VARIANTS OF HUMAN HEMOGLOBIN

Name(s)	Position	Substitution	Reference(s)
Tokuchi	2	his → tyr	622
S	6	glu → val	330
C	6	glu → lys	330
G San Jose	7	glu → gly	330
C Georgetown } these hemoglobins differ in electrophoretic mobility	7	glu → lys(?)	538
Siriraj	7	glu → lys(?)	691
Durham-1	βT-1		612c
J Baltimore, J Ireland, J Trinidad, N New Haven	16	gly → asp	330, 737
G Coushatta	22 or 26	glu → ala	612
E, Nagasaki	26	glu → lys	330, 304
D Gujerat	βT-3		612c
Miyada	βT-3		304
G Galveston, G Texas, G Port Arthur	43	glu → ala	330
K Ibadan	46	gly → glu	18
J Korat, J Meinung Taiwan	βT-5	phe or gly → asp	90a
Hikari, Ube-3	61	lys → asg	622
Yukuhashi I	βT-6		304
M Saskatoon, M Emory, M Chicago, M Kurume, M Radom, M Hita, M Arhus	63	his → tyr	330, 304, 322a
Zurich	63	his → arg	330
M Milwaukee-1	67	val → glu	330
Rambam	69 or 74	gly → asp	592a
Seattle	70 or 76	ala → glu	612c
G Accra	79	asp → asg	330
D Ibadan	87	thr → lys	735
Ube-1	93	cysSH → ?	304
Oak Ridge	94	asp → asg?	612c
N Baltimore, N Memphis	95	lys → glu	175, 612c
Köln	98	val → met	150a
D Punjab, D Cyprus (Greek), D Chicago, D Los Angeles, D Portugal, D North Carolina	121	glu → glm	330, 339b
O Arabia, O Bulgaria, O New York	121	glu → lys	330, 371, 46a
K Cameroon	130	ala → glu or asp	18
K Woolwich	132	lys → glm	18
Hope	136	gly → asp	480
Kenwood	143	his → glu or asp	60
St. Mary's			612c
D Frankfurt			612c
Nishiki IV			304
Tsukiji			304

TABLE 2 (Continued)
β-CHAIN VARIANTS OF HUMAN HEMOGLOBIN

Name(s)	Position	Substitution	Reference(s)
Hofu			304
Hiroshima-1			304
Hiroshima-2			304
New Haven-2			165
Chicago-1			165
Tacoma			57a
P Calabria			636
M Wales			407a
O Tel Hashomer			407a
M Milwaukee-2			612c
J Georgia			612c
J Jamaica			612c
C Harlem	6 or 7 73 or 79	glu → val asp → asg	99b

Hemoglobin synthesized in vivo always has two identical α-chains and two identical β-chains. Human α-chains contain a sequence of 141 amino acids, while human β-chains have 146. Fetal hemoglobin has been shown to have two α-chains identical to those of hemoglobin A, and two γ-chains that, like the β-chain, have a sequence of 146 amino acids. Hemoglobin A_2 has been found to have the same α-chains and two δ-chains which also contain 146 amino acids. In addition to being the same length, the β- and δ-chains differ in only ten amino acids out of the total of 146 positions in the sequence, while the β- and γ- chains differ by 37 (753). For one position of the six where they both differ from the β-chain, the γ- and δ-chains are the same, so that the γ- and δ-chains differ by forty amino acids. However, if the chains are arranged as Zuckerkandl (753) has done, then the α-chain differs from the β-chain in 83 positions if deletions and additions are included.

Most of the adult hemoglobin variants can now be described by the way in which they differ in amino acid structure from normal adult hemoglobin. The great majority differ by only one amino acid. Tables 1, 2, and 3 are as up-to-date a compilation as possible of all the known hemoglobin variants. In many cases the exact substitution is not known, but the abnormal peptide or polypeptide chain is. Whether the α- or β-chain is involved can be established by hybridization experiments (342a), while the abnormal peptide can be identified by fingerprinting.

Although most hemoglobin variants appear to be point mutations of the DNA controlling hemoglobin synthesis and hence differ by only one amino acid, others are either abnormal chain combinations or changes of more than one amino acid in some chain. Hemoglobin H is found in individuals with thalassemia and has been found to consist of four normal β-chains. Hemoglobin Lepore, which has been found in many populations,

TABLE 3
OTHER HEMOGLOBIN VARIANTS

Name(s)	Position	Substitution	Reference(s)
γ-Chain Variants			
Texas	γT-1	glm → lys	611
F Roma			635
Alexandria			330
Aegina			330
F Houston, F Warren		glu → ala	612a
δ-Chain Variants			
Sphakia	2	his → arg	362a
B_2, A_2'	16	gly → arg	362a
Flatbush	22	ala → glu	362a
Abnormal Chain Combinations			
α		α_4	163a
H		β_4	339b
Barts		γ_4	339b
δ		δ_4	330
Augusta I		β_4^s	331
Augusta II		β_4^c	331
Lepore Boston	δT-1 . . . δT-5 + (β or δ)T-6 . . . (β or δ)T-11 + βT-12 . . . βT-15		48b
Lepore Hollandia	δT-1 . . . δT-3 + βT-4 . . . βT-15		330
New Haven-1			165
Cyprus-1			330

has been discovered in two cases to be composed of two normal α-chains and two chains that contain varying parts of the normal β- and δ-chains (48b). This implies that hemoglobin Lepore is due to an unequal crossing-over of the DNA that controls the synthesis of these two chains, which further implies that the β- and δ- chains are under the control of adjacent or very close segments of DNA of the same chromosome. Further evidence for this interpretation is the fact that one end of the abnormal chain of hemoglobin Lepore is identical to the normal β-chain, and the other end is identical to the normal δ-chain.

Persons homozygous for the Lepore duplication have a clinical condition similar to forms of thalassemia. And in the absence of techniques such as electrophoresis, individuals homozygous for this hemoglobin variant would be diagnosed as having thalassemia. But for the overwhelming majority of individuals with thalassemia major or minor (or, respectively, homozygotes and heterozygotes for a thalassemia), no hemoglobin variant has been detected. Of course, many individuals are known who are simultaneously heterozygous for a thalassemia gene and a hemoglobin variant. Some combinations, such as hemoglobin S-thalassemia, are very serious while others, such as hemoglobin C-thalassemia, are milder conditions. Although the thalassemia genes do not produce an abnormal hemoglobin, they seriously impair the synthesis of hemoglobin. And since the discovery of the structure of hemoglobin, some genes have been found to impair the production of α-chains, and others the production of β-chains. Hemoglobin H, which has four β-chains, has thus been found in individuals with thalassemia major, in which the thalassemia gene impairs the production of α-chains. In addition, such individuals produce another type of hemoglobin called Barts which has subsequently been found to contain four γ-chains.

Thalassemia genes that affect the β-chain are much more common than these mutants, although "more common" is used here in the sense of having a higher frequency in the human species as a whole. In terms of the number of mutations that occur every generation there are probably as many α-chain mutants. By analogy with the α-chain mutants, we might expect that β thalassemias would be characterized by a hemoglobin with four α-chains. This hemoglobin has been detected (163a), but it is not common in β thalassemia. Most β thalassemias are characterized instead by increased amounts of hemoglobin A_2, which is $\alpha_2^A\delta_2^A$, and sometimes by increased amounts of fetal homoglobin, which is $\alpha_2^A\gamma_2^A$. Since hemoglobin A is $\alpha_2^A\beta_2^A$, it can be seen that in β thalassemia, the β-chain has been replaced by δ- and γ-chains.

Although the mechanics of thalassemia are known to a great extent, there are still many problems as to its inheritance. In all cases the thalassemia condition is inherited as a single gene, but as there are α and β thalassemias, it is obvious that these cases are not always the same gene in the sense of being the same change from the normal genotype. And despite the fact that we know how thalassemias affect the synthesis of hemoglobin, the specific structural difference associated with any thalassemia gene remains unknown, with the exception of the thalassemia associated with hemoglobin Lepore. This has given rise to the general idea that thalassemias are mutations of regulator, repressor, or controller genes which regulate the synthesis of α– or β-chains, and not mutations of the genes that control the structure of these chains.

However, the possibility that thalassemias are mutations in the structural genes has not been completely ruled out. At the time when family studies were beginning to show that some thalassemia genes appeared to be alleles of the sickle-cell gene, while others did not, Ingram and Stretton (339c) proposed that thalassemia genes may be "hidden" mutants of the genes controlling the structures of α- and β-chains. "Hidden" was meant in the sense that the mutations were amino acid substitutions which did not change the electrophoretic or other properties of the hemoglobin molecule and thus would not be detected by present techniques. Attempts to find hidden mutations (339b) and also to detect an abnormal chain in thalassemia have not been successful. However, Itano (340a) has recently emphasized that there is still a strong possibility that thalassemias are mutations of structural genes. Because of the degeneracy of the genetic code, it is possible to have a change in the DNA that controls hemoglobin structure without any change in the amino acid sequence. Since for the amino acids with more than one triplet codon of RNA it would seem reasonable for some of these codons to be more efficient than others, a mutation from one to another could result in a change in the rate of synthesis of the particular chain but no change in its structure.

In any case, the analysis of family data indicates that the α and β thalassemia genes are alleles or very closely linked to the α and β structural genes, respectively, although the α and β structural genes are independent or on different chromosomes. Thus, either one of the current hypotheses—a regulator gene closely linked to the α and β structural genes, or a non-detectable structural gene allelic to them—could prevail. But whether the genes are closely linked or allelic, the population genetics of the two possibilities are identical in the absence of a significant amount of crossing-over. Since this is true, the great majority of the data in this book are concerned with but two different genes, one controlling α-chain synthesis and the other β-chain synthesis. In addition, we can state that all the abnormal hemoglobin and thalassemia genes that attain appreciable frequencies in some human population are β-chain mutants; so that our efforts to explain the differences in the frequencies of these genes will be concerned for the most part with but one locus and several alleles.

In most cases, however, the detection of β thalassemia requires the identification of other hemoglobins. In particular, it requires the estimation of the amount of hemoglobin A_2, and perhaps also of hemoglobin F. For the detection of α thalassemia in a population, one of the most effective methods is the finding of a significant amount of hemoglobin Barts in cord blood. Since hemoglobins A_2 and F possess different polypeptide chains than hemoglobin A, there can obviously be mutations on these different chains. These hemoglobin variants are found in fewer individuals and in much lower quantities, so their analysis is more difficult. But some variants have been detected and for the sake of completeness are included in Table 3. Other hemoglobin variants that have been infrequently encountered are also included.

Now that the genetic code has been worked out to a very considerable degree, it is possible to analyze the hemoglobin mutations in terms of the base pair changes. The hemoglobin variants for which the exact amino acid substitution has been determined can be related to the implied changes in the codon as Ingram (339b), Beale and Lehmann (61), and more recently Vogel and Rohrborn (722a) have done. In Table 4 are shown the different kinds of amino acid substitutions known to occur in hemoglobin and their

TABLE 4
AMINO ACID SUBSTITUTIONS
OF ADULT HUMAN HEMOGLOBIN

Substitution (No. residues)	No. on α-chain →	No. on α-chain ←	No. on β-chain →	No. on β-chain ←	Total	Possible one-step code changes	Base pair change
gly ↔ asp	8	6	6	0	20	GGC ↔ GAC	G – A
(20) (19)						GGU GAU	G – A
his ↔ tyr	6	0	8	0	14	CAC ↔ UAC	C – U
(19) (6)						CAU UAU	C – U
glu ↔ lys	1	1	7	2	11	GAA ↔ AAA	G – A
(11) (22)						GAG AAG	G – A
glu ↔ glm	3	2	6	0	11	GAA ↔ CAA	G – C
(11) (5)						GAG CAG	G – C
asg ↔ lys	5	0	0	2	7	AAC ↔ AAA	C – A
(6) (22)						AAC AAG	C – G
						AAU AAA	U – A
						AAU AAG	U – G
glu ↔ ala	0	0	4	1	5	GAA ↔ GCA	A – C
(11) (36)						GAG GCG	A – C
glm ↔ arg	2	0	0	0	2	CAA ↔ CGA	A – G
(5) (6)						CAG CGG	A – G
asp ↔ his	1	0	0	1	2	GAC ↔ CAC	G – C
(19) (19)						GAU CAU	G – C
glu ↔ gly	0	0	1	1	2	GAA ↔ GGA	A – G
(11) (20)						GAG GGG	A – G
asp ↔ asg	0	0	2	0	2	GAC ↔ AAC	G – A
(19) (6)						GAU AAU	G – A
glu ↔ val	0	0	1	1	2	GAA ↔ GUA	A – U
(11) (31)						GAG GUG	A – U
lys ↔ asp	2	0	0	0	2	none	
(22) (19)							
his ↔ arg	0	0	1	0	1	CAC ↔ CGC	A – G
(19) (6)						CAU CGU	A – G
thr ↔ lys	0	0	1	0	1	ACA ↔ AAA	C – A
(16) (22)						ACG AAG	C – A
ala ↔ asp	1	0	0	0	1	GCU ↔ GAU	C – A
(36) (19)						GCC GAC	C – A
lys ↔ glm	0	0	1	0	1	AAA ↔ CAA	A – C
(22) (5)						AAG CAG	A – C

frequencies. One of the problems in determining the frequencies of these substitutions is which discoveries to count as separate mutations. When the same substitution occurs in a Japanese and in an English yeoman, they are most likely to be different mutations. But when the same mutation is found in American Negroes in different cities of the United States, the probabilities appear to be about the same as to whether these are separate mutations or descendants of the same one. For hemoglobin variants such as S and C which are rather frequent in American Negroes, most occurrences are almost certainly descendants of the same mutation, but it is impossible to determine whether this is true for any individual occurrence. For hemoglobin variants that are much rarer, and for which there is no definite indication of a possibility of relationship, multiple occurrences would appear to be due to separate mutations.

The interpretation of the frequencies of various mutations of the hemoglobin loci is further complicated by the great amount of selection for some of these mutants. Many hemoglobin mutants are discovered through hospital surveys or diagnoses, so that those with deleterious effects are much more likely to be detected. For example, the great number of substitutions of tyrosine for histidine are apparently due to the fact that these result in methemoglobinemia and cyanosis. There are no known histidine for tyrosine mutations, and this assymetry is perhaps due to the differential effects on fitness. However, there are nineteen histidine residues and only six tyrosine on the α- and β-chains; many other factors also affect the probability of mutation. On the other hand, for rare hemoglobin variants that are almost totally benign when heterozygous, there appear to be mutations in both directions. There are fourteen glycine to aspartic acid substitutions and six aspartic acid to glycine.

In Table 4 the RNA triplets that code for the various amino acids are shown. From these one can attempt to determine which substitutions are only a single change in base pairs and which require more. The genetic code used here is given in Jukes (367a). Several points are brought out by this table. First, the most common substitutions, gly-asp and his-tyr, can be accomplished in two different ways. For gly-asp both ways are a G-A change, and for his-tyr both are a C-U. According to Freese and Yoshida (262a), the most common type of point mutations are the substitution of the purines for one another or the pyrimidines for one another. Thus, the spontaneous mutations at the hemoglobin loci seem to be what would be predicted by the genetic code.

Most of the abnormal hemoglobin genes that are found in high frequencies occur on the β-chain. Two, hemoglobins C and E, are glu-lys substitutions; and hemoglobin O α Indonesia, which is the only α-chain variant found in many populations in appreciable frequency, is the same substitution. This substitution can occur in two different ways as a

G-A change and hence should be a relatively common mutation. It has been found in Bulgaria, Arabia, Thailand, and the United States, and in both directions. According to Zuckerkandl and Pauling (754), this is also a conservative substitution, which means that it should not change the functioning of the molecule very much; and this seems to be true.

Hemoglobin S, the remaining hemoglobin variant that is found in high frequencies and whose substitution has been determined, is the only glu to val change known for human hemoglobin, although hemoglobin Milwaukee-I is a val to glu change. Glu to val would most likely occur as GAU to GUU; and A to U is a purine-pyrimidine change, which is less probable. The change from glu to val is also labeled radical by Zuckerkandl and Pauling (754) since it occurs very infrequently and alters the functioning of the molecule.

From this analysis of the amino acid substitutions in human hemoglobin and the implied base pair alterations, I think we can make the following conclusions that are relevant to the population genetics of the abnormal hemoglobin genes. First, the hemoglobin S gene is a rather rare and radical mutation. Since all hemoglobin S genes are found in relatively contiguous human populations or those with known gene flow from these contiguous populations, hemoglobin S may well be due to a single ancestral mutation or at least to a very few mutations. Second, hemoglobins C and E, the only other abnormal hemoglobins found in frequencies approaching those of hemoglobin S, are the result of the more common substitution, glu to lys. There are other hemoglobins with the same substitution, and recently some hemoglobin N's have been found to be the reverse substitution. But with the exception of hemoglobin Nagasaki (304), hemoglobin E is the only one at position 26 on the β-chain, and hemoglobin C occurs with hemoglobin S at position 6 of the β-chain. Hemoglobins C and E are hence almost unique as to position, if not in substitution.

The isolated case of hemoglobin E from New Guinea may be a separate mutation (193), but it could just as well be the result of gene flow from Southeast Asian populations. The hemoglobin found in Nagasaki, Japan, could also be the result of a gene flow from the south, since hemoglobin E has apparently been present in Southeast Asia for centuries and the gene flow into the Nagasaki population could have occurred so long ago as to be undetectable today. As the center of Western trade in Japan, Nagasaki was perhaps the population most open to outside gene flow before the seventeenth century, when the country was closed to the outside. There are also rather significant frequencies of hemoglobin E in the Eti-Turks (7), and more isolated instances of this hemoglobin have been discovered in the Middle East (323a, 619, 693). These may be separate mutations, but peptide analysis of these hemoglobin E's has not been done to determine whether in fact they are the same substitution. In any case the great numbers of hemoglobin E genes in Southeast Asia are probably due to the same ancestral mutation as are the more restricted hemoglobin C genes in West and Northwest Africa. A detailed inspection of the frequencies of these two hemoglobin genes makes this more apparent and will be undertaken in the appropriate chapters.

Since hemoglobin D β Punjab was found to be different from hemoglobin D Gujerat, and since the hemoglobin D's found in a Turkish and a Greek Cypriot were also different, it appears to be difficult to attribute the occurrence of hemoglobin D in two populations to the same mutation. Since many hemoglobin D's are found in diverse populations, they would appear to be common mutants. However, the occurrence of gene flow between England and India, as demonstrated by Konigsberg et al. (387a), indicates that very diverse occurrences may be due to gene flow and not be separate mutations. Thalassemia as a clinical or morphological entity may also be due to many different mutations. Because of the many different point mutations that can result in the symptoms of thalassemia, the mutation rate to thalassemia includes both α- and β- varieties and is much higher than the mutation rate for any specific abnormal hemoglobin. Until the specific chemical change is known for any particular thalassemia, it is almost impossible to determine ancestral relationships or trace gene flow between populations on the evidence of this genetic trait.

III

THE GLUCOSE-6-PHOSPHATE DEHYDROGENASE DEFICIENCY

THE OTHER GENE loci with which we will be concerned have had a history similar to that of the hemoglobin and thalassemia loci. For years it had been known in the Mediterranean countries that many individuals were severely "allergic" to the fava bean. A quote from Pythagoras is frequently cited as evidence for this allergy, favism, having existed since antiquity (see 40 for an account of references to favism and the fava bean in classical literature). Fava beans have been found in Bronze Age excavations in Italy (681) and Palestine (243); so this bean has been a staple in the Mediterranean area for a long time. The cultivation of the bean spread eastward to China (40), but it has never been of great importance in Northern Europe, Africa, or India.

Favism was known to affect more males than females, and it also seemed to be confined to certain families. In some countries such as Sardinia it was a serious disease that afflicted a large percentage of the population. Crosby (191) estimated that there were annually 5 cases per 1000 of favism in Sardinia, and a death rate of 250 a year from the disease for the whole island. Favism was prevalent in many other countries in the Mediterranean and the Middle East and was also known in China (223), as well as elsewhere in individuals with Mediterranean ancestry.

The inheritance of favism had not been worked out by

the 1950's when another series of experiments and discoveries began to throw light on this condition. It had been known since the 1920's that some individuals have a sensitivity to certain anti-malarial drugs, notably pamaquine. In fact, it was also known that among certain "races," such as Asiatic Indians in the British Army, this sensitivity was quite frequent, while it was almost completely absent in soldiers from the British Isles. During World War II a similar drug, primaquine, was developed in the United States, and it was found that American Negroes were particularly sensitive to this drug. Several studies attempted to determine the prevalence of primaquine sensitivity in various populations by administration of the drug (for an extensive historical review, see Beutler [80]), but a series of laboratory tests was then developed that made the detection of susceptible individuals both easier and more accurate. The first of these was the glutiathione stability test (79). By this test the inheritance of primaquine sensitivity was first determined (168, 294); it is an accurate test but not adaptable to field conditions. Although a test for the determination of glucose-6-phosphate dehydrogenase was known (151), the development of a rapid screening test by Motulsky and Campbell (494a) permitted the widespread surveying of the world's populations. In the past few years two other tests have been developed by Brewer, Tarlov, and Alving (117a) and by Fairbanks and Beutler (242b).

These studies have shown that almost all cases of favism and primaquine sensitivity possess a gene that produces a deficiency of glucose-6-phosphate dehydrogenase activity. This gene is sex-linked, which explains the greater frequencies of favism and primaquine sensitivity in males. Since males have only one allele for a sex-linked locus, the frequency of males with the G6PD deficiency would be the same as the frequency of the deficiency allele in the population. But since females have two alleles for such a locus, to exhibit these conditions they must be homozygous for the deficiency allele. In a random-mating population the frequency in females will be approximately the square of the gene frequency. Although almost all individuals who develop favism or primaquine sensitivity are either hemizygous or homozygous for the G6PD deficiency alleles, the reverse is not true, and all such persons do not develop these conditions. This makes the use of favism or primaquine sensitivity for the estimation of the G6PD-deficiency genes somewhat inaccurate; so that they have been used only in the absence of other data.

Female heterozygotes for the G6PD deficiency alleles have a variable amount of enzyme activity. Some appear to have normal G6PD enzyme activity, and others seem to be deficient. The various screening tests differ in their ability to detect female heterozygotes, so that studies on G6PD deficiency that include females are difficult to interpret in terms of gene frequencies. However, the deficient and non-deficient males are very different, with practically no overlap between the two groups on any test. For this reason the data for G6PD deficiency specify whether the sample is male, female, or both.

Like thalassemia, the G6PD deficiency is widespread in the world's populations and also seems to result from many different mutations. Marks and Gross (462) found that American Negroes who are deficient for G6PD in their red cells were not deficient in their leukocytes, while most deficient white Americans were. Measurements of the G6PD enzyme activity indicated that deficient Negroes had some enzyme activity, but white males for the most part had none. This evidence indicated that different alleles were involved. With the development of starch gel electrophoresis and its application to G6PD, concrete proof for the inheritance of differences in G6PD was forthcoming. Boyer and his associates (104) showed that among American Negro males there were two types of G6PD, the most common, which they labeled B type, being electrophoretically slower than the less common variant, which they called A. Family data showed that these electrophoretic variants were inherited, but there was no direct association between electrophoretic type and G6PD enzyme activity. However, with few exceptions, all American Negro males who were G6PD deficient had type A. On the other hand, deficient American whites all had type B, and no type A has been found in any group without African ancestry (553).

The electrophoretic variants of G6PD have also been shown to be sex-linked. While American Negro males have either type A or type B, American Negro females are A, B, and AB. And the AB type appears in the frequency expected for heterozygotes. Although there is no one-to-one correspondence between electrophoretic type and enzyme activity, the data for Nigerians and American Negroes indicate that the loci controlling type and activity must be quite closely linked (553). Family studies from Sardinia have also shown that the G6PD deficiency locus is very closely linked to the deutan color-blind locus and somewhat less close to the protan color-blind locus (641a).

Most populations which have been studied so far have had almost 100 per cent type B. But relatively rare occurrences of other variants have been found in large-scale surveys of most populations. Most of these variants are slower on starch gel electrophoresis than type B and are frequently deficient in G6PD enzyme activity. In American Negroes there is a Baltimore variant that is slower than type B and does not result in enzyme deficiency, and an even slower variant has been found in Nigerians (553). In a survey of 172 American Negroes in Austin, Texas, two were found to have a slow variant, Austin-1, and two were found with another slow variant, Austin-2 (451). Both variants resulted in enzyme deficiency. In American whites there is a Seattle variant, which is deficient (384); two instances of a slow variant that is deficient were also found in Chicago (383), but these may be the Seattle type. There is also a slow Madison variant that is deficient (451). In Italians, a fast variant, which is moderately deficient, has been found in Northern Italy (460), while two slow variants, Sardinian-1 and Sardinian-2, have been found in Sardinia (553). The slow Baltimore variant has also been found in Sardinia as well as in New Guinea (553). Five Chinese male deficients had the same fast variant (470a). On the other hand no variants have been found among Japanese, Thais, Marshall Islanders, or Iraqi Jews, who have the highest frequency of the G6PD deficiency in the world. Other low-frequency variants have been found in Israel (562, 563) and in the United States (503).

Like the many rare abnormal hemoglobins found all over the world, these electrophoretic variants of G6PD are excellent examples of the process of mutation. In addition, each area with high G6PD-deficiency frequencies seems to have its own variant that causes the deficiency. To date, the only populations sampled enough to obtain a reasonable estimate for a G6PD variant are the Nigerians, for whom the estimate of type A is 62/141 or .44 (553); the American Negroes, for whom the estimates of type A are 105/311 or .34 in Baltimore, 47/135 or .35 in Oklahoma City, and 387/1276 or .30 in Dallas (553, 382, 450); and the Djukas of Surinam, for whom the estimate of type A is 93/242 or .38 (642a).

Compared with the deficient alleles, the electrophoretic variants do not have so much selection against them, a situation comparable to the α and β hemoglobin loci for which thalassemia alleles are invariably selected against while hemoglobin electrophoretic variants are not. The thalassemia and G6PD-deficiency alleles are also comparable in that both are recognized by an abnormal functioning of the protein and both can be produced by many different mutational changes. Hence both have selection against them, and higher mutation rates than any specific electrophoretic variant.

In the future the structure of G6PD will be known in detail; so that the structural changes resulting in enzyme deficiency can be specified. At present, the molecular weight seems to be about 190,000, and the molecule consists of at least two polypeptide chains (174). Chung and Langdon (174) have also shown that removal of the nucleotide (TPN) results in two inactive subunits with one-half the molecular weight of the enzyme. When the amino acid sequences of these peptide chains are worked out, the structural basis of enzyme deficiency will surely be forthcoming, just as the structural reasons for methemoglobinemia have been found (312). The great size of the enzyme and its two-chain structure raise the question of how many loci are involved in the G6PD deficiency. The G6PD-deficiency alleles that are found in appreciable frequencies in human populations throughout the world are all sex-linked. If two loci are involved, they must therefore both be on the X chromosome, or we have no frequent mutants for one of them. If there were two loci on the X chromosome that were closely linked, then, in the absence of appreciable crossing-over, the population dynamics would be similar to the one-locus case. The discovery of the structure of G6PD will also help solve this problem. At present, the data for the linkage of G6PD-deficiency alleles with other sex-linked loci in different human populations seem to result in different X-chromosome maps (641a). One possible explanation of these data is the existence in different populations of different sex-linked loci for the G6PD deficiency.

IV

THE POPULATION GENETICS OF THE RED CELL DEFECTS

ALL OF THE conditions that we have discussed are due to the presence of a single gene, and most of these genes, when heterozygous, are relatively benign. Of course, many loci are involved, and many alleles at each of these loci. Those involving the glucose-6-phosphate dehydrogenase deficiency are sex-linked, while the hemoglobin and thalassemia loci are autosomal. By "single gene" we mean that the condition or trait can be produced by a single change in the normal chromosome. These changes are all called mutations, and can be of two general types. The most common is a change in a single base pair of the chromosome, which is called a *point mutation.* The other kind of mutation, or *chromosomal mutation*, includes the many different ways by which an imperfect copy of the chromosomes can occur during the process of reproduction. Duplication, deletion, inversion, and translocation are the various kinds of chromosomal mutation. Although most hemoglobin variants are examples of point mutations, the Lepore hemoglobins are instances of chromosomal mutations.

Because these conditions are produced by a single gene, differences in them among a series of populations can be expressed as differences in gene frequencies. To apply to them the theory of gene frequency change, we begin by dividing the human species into breeding isolates, which are defined as the groups within which the members most often mate or marry. In many areas of the world, human mating behavior is such that it is impossible to divide the people into several discrete, exclusive groups. This indicates that our theory is only a rough approximation to reality, and raises the question as to how much the process of approximation has affected our conclusions. However, all sciences make simplifying assumptions and thus in a sense are only approximations to actuality. Mathematical theories are models of actuality, and those in population genetics are no exception. To indicate that any particular application of mathematics does not "fit the facts" is an irrelevant criticism. None do. It must be shown how the differences between the model and the data it is attempting to interpret affect the conclusions of the application and result in wrong ones. Nevertheless, the interaction between new measurements and old theories is the progress of science.

This aside into the philosophy of science can be considered either the rationalization or the rationale of the approach used in this book. All the interpretations of the gene frequency differences can be dismissed as not proven. This is true because many of the parameters necessary to predict future gene frequencies or interpret present ones are simply estimated and not measured from concrete data on human populations. Such data do not exist and, more importantly, I think never will. Data on the amount of gene flow among prehistoric populations or the amount of natural selection by malaria are gone for good. But this does not mean that historical problems are not valid ones for "science." The choice of one interpretation over another will not result from its being "proven" but from its being able to explain a greater array of data.

Returning to the theory of population genetics, for each breeding isolate we can calculate a gene frequency and then plot these geographically. Although some human breeding isolates occupy the same geographical areas or are interdispersed together, most human genetic variation can be described as variation between geographically separate isolates. Genetic variation among these isolates can be expressed in terms of the concepts of isogene and genocline. Like the isobars of a weather map which express areas of equal pressure, isogenes are lines that indicate equal gene frequencies among the breeding isolates along them. On the other hand, the concept of *cline* implies change in gene frequency. In a restricted sense, it means a gradual change in gene frequency in one direction among a linear series of adjacent isolates, but in this book *genocline* (or *cline* for short) will be used to express any kind of gene frequency change among a linear series of adjacent populations. If we assume that gene flow occurs only between adjacent isolates and that it is equal for all such isolates, then, if the sequence of isolates are represented on the x-axis of a two-dimensional graph and their gene frequencies for a particular locus on the y-axis, the resulting curves are the clines for this particular locus. An illustration is shown in Figure 1.

For many specific series of human populations, it is obvious that the clines for different loci are not the same. And since the populational phenomena, gene flow and gene drift, are the same for all loci, much of the differences in these clines must be due to the forces of selection and mutation, particularly if the clines are stable and hence presumably close to equilibrium. When gene frequency differences are described in this way, the explanation of them becomes an analysis of how the factors that can change gene frequencies determine the shape of these clines or curves. Haldane (302a) first attempted this kind of analysis and showed how a cline for a single gene with a specific type of variation in the fitness of the genotypes could be approximated. But because this model is greatly simplified and because there are a great many factors which can influence gene frequencies, it is at present very difficult, if not impossible, to apply this type of analysis to most human gene frequency differences. In this respect human population genetics is in a position similar to weather forecasting: we know all the forces that affect weather but are still unable to predict it in many cases.

Although the analysis of clines has barely begun and has many difficult problems associated with it, we can start with a single isolate and consider

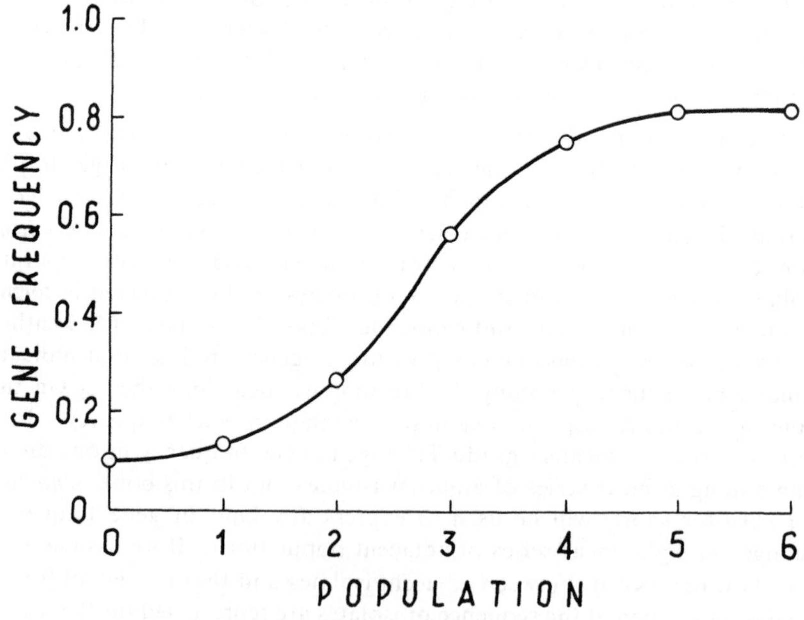

Figure 1. A Theoretical Example of a Cline.

the effects of the forces of gene frequency change within it. To begin with mutation, which has already been discussed to some extent, the many rare hemoglobin and G6PD electrophoretic variants are excellent examples of recurrent mutation for their respective loci. The rate of mutation, which is expressed as the amount of change to a specific mutant per gene per generation, to any specific hemoglobin or G6PD variant is obviously much less than the usual mutation rates discussed in genetics textbooks for human loci. These rates are for clinical conditions such as hemophilia or achondroplasia, and average something greater than 10^{-5}. But such conditions are known to result from mutation at many different loci, which accounts for their greater rates, although the possibility that these loci are more mutable cannot be ruled out. For this reason, the entities thalassemia and G6PD deficiency probably have higher rates than any specific electrophoretic variant and approach the classical mutation rates, which, as the first mutation rates to be measured, are about as great as any known. Both thalassemia and the G6PD deficiency are detected by the function, not the structure, of a specific protein. In this way they are like albinism and hemophilia, and since many different structures can be approximately the same functionally, many different specific mutants will be included in the same entity. The very widespread distributions of thalassemia and the G6PD deficiency in the world's populations are due in part to their higher mutation rates.

On the other hand, the distributions of the specific abnormal hemoglobins seem to be due to the spread of very few mutants. This seems reasonable because these hemoglobin variants are found in contiguous populations and have relatively restricted distributions. Hemoglobin K in Northwest and West Africa and the same hemoglobin in the Madras area of India are instances of the spread of a single or a few mutant genes. Hemoglobin O Indonesia in the Celebes and some of the hemoglobin D's seem to be similar instances of such a spread. The three hemoglobin variants that attain very appreciable frequencies and are somewhat more widespread are hemoglobins S, C, and E. But their distributions are also contiguous and seem to be due to the spread of a few mutant genes. However, the deleterious effects of these hemoglobins when homozygous indicates that natural selection plays an important role in determining their high frequencies, and we will consider this factor next.

Natural selection is expressed by the concept of *fitness*. By definition, fitness is the contribution of the genotype to the next generation, and hence a measure of its capacity to survive and to reproduce. To include both these aspects it is measured at the same time in the life cycle. A constant population size is usually assumed, so that "normal" fitness would be 1.0, meaning that the genotype is just reproducing itself.

At times it is easier to use another measure of natural selection, the selection coefficient, which measures the amount by which the genotype's fitness is decreased in comparison with the optimum genotype's fitness. If w is the fitness of a genotype and s its selection coefficient, then $w = 1 - s$, although this does not hold when the fitness is greater than 1.0. Although the selection coefficient can be used to measure selection against the genotype, it is difficult to use it to indicate a fitness superior to normals.

The range of fitness for the hemoglobin genotypes is perhaps as great as for any set of human loci. Many of the rare hemoglobin variants have yet to be detected in homozygous form, but will probably be found to be intermediate in fitness. Homozygosity for the hemoglobin S gene or for many of the thalassemia genes is extremely severe; and in the medical conditions in the African bush today, or in most of the world prior to the twentieth century, such homozygosity could be considered to be lethal. For example, among the Bwamba, who have about a 40 per cent frequency of hemoglobin S heterozygotes, no homozygotes were found among adults (413). If we assume that some of the high frequencies of these lethal genes are close to equilibrium, then if the balancing factor is an increased fitness of the heterozygote, these heterozygotes must have a fitness of about 1.25, which is the highest known fitness for any human genotype.

The other abnormal hemoglobin genes do not have as severe complications when homozygous as hemoglobin S or most thalassemias do. Homozygosity for either hemoglobin E, C, or D does have some adverse effects; the range in fitness is from perhaps .5 to .9. In the discussion of the areas where these genes are frequent, attempts will be made to estimate fitness more precisely. Not only homozygosity for one hemoglobin gene, but also simultaneous heterozygosity for two abnormal hemoglobin genes affects fitness adversely. This is particularly true when the two hemoglobin variants affect the same chain. So few frequent variants of the α-chain are known, however, that two different variants for this chain are unknown in one person. But the inheritance of one α-chain variant and one β-chain variant seems to result in a milder condition than two β variants, although it of course depends to a great extent on the specific variants involved. The combinations that are relatively frequent, so that their fitnesses are of significance for population genetics, are hemoglobin S-β thalassemia, which is the most severe; hemoglobin E-β thalassemia, which is more severe than homozygosity for hemoglobin E; hemoglobin C-β thalassemia, which is also more severe than homozygosity for hemoglobin C; and hemoglobin S-hemoglobin C disease, which is very deleterious, despite the relatively benign nature of hemoglobin C. However, Fullerton et al. (264) estimate that the mortality during pregnancy for SC females is only 10 per cent, while Edington and Laing's (228) statistics indicate that the SC genotype survives as well as normals. Besides this demonstrated selection against the SC heterozygotes and the heterozygotes for thalassemia and an abnormal hemoglobin, these genotypes in most cases seem to have an anemia that, though perhaps slight, is nevertheless almost always present. Hence they would seem to be at some disadvantage, although not one striking enough to be observed as a clinical syndrome.

Although not as severe as the more common abnormal hemoglobins, the G6PD deficiency also has some selection against it. And since it is sex-linked, males with deficient genotypes will be very frequent in the population. The G6PD deficiency has been shown to cause neonatal jaundice in some populations, such as Greece (750,216) or Southeast Asia (153a, 431a, 644a, 748), but this has not been a constant finding. In Thailand (255), Nigeria (147), and Israel (668) neonatal jaundice does not seem to be as important a selective factor. This could be due to different enzyme activity levels in the populations, since Caucasians are known to have the lowest levels of enzyme activity.

The survival of G6PD-deficient genotypes must also be affected by their known drug reactions, perhaps not so much by their ingestion of these drugs as by their encountering similar chemicals in nature. There is also some evidence that deficient individuals are more susceptible to some bacterial and viral infections (494a, 746a, 662a), and of course there is selection due to favism in areas where the bean is found. This selection must have been quite severe at one time; it is curious that high frequencies of the G6PD-deficiency genes are found in areas where the fava bean is a common staple. For Sardinia, Crosby (191) estimated that there were 5 cases per 1000 annually, and a 10 to 40 per cent mortality. If we estimate the frequency of the G6PD-deficiency gene in Sardinia as 20 per cent, and the total population is about one million, then there are 500,000 males of which 100,000 are deficient. With 40 per cent mortality, two people out of very 1000 die from favism each year, or 2000 for the whole island. If a generation is 25 years, then in that time 50,000 will die. Since the males per generation must be less than half the total males, there would be less than 50,000 deficients per generation. Assuming all deaths are males, this would indicate a selection coefficient of about .5. If 10 per cent mortality is assumed, the selection coefficient would be somewhat greater than .1. These are obviously rough estimates, but they do indicate that there should be significant differences in the frequency of the G6PD deficiency in infants and in adults, but these so far have not been detected. And with this selection against the G6PD deficiency, it is even more curious that Sardinia has some of the highest frequencies of the gene in the world.

Thus far we have discussed only selection against the hemoglobin and G6PD genes. This selection usually occurs when the individual has only abnormal genes for some particular locus, but there is evidence that the simple sickle cell trait may also be deleterious in particular circumstances (see Rucknagel and Neel [586] for a review of this problem). For the most part this selection can be considered dysfunctional in the sense that the genotype cannot function in any environment, and environmental changes do not affect the fitness of the genotypes to any great extent. If this were the only kind of selection operating on the hemoglobin and G6PD loci, it would be difficult to explain the high frequencies of the deleterious alleles in many populations. But where there are not high frequencies of these alleles and where there does not seem to be any selection increasing them, this dysfunctional selection is the major determinant of gene frequency change.

If there is only selection against these deleterious alleles, then their frequencies will be due to a balance between the selection against them and the mutations to them from other alleles. If the allele in question is autosomal and recessive, which means that there is only selection against homozygotes for it, then at equilibrium the frequency of the deleterious allele will be:

$$\hat{q}_x = \sqrt{\frac{m}{s_{xx}}} \qquad (1)$$

where $\hat{q}_x$ is the frequency of the gene, m is the mutation rate to it per gamete per generation from other alleles, and s_{xx} is the selection coefficient of homozygotes for the deleterious gene.

If, on the other hand, the gene is dominant, or there is selection against heterozygotes for it, then:

$$\hat{q}_x = \frac{m}{s_{ax}} \qquad (2)$$

where s_{ax} is the selection coefficient of the heterozygotes. If the deleterious allele is sex-linked, then its frequency will be:

$$\hat{q}_x = \frac{3m}{s_x} \qquad (3)$$

where s_x is the selection coefficient for male hemizygotes for the x gene. All these formulas are approximations in which the selection coefficients must be very different from 0 and close to 1.0, but they are as accurate as any data we have for the hemoglobin and G6PD genes.

If we take 10^{-5} as the maximum mutation rate possible for these deleterious alleles, then the highest equilibrium frequency that a recessive lethal could attain would be .003. This is far below the observed frequencies of hemoglobin S and β thalassemia for many populations. If the selection against homozygotes were .1, then the equilibrium frequency would be .01. The finding of an occasional abnormal hemoglobin in England, where the frequency is perhaps .001, or in Japan, where it is about the same, seems to be within the range predicted by these formulas. In Japan the frequency of the β-thalassemia gene seems to be about .0001 which, assuming $s_{tt} = 1.0$, indicates a mutation rate of about 10^{-8}. The data for the abnormal hemoglobins in Japan shows a frequency for all variants as about .0003 which, assuming an average selection against homozygotes of .5, gives a mutation rate of about 4×10^{-8}. Both of these estimates are far below the maximum human mutation rates.

Most of the hemoglobin genes are relatively recessive, and so would conform to the first formula. However, the hemoglobin M genes do produce a mild cyanosis when heterozygous. Today there does not appear to be much selection against heterozygotes for these genes, but in more primitive conditions the easy fatigability of hemoglobin M heterozygotes may have been more deleterious. Scott and Hoskins (615) have found a focus of an enzyme deficiency among Alaskan Eskimos and Indians which produces the same methemoglobinemia as hemoglobin M. In the severe Arctic environment the gene seems to have spread. The condition here is recessive and seemingly has no selective advantage, but still attains a frequency of about .07. This seems to indicate that deleterious genes can become relatively common by simple chance or random gene drift.

With regard to the G6PD-deficiency alleles, it can be seen from the formulas that sex-linked genes would be expected in higher frequencies than autosomals with the same amount of selection against them. But even if we estimate the selection against hemizygotes as .05, with the maximum mutation rate of 10^{-5} we would only expect a gene frequency of .03. If we use the mutation rate of 10^{-8} that we found for the abnormal hemoglobins in Japan, then with a selection of .1 against hemizygotes for the G6PD deficiency, we would expect a frequency of .0006. The occasional cases of G6PD deficiency found in Northern Europe would be anticipated with this formula, but the great clustering of high frequencies of the G6PD-deficiency genes in the tropical regions of the Old World require another explanation.

Although recurrent mutation balanced by selection may not explain the high frequencies of G6PD and hemoglobin variants, there is no doubt that among many present-day populations the frequencies of these genes are decreasing to the levels predicted by these formulas. Interpretation of many of the observed frequencies requires knowing how long it would take to reach these low levels, and for this problem we must consider the equations of gene frequency change.

The basic equation for gene frequency change at an autosomal locus with two alleles is:

$$\Delta q_2 = \frac{W_{22}q_2^2 + W_{12}q_2(1 - q_2)}{W_{11}(1 - q_2)^2 + 2W_{12}q_2(1 - q_2) + W_{22}q_2^2} - q_2$$

where the W's are the respective fitnesses of the genotypes, and q_2 the frequency of the gene in question. Also q_1, the frequency of the other allele equals $(1 - q_2)$. If we treat this as an ordinary differential equation, then separating the variables we get:

$$\int dt =$$

$$\int \frac{W_{11}(1 - q_2)^2 + 2W_{12}q_2(1 - q_2) + W_{22}q_2^2}{W_{22}q_2^2 + W_{12}q_2(1 - q_2) + W_{11}q_2(1 - q_2)^2 + 2W_{12}q_2^2(1 - q_2) + W_{22}q_2^3}\, dq_2$$

Integration yields:

$$t \Big|_{t_0}^{t_1} = \Bigg| \frac{W_{11}}{W_{12} - W_{11}} \log q_2 + \frac{W_{22}}{W_{12} - W_{22}} \log (1 - q_2) +$$

$$\frac{W_{11}W_{22} - W_{12}^2}{(W_{12} - W_{11})(W_{12} - W_{22})} \log [W_{12} - W_{11} + q_2(W_{11} + W_{22} - 2W_{12})] \Bigg|_{q_0}^{q_1} . \tag{4}$$

This formula obviously cannot be used when $W_{12} = W_{11}$ or $W_{12} = W_{22}$ (if these had been set equal at the beginning the integration would have been much easier), but by making the difference between the two similar fitnesses as small as is necessary, we can get close estimates for these situations.

For populations no longer in the circumstances that increased the frequencies of abnormal hemoglobin genes, it is of interest to determine how long it will take these deleterious recessives to decrease to practically 0. If we set the fitness of the abnormal hemoglobin homozygote, $W_{22} = .05$, and $W_{11} = 1.0$, and $W_{12} = .99$, then it would take about 70 generations for the frequency to go from .20 to .01. If we set $W_{22} = .5$ with the same values for W_{11} and W_{12}, it would take 107 generations, which is a considerably longer time, but not so long as equivalent changes in heterozygote fitness would require. If, for example, the fitnesses of the two surviving genotypes are reversed so that $W_{12} = 1.0$ and $W_{11} = .99$, then it would take 465 generations. With $W_{22} = 0$, if $W_{11} = .9999$ and $W_{12} = 1.0000$, then it would take 99 generations for the gene frequency to go from .2 to .01. This is close to the value obtained by Smith (32), whose methods permit the two surviving genotypes to have equal fitnesses; so that our formula seems to be converging to the same value.

For a multi-allelic autosomal or a sex-linked locus, the equations for gene frequency change are not solvable by classical methods. But we can still get an expression for the change in one generation; by continuous substitution of the new value on a computer, the solution for any set of numerical values for the fitnesses and the gene frequency at the start can be obtained. For three autosomal alleles we have:

$$\Delta q_1 = \frac{W_{11}q_1^2 + W_{12}q_1q_2 + W_{13}q_1q_3}{W_{11}q_1^2 + W_{22}q_2^2 + W_{33}q_3^2 + 2W_{12}q_1q_2 + 2W_{13}q_1q_3 + 2W_{23}q_2q_3} - q_1$$

and similarly for the other two alleles. The general case can be written as:

$$\Delta q_i = \frac{\sum_{j=1}^{n} W_{ij}q_iq_j}{\sum_{i=1}^{n}\sum_{j=1}^{n} W_{ij}q_iq_j} - q_i \tag{5}$$

For a sex-linked locus the general case for the change in gene frequency in males in one generation is:

$$\Delta q_{2m} = \frac{W_{2-}\,q_{2f}}{W_{1-}(1 - q_{2f}) + W_{2-}\,q_{2f}} - q_{2m} \tag{6}$$

and for the females it is:

$$\Delta q_{2f} = \frac{.5W_{12}q_{2m} + .5W_{12}q_{2f} + (W_{22} - W_{12})q_{2m}q_{2f}}{W_{11} + (W_{12} - W_{11})q_{2m} + (W_{12} - W_{11})q_{2f} + (W_{11} + W_{22} - 2W_{12})q_{2m}q_{2f}} - q_{2f} \tag{7}$$

where W_{1-} and W_{2-} are the fitnesses of the two male hemizygotes, and W_{11}, W_{22}, and W_{12} are, respectively, the fitnesses of the female homozygotes and heterozygote.

A related problem is to compute the equilibrium frequencies, and again the simplest case is an autosomal locus with two alleles. For this case the two equilibrium gene frequencies are given by:

$$\hat{q}_1 = \frac{W_{22} - W_{12}}{W_{11} + W_{22} - 2W_{12}} \qquad \hat{q}_2 = \frac{W_{11} - W_{12}}{W_{11} + W_{22} - 2W_{12}} \tag{8}$$

For the tri-allelic autosomal case, I find the equations in Li (424) the easiest to use. First we define the three 2 × 2 determinants:

$$D_1 = \begin{vmatrix} (W_{33} - W_{13}) & (W_{12} - W_{23}) \\ (W_{33} - W_{23}) & (W_{22} - W_{23}) \end{vmatrix} \qquad D_2 = \begin{vmatrix} (W_{11} - W_{13}) & (W_{33} - W_{13}) \\ (W_{12} - W_{13}) & (W_{33} - W_{23}) \end{vmatrix}$$

and

$$D_3 = \begin{vmatrix} (W_{11} - W_{13}) & (W_{12} - W_{23}) \\ (W_{12} - W_{13}) & (W_{22} - W_{23}) \end{vmatrix} .$$

Then if $D = D_1 + D_2 + D_3$, the three equilibrium frequencies can be written as:

$$\hat{q}_1 = \frac{D_1}{D} \quad \hat{q}_2 = \frac{D_2}{D} \quad \text{and} \quad \hat{q}_3 = \frac{D_3}{D} \tag{9}$$

For sex-linked genes there are two equilibria, one for the frequency in males, and the other for females; and these can be quite different if selection is acting in opposite directions for the two sexes. For males the equilibrium frequencies are:

$$\hat{q}_{1m} = \frac{W_{1-}[W_{12}(W_{1-} + W_{2-}) - 2W_{22}W_{2-}]}{W_{12}(W_{1-} + W_{2-})^2 - 2W_{1-}W_{2-}(W_{11} + W_{22})}$$

and

$$\hat{q}_{2m} = \frac{W_{2-}[W_{12}(W_{1-} + W_{2-}) - 2W_{11}W_{1-}]}{W_{12}(W_{1-} + W_{2-})^2 - 2W_{1-}W_{2-}(W_{11} + W_{22})} \cdot \tag{10}$$

For the females, they are:

$$\hat{q}_{1f} = \frac{W_{12}(W_{1-} + W_{2-}) - 2W_{22}W_{2-}}{2[W_{12}(W_{1-} + W_{2-}) - W_{22}W_{2-} - W_{11}W_{1-}]}$$

and

$$\hat{q}_{2f} = \frac{W_{12}(W_{1-} + W_{2-}) - 2W_{11}W_{1-}}{2[W_{12}(W_{1-} + W_{2-}) - W_{22}W_{2-} - W_{11}W_{1-}]} \tag{11}$$

where the W's are the respective fitnesses as previously defined.

In many cases it is of value to know whether a third allele will increase when introduced into a population. The autosomal case is outlined in Bodmer and Parsons (98), whose primary conclusion is that a third allele (3) will increase when introduced at a small frequency if

$$k = \frac{W_{13}(W_{12} - W_{22}) + W_{23}(W_{12} - W_{11})}{W_{12}^2 - W_{11}W_{22}} \tag{12}$$

is greater than 1.0.

Although both the hemoglobin and G6PD loci are now known to be multi-allelic, the equations for these more complicated conditions will not be utilized. Most abnormal hemoglobin genes that are found in appreciable frequencies in some population occur alone or with at most one other abnormal gene. Thus, the existence of three hemoglobin alleles—including the normal one—in appreciable frequencies seems to be the most complicated equilibrium condition that is at all common. In the discussions of specific geographical areas it will be shown that the condition of even two abnormal genes in equilibrium does not seem to be a usual state of affairs. For the G6PD alleles, there is a question whether an extreme deficiency allele can replace a less severe variant or vice versa.

However, in most populations with a high frequency of a G6PD-deficiency gene, one variant seems to be involved.

The final deterministic force of evolution to be considered is gene flow or migration. Migration between isolates tends to equalize their gene frequencies. Although this force cannot explain the presence of deleterious genes in the human species, for any specific set of contiguous populations it is a major determinant of the variation in gene frequency. Where the fitnesses of the hemoglobin or G6PD genotypes are such that an equilibrium exists in the presence of an abnormal allele (or, in other words, endemic malaria is present), migration will have little effect on the gene frequencies. But when the abnormal genes are present in a population because of migration from a malarious area, the effect can be pronounced.

For an autosomal locus with two alleles, if we approximate the selection against homozygotes for the abnormal allele as $-sq^2$, where s is the selection coefficient of the homozygotes, and the amount of gene change due to migration is $m(Q - q)$ where m is the frequency of migration and Q is the gene frequency of the immigrants, then the two forces will balance each other at equilibrium so that:

$$\Delta q = -sq^2 + m(Q - q) = 0$$

and the equilibrium gene frequency is:

$$\hat{q} = \frac{-m \pm \sqrt{m^2 + 4msQ}}{2s} \qquad (13)$$

If this equation is considered as a differential equation, the time it would take to approach equilibrium can be approximated. In integral form the equation is.

$$\int dt = \int \frac{dq}{-sq^2 - mq + mQ}$$

Integrating we get:

$$t\Big|_{t_0}^{t_1} = \Big| -\frac{1}{\sqrt{m^2 + 4msQ}} \log \frac{2sq + m - \sqrt{m^2 + 4msQ}}{2sq + m + \sqrt{m^2 + 4msQ}} \Big|_{q_0}^{q_1} \qquad (14)$$

For any numerical estimates of m, s, and Q, the time it would take for any specific gene frequency change can be calculated from this equation.

The other two factors that can influence gene frequency change—random genetic drift and the mating system of the population—will not be considered separately. All the previous equations and the models yet to be discussed assume that the population undergoes random mating. Many small human isolates have a considerable amount of inbreeding

```
        $COMPILE MAD,EXECUTE,DUMP,PRINT OBJECT                                          001421   05/17/66      8 00 43.4 PM

     MAD (03 JAN 1966 VERSION) PROGRAM LISTING ... ... ..,

        AGAIN      READ FORMAT CARD, GDM, GRM, GDF, GRF, MM, FA, SDM, SRM, SDF,              *001
                 1  SRF, SHF, GEN, COMP, POP                                                 *001
                   PRINT FORMAT TITLE, GDM, GRM, GDF, GRF, MM, FA, SDM,SRM, SDF,             *002
                 1  SRF, SHF, GEN, COMP, POP                                                 *002
                   READ FORMAT MIGT, MIG, TR, FDM, FRM, FDF, FRF                             *003
                   PRINT FORMAT MIGR, MIG, TR, FDM, FRM, FDF, FRF                            *004
                   INTEGER FR,FH,FD,MD,MR,IND,N,POP,NP                                       *005
                   DIMENSION XG(500),XFRAM(500),XFRAF(500)                                   *006
                   PLTXMX.(GEN/5.0 + 3.0)                                                    *007
                   NP=0                                                                      *008
                   G=0                                                                       *009
        START      G=G+1.0                                                                   *010
                   WHENEVER G.G.GEN, TRANSFER TO PLOT                                        *011
                   FR=0                                                                      *012
                   FH=0                                                                      *013
                   FD=0                                                                      *014
                   MD=0                                                                      *015
                   MR=0                                                                      *016
                   IND=0                                                                     *017
        BEGIN       X=RANDOM.(RNO)                                                           *018
                   WHENEVER X .LE. GDM, H=78                                                 *019
                   WHENEVER X .G. GDM, H=79                                                  *020
                    X=RANDOM.(RNO)                                                           *021
                   WHENEVER H .E. 78 .AND. X.G. MM, GAM=7                                    *022
                   WHENEVER H .E. 78 .AND. X .LE. MM, GAM=8                                  *023
                   WHENEVER H .E. 79 .AND. X .G. MM, GAM=7                                   *024
                   WHENEVER H .E. 79 .AND. X .LE. MM, GAM=9                                  *025
                    X=RANDUM.(RNO)                                                           *026
                   WHENEVER X.LE. GDF, C=88                                                  *027
                   WHENEVER X.G.GDF.AND. X.LE. GDF + GRF, C=99                               *028
                   WHENEVER X.G. GDF + GRF, C=89                                             *029
                   WHENEVER C.E. 88                                                          *030
                   GAMF= 8                                                                   *031     01
                   OR WHENEVER C.E. 99                                                       *032     01
                   GAMF = 9                                                                  *033     01
                   END OF CONDITIONAL                                                        *034     01
                    X=RANDOM.(RNO)                                                           *035
                   WHENEVER C.E.89 .AND. X.LE. FA, GAMF=8                                    *036
                   WHENEVER C .E.89 .AND. X .G. FA, GAMF=9                                   *037
                   WHENEVER GAMF .E. 8 .AND. GAM .E. 7, Z=78                                 *038
                   WHENEVER GAMF .E. 8 .AND. GAM .E. 8, Z=88                                 *039
                   WHENEVER GAMF .E. 8 .AND. GAM .E. 9, Z=89                                 *040
                   WHENEVER GAMF .E. 9 .AND. GAM .E. 7, Z=79                                 *041
                   WHENEVER GAMF .E. 9 .AND. GAM .E. 8, Z=89                                 *042
                   WHENEVER GAMF .E. 9 .AND. GAM .E. 9, Z=99                                 *043
                    X=RANDOM.(RNO)                                                           *044
                   WHENEVER Z.E. 78 .AND. X.G. SDM                                           *045
                   MD=MD+1                                                                   *046     01
                   OR WHENEVER Z .E. 79 .AND. X.G. SRM                                       *047     01
                   MR=MR+1                                                                   *048     01
                   OR WHENEVER Z.E.88.AND.X.G.SDF                                            *049     01
                   FD=FD+1                                                                   *050     01
                   OR WHENEVER Z.E.89.AND.X.G.SHF                                            *051     01

                   FH=FH+1                                                                   *052     01
                   OR WHENEVER Z.E.99.AND.X.G.SRF                                            *053     01
                   FR=FR+1                                                                   *054     01
                   OR WHENEVER COMP .E.1.0                                                   *055     01
                   TRANSFER TO BEGIN                                                         *056     01
                   END OF CONDITIONAL                                                        *057     01
                   IND=IND+1                                                                 *058
                   WHENEVER IND .G. POP, TRANSFER TO GNFL                                    *059
                   TRANSFER TO BEGIN                                                         *060
        GNFL       N=0                                                                       *061
        MILOP       X=RANDOM.(RNO)                                                           *062
                   N=N+1                                                                     *063
                   WHENEVER N.G. POP, TRANSFER TO PRINT                                      *064
                   WHENEVER X .LE. MIG, TRANSFER TO SUB                                      *065
                   WHENEVER X .G. MIG, TRANSFER TO MILOP                                     *066
        SUB         X=RANDOM.(RNO)                                                           *067
                   WHENEVER X.LE. TR, TRANSFER TO MMIG                                       *068
                   WHENEVER X .G. TR, TRANSFER TO FMIG                                       *069
        MMIG        X=RANDOM.(RNO)                                                           *070
                   WHENEVER  X .LE. FDM, MD=MD+1                                             *071
                   WHENEVER X .G. FDM, MR=MR+1                                               *072
                   TRANSFER TO MILOP                                                         *07
        FMIG        X=RANDOM.(RNO)                                                           *074
                   WHENEVER X .LE. FDF, FD=FD+1                                              *075
                   WHENEVER X .G. FDF.AND. X.LE. FDF+FRF, FR=FR+1                            *076
                   WHENEVER X.G. FDF+FRF, FH=FH+1                                            *077
                   TRANSFER TO MILOP                                                         *078
        PRINT      GDM=(1.0*MD)/ (1.0*MD+MR)                                                 *079
                   GRM=(1.0*MR)/(1.0*MD+MR)                                                  *080
                   FRAM=GRM                                                                  *081
                   GDF=(1.0*FD)/(1.0*FD+FH+FR)                                               *082
                   GRF=(1.0*FR)/(1.0*FR+FH+FD)                                               *083
                   FRAF=(2.0*FR+FH)/(2.0*FR+2.0*FH+2.0*FD)                                   *084
                   NP=NP+1                                                                   *085
                   XFRAM(NP)=FRAM                                                            *086
                   XFRAF(NP)=FRAF                                                            *087
                   XG(NP)=G                                                                  *088
                   TRANSFER TO START                                                         *089
        PLOT       PLTOFS.(0.0,5.0,0.0,0.1,2.0,2.0)                                          *090
                   PLINE.(XG(1),XFRAF(1),NP,1,0,0,1)                                         *091
                   POSHLN.(XG(1),XFRAM(1),NP,1,0.1,1)                                        *092
                   PAXIS.(2.0,2.0,XCOM,-10,GEN/5.0,0.0,0.0,5.0,1.0)                          *093
                   PAXIS.(2.0,2.0,YCOM,14,10.0,90.0,0.0,0.1,1.0)                             *094
                   PLTEND.                                                                   *095
                   TRANSFER TO AGAIN                                                         *096
                     VECTOR VALUES  RNO=0.                                                   *097
                   VECTOR VALUES CARD=$13F5.3,115*$                                          *098
                   VECTOR VALUES TITLE=$ 12H POPULATION  13F7.3,117*$                        *099
                    VECTOR VALUES MIGT=$ 6F10.6 *$                                           *100.
                    VECTOR VALUES MIGR=$ 15H MIGRATION DATA  6F10.6 *$                       *101
                   VECTOR VALUES XCOM=$GENERATIONS$                                          *102
                   VECTOR VALUES YCOM=$GENE FREQUENCY$                                       *103
                   END OF PROGRAM                                                            *104
```

Figure 2. A MAD Program for the Simulation of Genetic Reproduction at a Sex-linked Locus with Two Alleles.

```
START      READ FORMAT INPUT, MA,MB,MO,FA,FB,FO,NM,NF
           PRINT FORMAT IN,   MA,MB,MO,FA,FB,FO,NM,NF
           READ FORMAT SELT,SAA,SAB,SAO,SBB,SBO,SOO,COMP,GEN
           PRINT FORMAT SE, SAA,SAB,SAO,SBB,SBO,SOO,COMP,GEN
           READ FORMAT MIGT,  MIG, TR, GAA,GAB,GAO,GBB,GBO,GOO
           PRINT FORMAT MIGR, MIG, TR, GAA,GAB,GAO,GBB,GBO,GOO
           DIMENSION IMAGE(10000)
           PLOT1.(0,GEN/10,10,10,10)
           PLOT2.(IMAGE,1.0,0.0,0.0,GEN)
           G=0
 START1    G=G+1.0
           WHENEVER G.G.GEN,TRANSFER TO GRAPH
           MAA=0
           MAB=0
           MAO=0
           MBB=0
           MBO=0
           MOO=0
           FAA=0
           FAB=0
           FAO=0
           FBB=0
           FBO=0
           FOO=0
           IND=0
GAMLP       X=RANDOM.(RNO)
           WHENEVER X.LE.MA,SPM=7
           WHENEVER X.G.MA.AND.X.LE.MA+MB,SPM=8
           WHENEVER X.G.MA+MB,SPM=9
            X=RANDOM.(RNO)
           WHENEVER X.LE.FA,OVA=7
           WHENEVER X.G.FA.AND.X.LE.FA+FB,OVA=8
           WHENEVER X.G.FA+FB,OVA=9
           WHENEVER SPM.E.7.AND.OVA.E.7,OFSP=77
           WHENEVER SPM.E.7.AND.OVA.E.8,OFSP=78
           WHENEVER SPM.E.7.AND.OVA.E.9,OFSP=79
           WHENEVER SPM.E.8.AND.OVA.E.7,OFSP=78
           WHENEVER SPM.E.8.AND.OVA.E.8,OFSP=88
           WHENEVER SPM.E.8.AND.OVA.E.9,OFSP=89
           WHENEVER SPM.E.9.AND.OVA.E.7,OFSP=79
           WHENEVER SPM.E.9.AND.OVA.E.8,OFSP=89
           WHENEVER SPM.E.9.AND.OVA.E.9,OFSP=99
            X=RANDOM.(RNO)
           WHENEVER OFSP.E.77.AND.X.G.SAA,TRANSFER TO STORE
           WHENEVER OFSP.E.78.AND.X.G.SAB,TRANSFER TO STORE
           WHENEVER OFSP.E.79.AND.X.G.SAO,TRANSFER TO STORE
           WHENEVER OFSP.E.88.AND.X.G.SBB,TRANSFER TO STORE
           WHENEVER OFSP.E.89.AND.X.G.SBO,TRANSFER TO STORE
           WHENEVER OFSP.E.99.AND.X.G.SOO,TRANSFER TO STORE
           WHENEVER COMP.E.0.0, IND=IND+1.0
           WHENEVER IND.G.NM+NF, TRANSFER TO OUT
           TRANSFER TO GAMLP
 STORE     IND=IND+1.0
           WHENEVER IND.LE.NM,TRANSFER TO MALE
           TRANSFER TO FEMALE
 MALE      WHENEVER OFSP.E.77,MAA=MAA+1.0
           WHENEVER OFSP.E.78,MAB=MAB+1.0
           WHENEVER OFSP.E.79,MAO=MAO+1.0
           WHENEVER OFSP.E.88,MBB=MBB+1.0
           WHENEVER OFSP.E.89,MBO=MBO+1.0
           WHENEVER OFSP.E.99,MOO=MOO+1.0
           TRANSFER TO GAMLP
 FEMALE    WHENEVER OFSP.E.77,FAA=FAA+1.0
           WHENEVER OFSP.E.78,FAB=F/B+1.0
           WHENEVER OFSP .E.79,FAO=FAO+1.0
           WHENEVER OFSP.E.88,FBB=FBB+1.0
           WHENEVER OFSP.E.89,FBO=FBO+1.0
           WHENEVER OFSP.E.99,FOO=FOO+1.0
           WHENEVER IND.G.NM+NF,TRANSFER TO OUT
           TRANSFER TO GAMLP
OUT        WHENEVER MIG.E.0.0, TRANSFER TO FLOW
           N=0
MILOP       X=RANDOM.(RNO)
           N=N+1.0
           WHENEVER N.G. NM+NF, TRANSFER TO FLOW
           WHENEVER X .LE. MIG, TRANSFER TO SUB
           WHENEVER X .G. MIG, TRANSFER TO MILOP
SUB         X=RANDOM.(RNO)
           WHENEVER X .LE. TR, TRANSFER TO MMIG
           WHENEVER X .G. TR, TRANSFER TO FMIG
MMIG        X=RANDOM.(RNO)
           WHENEVER X.LE. GAA, MAA=MAA+1.0
           WHENEVER X.G.GAA.AND.X.LE.GAA+GAB,MAB=MAB+1.0
           WHENEVERX.G.GAA+GAB.AND.X.LE.GAA+GAB+GAO,MAO=MAO+1.0
           WHENEVERX.G.GAA+GAB GAO.AND.X.LE.GAA+GAB+GAO+GBB,MBB=MBB+1.0
           WHENEVER X.G.GAA+GAB+GAO+GBB.AND.X.LE.GAA+GAB+GAO+GBB+GBO,
          1MBO=MBO+1.0
           WHENEVER X .G. GAA+GAB+GAO+GBB+GBO, MOO=MOO+1.0
           TRANSFER TO MILOP
FMIG        X=RANDOM.(RNO)
           WHENEVER X.LE. GAA, FAA=FAA+1.0
           WHENEVER X.G.GAA.AND.X.LE.GAA+GAB, FAB=FAB+1.0
           WHENEVERX.G.GAA+GAB.AND.X.LE.GAA+GAB+GAO,FAO=FAO+1.0
           WHENEVERX.G.GAA+GAB+GAO.AND.X.LE.GAA+GAB+GAO+GBB,FBB=FBB+1.0
           WHENEVER X.G.GAA+GA2+GAO+GBB.AND.X.LE.GAA+GAB+GAO+GBB+GBO,
          1FBO=FBO+1.0
           WHENEVER X .G. GAA+GAB+GAO+GBB+GBO, FOO=FOO+1.0
           TRANSFER TO MILOP
FLOW       MTOT=MAA+MAB+MAO+MBB+MBO+MOO
           FTOT=FAA+FAB+FAO+FBB+FBO+FOO
           MA=((MAA*2.0)+MAB+MAO)/(2.0*MTOT)
           MB=((MBB*2.0)+MAB+MBO)/(2.0*MTOT)
           MO=1.0-(MA+MB)
           FA=((FAA*2.0)+FAB+FAO)/(2.0*FTOT)
           FB=((FBB*2.0)+FAB+FBO)/(2.0*FTOT)
           FO=1.0-(FA+FB)
           FRA=((MTOT*MA)+(FTOT*FA))/(MTOT+FTOT)
           FRB=((MTOT*MB)+(FTOT*FB))/(MTOT+FTOT)
           FRO=1.0-(FRA+FRB)
           PLOT3.($A$,FRA,G,1)
           PLOT3.($B$,FRB,G,1)
           PLOT3.($O$,FRO,G,1)
           WHENEVER FRA.GE.1.0,TRANSFER TO GRAPH
           WHENEVER FRB.GE.1.0,TRANSFER TO GRAPH
           WHENEVER FRO.GE.1.0,TRANSFER TO GRAPH
           TRANSFER TO START1
GRAPH      EXECUTE PLOT4.(0,0)
           VECTOR VALUES RNO=0.
           VECTOR VALUES INPUT=$8F10.4*$
           VECTOR VALUES IN=$19H INPUT POPULATION    8F10.4*$
           VECTOR VALUES SELT=$8F10.5*$
           VECTOR VALUES SE=$ 18H SELECTION VALUES   8F10.5*$
            VECTOR VALUES MIGT=$ 8F10.6 *$
            VECTOR VALUES MIGR=$ 15H MIGRATION DATA  8F10.6 *$
           END OF PROGRAM
```

126

Figure 3. A MAD Program for the Simulation of Genetic Reproduction at an Autosomal Locus with Three Alleles.

which would affect their gene frequencies; and even some isolates with high frequencies of the genes under consideration, such as the Kurdish Jews, apparently have a significant amount of inbreeding. But the problems associated with the G6PD and hemoglobin genes have not seemed to require a consideration of inbreeding. Generally it can be stated that inbreeding increases the frequency of homozygotes, so that for the hemoglobin genes it would increase the frequency of the deleterious genotypes, thus increasing the selection against these genes.

In order to include the effects of random gene drift, two programs have been written for the Michigan 7090 computer to simulate the reproduction of a single population. One is for sex-linked genes and the other for autosomal genes. The population size can be varied, but it is the same for all generations. The effects of selection and migration are included in the models, and mutation can be considered as a very small amount of migration. However, the genotypes are not actually mated, so that the variation in family size cannot be included. An attempt has been made to include compensation in the programs, but in the absence of specific families it is not a very close approximation to reality. Since the population size is constant in all generations, with compensation another genotype is generated for those selected out. This actually changes the fitness values. Many programs were run both with and without compensation, and it did not affect the results greatly. Most of the runs which are discussed in the chapters on specific populations and geographic regions were run without compensation. For the problems associated with the abnormal hemoglobins and the G6PD deficiency, this concept does not seem to be important. The programs are shown on Figures 2 and 3. They are written in the MAD language, which does not add to their general utility, but translations to FORTRAN are not difficult. Both programs have been run with the two different graphing systems, but for illustrative purposes the program for the graph of Figure 5 is shown on Figure 3, and that of Figure 11 on Figure 2.

V

SELECTION FOR THE RED CELL DEFECTS

AS WAS pointed out previously, the selection against the abnormal hemoglobin, thalassemia, and glucose-6-phosphate dehydrogenase deficiency genes is dysfunctional and quite obvious. Most homozygotes for an abnormal hemoglobin or thalassemia gene, or heterozygotes for two such genes, have an anemia, that, however severe, decreases fitness to some extent. This decreased fitness has certainly been present for most of human history. During the great majority of this time man was a hunter, and strenuous activity by the entire group was essential. The relative absence of deleterious genes in the Australian Aborigines is evidence for this "pristine condition." Although the G6PD deficiency genotypes do not have so severe a handicap, neonatal jaundice and susceptibility to infection would have selected against these genes.

The fact that there is so much selection against these genes raises the question of why they are so frequent in many populations in some parts of the world. With only this selection against them, their equilibrium frequencies would be zero or very close to it. In this case the formula for recurrent mutation balancing selection would be appropriate. Many isolated cases of these genes, such as α-thalassemia in Sweden (642), are most likely due to recurrent mutation, but the very high frequencies of hemoglobins S, C, and E and thalassemia cannot be explained by recurrent mutation. Theoretically it would be highly unlikely for populations to vary so much in their frequencies of these genes if recurrent mutation were the explanation for the high frequencies. This implies that there must be some selection for these genes. Furthermore, for the hemoglobin S and β-thalassemia genes, which are the most widespread, this selection must be for the heterozygotes for either of them and the normal allele, since it would be impossible for any selection for homozygotes for these genes to overcome their very severe and almost invariably lethal anemia. Even so, it seems curious that the two hemoglobin genes with the most selection against them are the most widespread.

For an autosomal locus with two alleles, when the heterozygote has an increased fitness over both homozygotes, a stable equilibrium with both alleles present can exist; it is called a balanced polymorphism. The more common abnormal hemoglobins and thalassemia are undoubtedly balanced polymorphisms, but this is not necessarily true for some of the more uncommon hemoglobins or the G6PD deficiency. For many uncommon hemoglobins homozygotes are unknown, but the decrease in fitness for these homozygotes or for homo- and hemizygotes for the G6PD deficiency is not likely to be very great. Thus it would be possible, and within the range of mortality rates for diseases like malaria, for the slightly decreased fitness of these individuals to increase to that of the normal genotypes in a malarious environment, and perhaps even to increase to a value greater than normals. In these cases the abnormal alleles would be more frequent than the normal alleles at equilibrium, but if the heterozygotes were still the most fit, both normal and abnormal genes would persist in the population. Strictly speaking, these would still be balanced polymorphisms, but the normal allele might be completely replaced, in which case it would be a transient polymorphism during this replacement.

If there is selection for heterozygotes for the hemoglobin and G6PD deficiency genes, then the question arises as to the physical basis of this selection. It is probably clear to the reader at this point that the major factor concerned in this selection seems to be malaria. But it behooves us to examine now the specific data on which this generalization is based.

Although Haldane (302b) had suggested earlier that malaria may account for the high frequencies of thalassemia, and others had discussed a similar possibility for the sickle cell gene, Allison first posed the problem and provided evidence for his conclusion. Allison (23) first showed that among schoolchildren in Kampala, Uganda, those with the sickle-cell trait had a lower malaria parasite rate, which is simply the proportion infected at any one time. In the same paper he also showed that among adults of the Luo tribe who were inoculated with malaria, the sicklers showed parasites in their blood far fewer times than non-sicklers (two out of fifteen sicklers showed parasites, but fourteen out of fifteen non-sicklers).

Allison (22) then showed that the frequency of the sickle-cell trait in many tribes of East Africa is closely correlated with the endemicity of malaria.

This evidence by itself was not conclusive, but it did provide a reasonable basis for an explanation of the high frequencies of the sickle-cell gene. Since then other investigations have demonstrated more conclusively the operation of selection by malaria. Raper (565), in a larger series, found the same lower parasite rate in sicklers and also showed that they do not have as many heavy infections as non-sicklers. He also (566) later provided conclusive evidence that sicklers do not die as frequently from cerebral malaria, which is the common lethal complication of falciparum malaria. Many studies have shown that sicklers have a lower malaria parasite rate, though others (84, 491, 730) have failed to demonstrate such a relationship. The Lambotte-Legrands (396) in Kinshasa, Congo Republic, and more recently Edington and Watson-Williams (231) in Ibadan, Nigeria have published data on postmortems that support Raper's conclusion that sicklers do not die as frequently from malaria.

These data indicate that selection for the sickle-cell gene operates through differential survival, but the possibility also exists that sicklers may have a greater fertility which in some way is caused by malaria. Not so much data exists on this aspect of the problem, but an advantage for sicklers has been reported in several cases. Delbrouck (199) and Allard (19) in the Congo both found sicklers to have a slightly higher fertility, but in the first study the female sicklers had the increased fertility, while in the second the males did. In West Africa, Roberts and Boyo (575) found the marriage of a sickler and a normal homozygote to have a slightly higher fertility; and in addition, the marriage of a hemoglobin C heterozygote and a normal homozygote had the same higher fertility. Finally, Firschein's (250) study of the Black Carib in British Honduras found striking fertility differences among women, with the sicklers having a greatly increased number of offspring. If female sicklers had a resistance to placental malaria, which is a major cause of pregnancy wastage, then they might be expected to have a higher fertility, while male sicklers would not (441). Firschein's data accord with this hypothesis, but the study by Cannon (146) which examined sicklers and non-sicklers for the frequency of placental malaria and of premature births did not find any differences. However, Cannon only found 10 per cent sicklers among pregnant women, while another study in the same area around Ilesha, Nigeria, by Roberts and Boyo (576) found 25 per cent hemoglobin S. This discrepancy is unexplained and may have influenced the malarial results.

There is thus considerable evidence that heterozygotes for the hemoglobin S gene have a greater resistance to malarial infections and perhaps have a greater fertility in a malarious environment. Investigations testing different age groups for sickling in a malarious environment have been reviewed recently by Allison (27) and by Rucknagel and Neel (586). As a group these studies are somewhat contradictory, but they do provide further indirect evidence for sicklers surviving at a greater rate in malarious environments.

Although many of the investigations testing the relationship between sickling and malaria have not distinguished the various species of human malaria, those that have indicate that sicklers have a lower parasite rate for falciparum malaria if they have a lower rate at all. This form of malaria is due to *Plasmodium falciparum*, or *Lavarania falciparum* in the recent terminology of Bray (115a). Bray has separated the falciparum parasite from the other human malaria parasites, *P. vivax*, *P. malariae*, and *P. ovale*, because recent discoveries have shown it to be quite different in its pre-erythrocytic and exo-erythrocytic cycles.

Falciparum and vivax malaria are the two most common and most widespread forms of the disease, although quartan malaria, which is due to *P. malariae*, is widely distributed in the Old World. Falciparum malaria is particularly common in the tropical regions, while vivax, although also endemic in the tropics, is found much further north than other malaria parasites. For example, malaria in Korea, Russia, and the Netherlands is due primarily to *P. vivax*; and in the Po River Valley of northern Italy *P. vivax* is more common than *L. falciparum* (482). On the other hand, malaria parasite surveys in Africa, India, Southeast Asia, and New Guinea usually find more than 50 per cent of the infections to be due to *L. falciparum*, and in most cases 90–100 per cent. According to the tropical area surveyed, the other 10 per cent of the infections will be either *P. vivax* or *P. malariae*. *P. ovale* is most common in West Africa, but it never attains sufficient frequency to be an important selective factor.

In a village with holoendemic malaria everyone is continuously reinfected with the disease. In these conditions the average individual is bitten by a mosquito carrying malaria about once every thirty days. By the time he reaches adulthood the individual has built up a solid immunity to malaria. Parasite surveys of adults will usually find 20–40 per cent infected at any one time, but with low-density infections. While among adults there is still a great amount of sickness due to malaria (477a), the children of the village are engaged in a lethal struggle with the parasite. The group from two-to-five-years old will be almost 100 per cent infected and will have enlarged spleens, which is a symptom of blood destruction and perhaps immunity-building. Under these conditions much of the mortality is either directly or indirectly due to malaria, but there is some dispute among malariologists as to whether mortality from malaria is closely correlated with endemicity (744a). There is some question as to whether malaria is not more lethal when this continuous reinfection is interrupted, thus also interrupting the process of immunity-building. Malaria as a selection agent will vary with the amount of mortality, so that the question arises whether the hemoglobin S gene would not be more frequent in populations in which the transmission of malaria is interrupted. In Africa, hemoglobin S is found in high frequencies in both situations. However, one of the highest hemoglobin S frequencies is found among the Bwamba. The parasite rate in children was about 80 per cent, which is close to being holoendemic, but about 50 per cent of the malaria was due to *P. malariae.* Most studies in Africa (23, 177, 448, 565) have found sicklers to have as high a parasite rate for *P. malariae* as non-sicklers, but Garlick (268) has found sicklers to have a lower rate and suggests that they may also have a resistance to *P. malariae.* The Bwamba data may support this hypothesis, but my own view as to the physiological basis of the resistance of sicklers to falciparum malaria argues against this possibility.

In view of the great number of red blood cell defects that are found in high frequencies and hence seem to provide some advantage to the individual carrier in resisting malaria, the hemoglobin S gene, as one of these defects, probably does provide some resistance to any malaria. The malaria parasites are adapted to the environment of the normal human red blood cell, and any change in that environment would seem to alter at least slightly the ability of the parasite to survive and reproduce. But hemoglobin S does seem to have a much more marked resistance to one malaria parasite, *L. falciparum.* As suggested by Miller, Neel, and Livingstone (477b), this resistance seems to be due to both the peculiar characteristic of hemoglobin S, the sickling of the red cells in an anoxic environment; and the peculiar characteristic of the life cycle of *L. falciparum*, its adherence to the walls of the small blood vessels during its maturation. This is a relatively anoxic environment, and the sickling of the infected cells would surely have adverse effects on the survival of the parasite. The placenta would also be an anoxic environment, so that these two characteristics of the hemoglobin and the parasite could also explain the possible higher fertility of female sicklers.

Although hemoglobin S and malaria have been investigated in some detail, there have been relatively few studies that attempt to test the relationship between malaria and the other hemoglobin abnormalities. In Northern Ghana, Edington and Laing (228) could find no evidence for hemoglobin C carriers having a resistance to falciparum malaria since the parasite rates and parasite densities were similar for all genotypes; however, the number of hemoglobin C heterozygotes was rather small. More recently Thompson (673) has found hemoglobin C carriers in Accra, Ghana, to have a lower parasite density. On the other side of the world, Kruatrachue et al. (391) could find no difference in parasite rate between hemoglobin E carriers and normals. In another investigation, hemoglobin E carriers and hemoglobin

E-thalassemia heterozygotes seemed to develop vivax infections as severe as normals on inoculation. But the numbers were small in both cases. Only thirty AE children were examined for parasitemia; and only three AE adults, four E-thalassemia children, and six AA adult controls were inoculated intramuscularly. Ray et al. (571) also inoculated several individuals with vivax malaria. The only two groups with appreciable numbers were AA normals and E-thalassemias, and the latter did not develop infections as frequently (13 out of 14 for AA's; 2 out of 11 for E-thalassemias).

In an attempt to duplicate Allison's original experiment, Beutler et al. (81) inoculated sicklers and non-sicklers among American Negroes with falciparum malaria. They did not find any differences. This could be considered as evidence against any relationship between sickling and malaria. But as later investigations of mortality from malaria have shown that such a relationship does exist, this experiment indicates how difficult it is to find evidence for selection even for the hemoglobin S gene. And since the differences in fitness for other hemoglobin genes and for just about all other human loci are much less than those for hemoglobin S, evidence for selection will be all the more difficult to find. The experiment of Beutler et al. also shows that just about all non-immune humans will become infected with falciparum malaria, particularly if inoculated with heavy doses of the parasite. During the first rapid increase in parasites, no hereditary factor within a species could produce the total suppression of their growth. However, if any red blood cell defect could decrease the rate of growth by as little as 5 per cent, it would be a significant factor during the period when the individual was acquiring an immunity to the parasite. These slight differences in the ability of the parasite to increase in the various hemoglobin genotypes may well be the basis of selection for these genes by malaria (444). Finally, Beutler et al. obviously had to stop the infections before they became lethal, so that the experiment was not a direct test of the operation of natural selection.

Although no studies have demonstrated by parasite rates, parasite densities, or mortality from malaria that any of the other abnormal hemoglobins or thalassemia have a resistance to malaria, it is difficult to explain the distributions of these deleterious genes without assuming that they do have some such resistance. There are also the correlations between malaria and high frequencies of these genes. Exceptions exist, but the few populations whose frequencies of abnormal hemoglobins or thalassemia seem to be too high for the amount of malaria to which they have been subjected are near enough to populations with high frequencies in malarious regions that the malaria hypothesis can still apply. It should be noted that the malaria hypothesis as an attempt to explain high frequencies of deleterious genes postulates only that wherever such high frequencies are found there should be or have been endemic malaria. It does not postulate that wherever endemic malaria occurs there should be high frequencies of abnormal hemoglobin genes.

The correlations between malaria and the abnormal hemoglobins, thalassemia, and the G6PD deficiency will be discussed in detail in the chapters on the geographical regions and their populations. Generally, one can say that hemoglobin E in Asia, hemoglobin C in West Africa, and hemoglobin S, thalassemia, and the G6PD deficiency in all the areas where they are found occur in the most malarious parts of these areas. The evidence for an association between the G6PD deficiency and malaria is at about the same stage as that for the abnormal hemoglobins other than S, although a few more studies have been done on the former trait. All these investigations have been examinations of the parasite rate in normals and G6PD deficients. Some have found differences in favor of deficients (31, 281), while others have not (389, 494, 601). In addition, Motulsky (494) has shown that the frequency of G6PD deficiency is correlated with that of hemoglobin S in the Congo; and Siniscalco et al. (641) have shown it to be correlated with thalassemia in Sardinia. A very recent study (389a) has shown that the red cells of deficients with normal enzyme levels have a significantly greater number of malaria parasites than deficient cells, which is the best evidence that the G6PD deficiency interferes with parasite multiplication.

In the succeeding chapters the malaria hypothesis in general will be assumed. But this does not mean that all species of human malaria are resisted equally by all abnormal hemoglobins, thalassemia, and the G6PD deficiency. Hemoglobin S seems to confer a marked resistance to falciparum malaria, but the other hemoglobins, thalassemia, or the G6PD deficiency may not be so specific. Hemoglobin S causes more physiological changes in red cell function than other red cell defects; and one of these changes, the sickling phenomenon, seems to be the reason for its specific resistance to falciparum malaria. There seems to be no specific interaction like this between any of the other red cell defects and one of the malaria parasites, although there are some possibilities (444). For example, most thalassemias result in smaller mean red cell size, while *P. vivax* enlarges the red cell during maturation; so that this characteristic of thalassemia may interfere with the parasite's reproduction. If specific interactions such as this exist, the great variation in the frequencies of the human malaria parasites may be one of the principle causes of the great variation in the frequencies of red cell defects in the world's populations.

VI

EASTERN ASIA AND THE PACIFIC

MOST OF THE major island groups of Polynesia, Micronesia, and Melanesia have been examined for hemoglobin variants, but, as would be expected in the absence of malaria, none have been found in high frequencies. However, some populations on New Britain and New Guinea in western Melanesia have high frequencies of thalassemia and/or the G6PD deficiency; and the westernmost islands of Micronesia, the Palaus, have been found to have almost 10 per cent G6PD deficiency. An absence of red cell defects is also characteristic of the Australian Aborigines. In recent years malaria has been known to be spreading through Australasia (394a), but the absence of Anopheline vectors in Polynesia, Micronesia, and eastern Melanesia has prevented its spread to these areas, and the nomadic life of the Australian Aborigines would seem to preclude any intense endemic malaria among them. The eastern limit of malaria is in the New Hebrides, where malaria intensity seems to have increased in the past forty years (134a, 469c); and malaria has become endemic in some of the outlying Solomon Islands, such as Tikopia and Rennell Islands, only since World War II.

The Pacific islands were peopled for the most part from mainland Asia, and to a great extent from areas where populations now have high frequencies of hemoglobin E. Since hemoglobin E is unknown in the Pacific east of Indonesia, it would seem that the ancestors of the Pacific populations must have left Asia before the hemoglobin

E gene become frequent. On the other hand, if we assume that their ancestors left mainland Asia with a hemoglobin E frequency like that of the hill tribes of Southeast Asia today, then we can estimate how long it would take for this gene to be reduced to practically zero in the absence of malaria. If the fitness of the EE homozygote is estimated as 0.5 and that of the AE heterozygote as .99, then, according to equation (4) of Chapter IV it would take 107 generations for the hemoglobin E frequency to go from .2 to .01, and another 61 generations for it to decrease further to .005. Using a generation length of twenty years for the human species, these decreases would take about 2000 and 3300 years. Since radiocarbon dates for some Pacific islands fall within this time range, it is possible that the Pacific islanders have lost the hemoglobin E gene since coming from Asia. Since most of these islands were settled by small groups, gene drift would have been an important factor and would have increased the probability of the loss of the hemoglobin E gene. But the other possibility, that the hemoglobin E mutation had not built up to high frequencies in Southeast Asia 2000 to 3000 years ago, seems equally reasonable; and the fact that the aboriginal peoples of Taiwan do not have any hemoglobin E strongly supports this second possibility. The population genetics of hemoglobin E in Thailand would seem to support the second alternative, but this will be discussed later in the chapter.

Although the abnormal hemoglobins are absent from the aboriginal Pacific populations, the G6PD deficiency has been found on Guam and the Palau Islands. The single male deficient found on Guam among the Chamorros may be due to recent gene flow from the Philippines or Spain, but the finding of 8 per cent on two Palau Islands and 6 per cent on the Yap Island of Ifalik would seem to be too high for such an explanation. Since there has never been any malaria on these islands, and they appear to have been inhabited for a long time, these frequencies do not seem to be explained by the malaria hypothesis. Figure 4 shows the decrease in the G6PD deficiency with various fitnesses for the homozygous and hemizygous deficients. Even with fitnesses of .95 for these genotypes, the frequency would have been very high 1000 years ago, but the Palauans have been on Palau for much longer. However, Riesenberg's recent study (573b) indicates considerable contact with the Philippines, which could have resulted in some gene flow. If this gene flow is estimated as .005 from a population with 10 percent G6PD deficiency, then the Palau frequencies could be maintained by it. The migrants were estimated to be 90 per cent males, which seems reasonable in view of the long distances but which decreases the amount of gene flow for a sex-linked gene. The fitnesses of the homozygous and hemizygous deficients were estimated as .95. Starting with 10 per cent G6PD deficiency and a population of 1000, there was still 7 per cent G6PD deficiency after sixty generations for one computer run, but most other runs were below this.

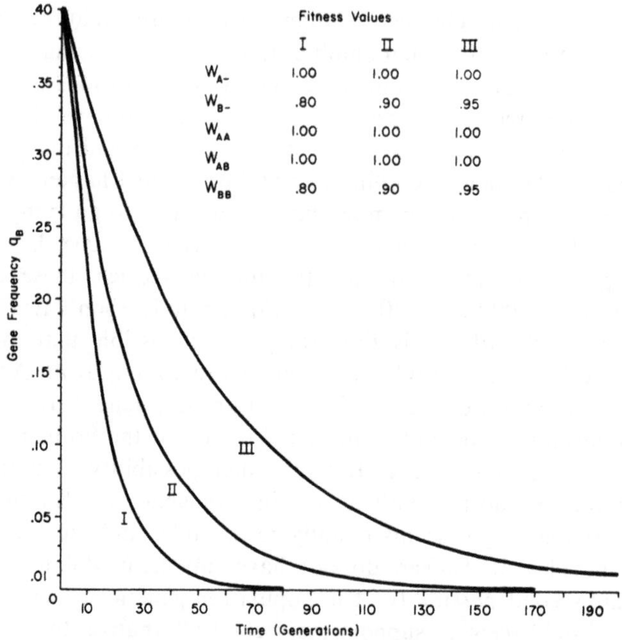

Figure 4. The Decrease in a Deleterious Sex-linked Allele. (From F. B. Livingstone, 1964, *American Journal of Human Genetics* 16:435-450, by permission).

With a population of 200 there were runs with over 10 per cent G6PD deficiency after 100 generations, and, as would be expected, the G6PD deficiency disappeared rather quickly in several runs. Figure 5 shows the extremes for the runs with the population sizes of 1000 and 200; and since the population of Palau has probably been between these limits, the G6PD-deficiency frequency there could be maintained.

In Australian New Guinea and New Britain the frequencies of the G6PD deficiency have prompted Kidson and Gorman (378) to question the role of malaria in determining high G6PD deficiency in some populations in malarious areas. In New Guinea there is a good correlation between the highlands with no malaria and no G6PD deficiency, and the lowlands with both; but on New Britain the Tolai have a very low frequency while neighboring groups with the same endemic malaria have high frequencies. In Indonesian New Guinea there is also a correlation between altitude and G6PD-deficiency frequency (Figure 6). In groups such as the Kapauka or Dani, who have been isolated for a long time in the mountains, malaria and the G6PD deficiency are practically absent. But there are neighboring groups on the North Coast with similar environments but with quite different frequencies. Nevertheless, wherever there are high frequencies of the G6PD deficiency there is evidence of endemic malaria, so that the data from New Guinea do not disprove the malaria hypothesis. In order to determine how fast the G6PD deficiency would increase in a population after introduction at a small percentage, several runs were made with the fitnesses, A- = 1.0, B- = .95, AA = .90, AB = 1.0, and BB = .85, where A is the normal allele and B the deficient allele. When introduced at a frequency of .02 or greater, the G6PD deficiency allele invariably increased, but after 100 generations varied in frequency from .15 to .30 with a population size of 1000. On the other hand, with a starting frequency of .01, the G6PD deficiency was unable to increase toward equilibrium most of the time. Many other runs with similar sets of fitness values seem to indicate the same conclusion. Since the establishment of the G6PD deficiency after it is introduced into a population is not certain, the presence in the Southwest Pacific of many populations with endemic malaria but low frequencies of this gene seems expectable.

Thalassemia is found in the same populations of New Guinea and New Britain as the G6PD deficiency. Thus it too is correlated with the distribution of malaria, except that no studies on thalassemia incidence have been done in Indonesian New Guinea. The frequencies of thalassemia in the Southwest Pacific are somewhat lower than in other areas of endemic malaria. On New Britain they range from 4 per cent to 8 per cent, with the Tolai having the lowest thalassemia frequency (4 per cent), as they have also for the G6PD deficiency. On the other hand, in the Sepik River region of New Guinea the Sause have a lower G6PD deficiency frequency than the Abelam (1 per cent vs. 8 per cent) but they have a higher thalassemia frequency (8 per cent vs. 2 per cent). And in the Markham River Valley, the G6PD deficiency has spread further up the valley than thalassemia, since at Wampur they are 21 per cent and 2 per cent respectively.

The spotty distributions of the G6PD deficiency and thalassemia in the malarious areas of New Guinea are what one would expect if malaria had only recently become an important selective factor in the area. If the disease has been spreading through the area, it would do so in a somewhat erratic fashion. This seems to be characteristic of most epidemic spreads of disease. And as the disease began to take its toll of life, it would begin to select for genes that provide some resistance to the disease. But it would not be expected that all the populations would acquire the same resistant genes or that these would increase at the same rate at the same time in all populations. Even if the resistant genes were acquired by gene flow, the frequencies in the populations would be quite different during the early encounter with the disease. At equilibrium one would expect the same frequencies in all populations with the same amount of malaria, but the populations would not be expected to attain equilibrium at the same time. As was pointed out

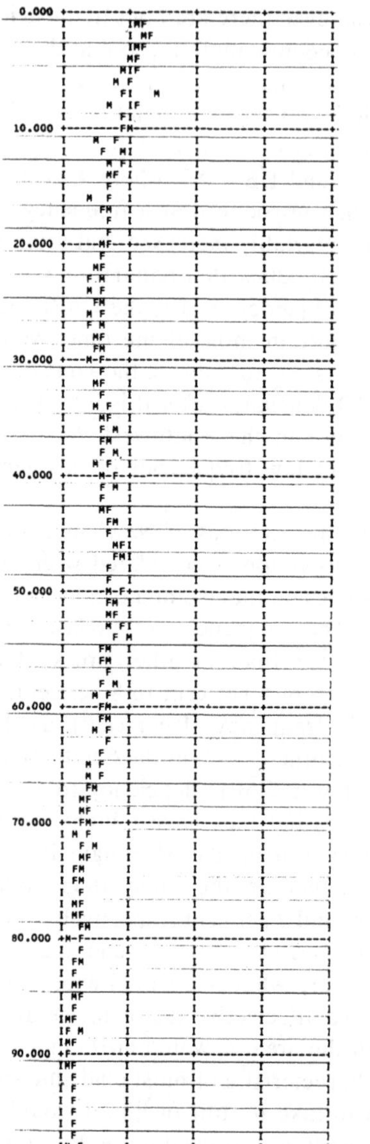

(a)

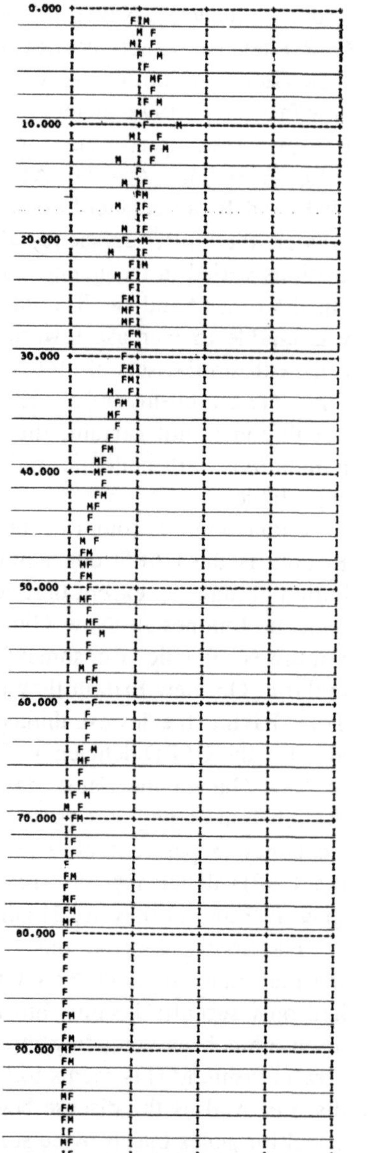

(b)

Figure 5. The maintenance of a deleterious sex-linked gene in a population by gene flow, when m = .005, $W_{1-} = W_{11} = .95$, $W_{2-} = W_{22} = W_{12} = 1.0$, and the population size is 1000 (a and b) or 200 (c

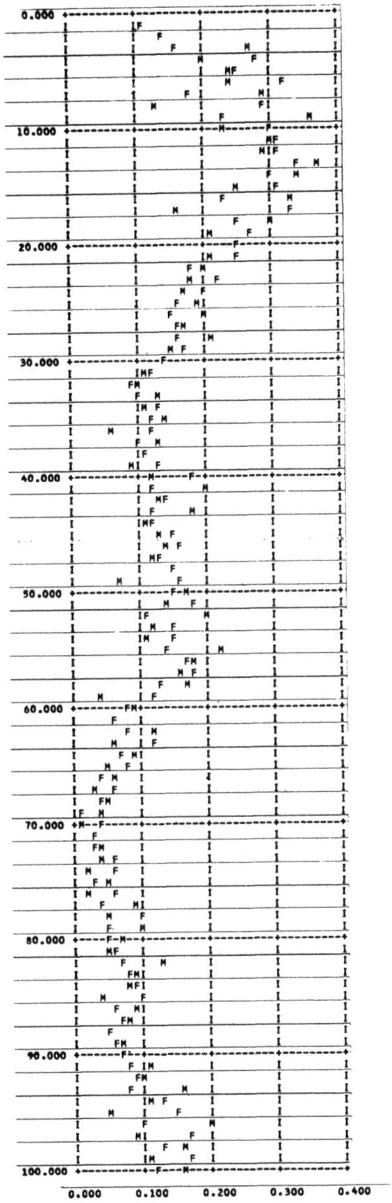

(c)

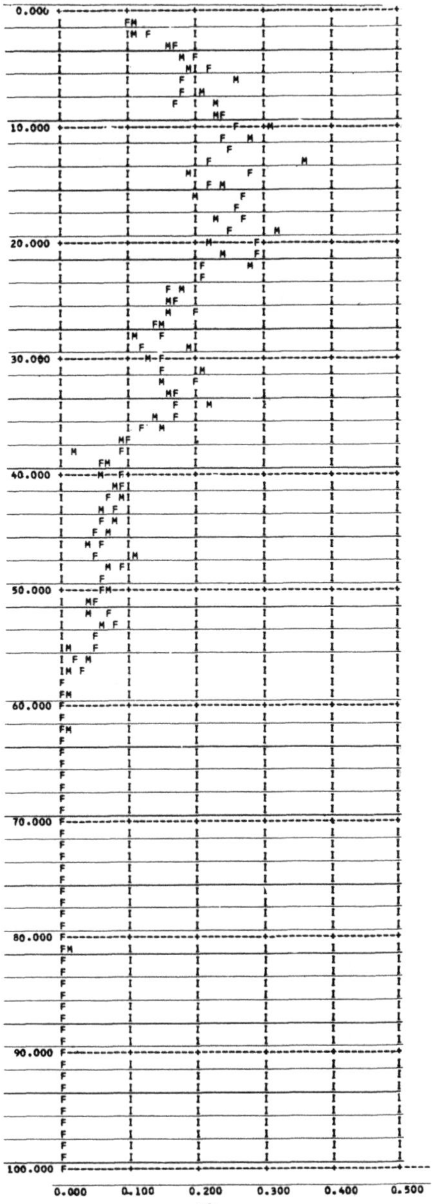

(d)

and d). M and F are the frequencies of the deleterious gene (1) in males and females respectively, and each population was reproduced for 100 generations.

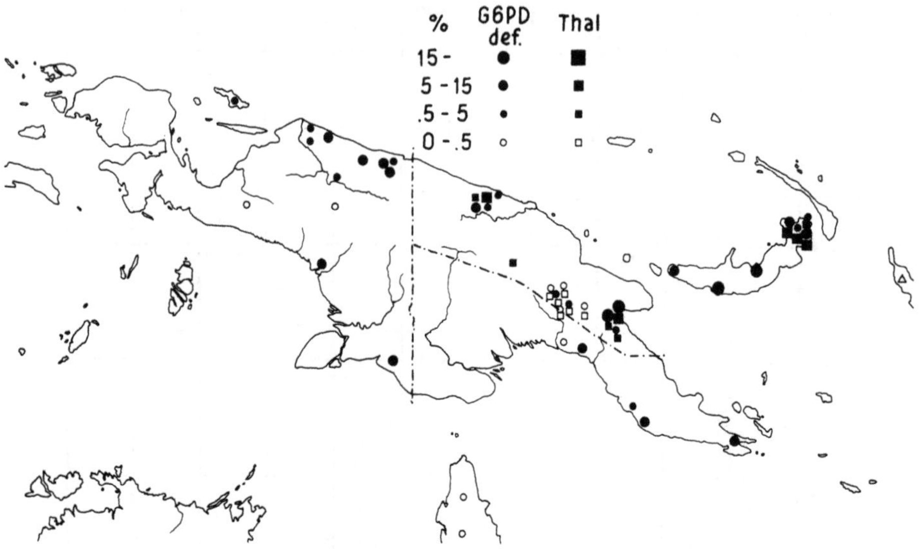

Figure 6. The Percentage Incidence of the Red Cell Defects in New Guinea.

in Chapters II and III, thalassemia and the G6PD deficiency are undoubtedly due to many different genes, in the sense of different alterations in the base pair arrangement of the DNA that controls G6PD or hemoglobin synthesis. These two genetic conditions probably have a much higher mutation rate than specific hemoglobins such as S, C, or E. When malaria became an important selective factor, it would be much more likely to encounter one of these two common mutants and begin to increase their frequency than to meet one of the more specific mutants. But in the small populations of New Guinea some may have a G6PD or thalassemia gene present and others not. When malaria began selecting for these genes, an erratic distribution of high frequencies is what would be expected. It thus seems possible for the G6PD deficiency and thalassemia genes in the Southwest Pacific to be different mutants in many populations. Or they could be due to erratic gene flow of one or a very few mutants. When we can describe thalassemia and G6PD structure completely, this question will be answerable.

To the north of New Guinea there has been greater contact with mainland Asia, and this is reflected in the presence of hemoglobin E there (653), in addition to thalassemia and the G6PD deficiency. However, it has rarely been detected on surveys. But very little survey data exists for the Philippines, and the Negritos and other more isolated primitive peoples have not been examined. In view of the high frequency of hemoglobin E in the hunters and gatherers of Malaya (430) and Thailand (252), such investigations would be of great anthropological value. The only large survey for the G6PD deficiency (496) indicates that it is found throughout the Philippines but varies greatly in frequency. Malaria is present in much of the Philippines and seems to vary in the same way, but there is too little data to be conclusive.

Since the aborigines of Taiwan to the north of the Philippines do not have any hemoglobin E (92), it has most likely been introduced into the Philippines from Borneo or directly from mainland Southeast Asia. But of the major islands of Indonesia (Figure 7), Borneo has the lowest frequencies of hemoglobin E. The Muruts of Sạbah have about 5 per cent hemoglobin E, while the Dyaks, Iban, and people of Indonesian Borneo (Kelimantan) have practically zero per cent of this hemoglobin. The rest of Indonesia has somewhat higher frequencies of hemoglobin E, but they do not approach those found in some populations on mainland Southeast Asia. This is expectable because malaria endemicity is quite erratic in Indonesia. The major vector of malaria there seems to have been *Anopheles sundaicus*, which breeds in brackish water. Most of the malaria occurs along the coast, but even here it is spotty. While the north coast of Java and Madura was quite malarious, the east coast of Sumatra was not.

Beyond Celebes (Sulawesi) the Anopheline fauna of Indonesia changes abruptly to the Australasian mosquito fauna. In contrast the Indonesian people are found in Ceram, Halmahera, and Amboina to the east of Celebes.

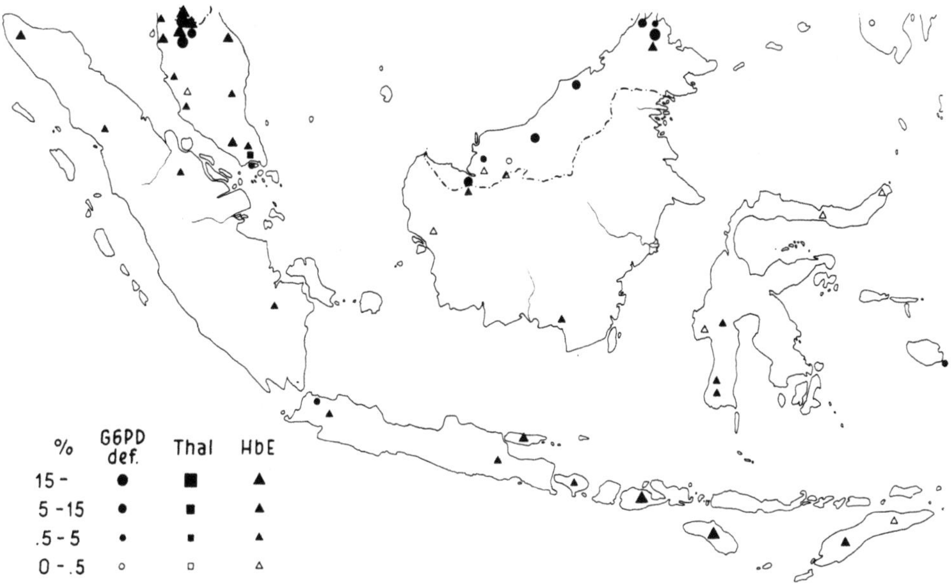

Figure 7. The Percentage Incidence of the Red Cell Defects in Indonesia.

The eastern border of hemoglobin E is at the Celebes, where the mosquitos change, and not further east where the people change. Hemoglobin E seems to be somewhat higher on Java than on Sumatra and is apparently even higher on the small islands except Bali to the east of Java. The vector, *A. sundaicus*, becomes prevalent only after considerable alteration of the landscape by man's activity, particularly farming. As the evolution of culture in Indonesia and its subsequent increase in population has changed the Anopheline fauna, they have also brought in malaria and, in its wake, hemoglobin E. In Borneo the vector of malaria is *A. leucosphyrus*, which is found in the jungle. There is malaria among the Dyaks, but they have not changed the landscape so drastically, so that malaria has never become intensely endemic everywhere. But the fact that jungle mosquitos can transmit human malaria in Southeast Asia implies that quite primitive hunters and gatherers could have been subjected to it. The additional fact that the monkeys of Southeast Asia have many similar malaria parasites makes this possibility even more likely (732, 742).

On Celebes, where the frequency of hemoglobin E decreases, there are also appreciable frequencies of hemoglobin O Indonesia. This hemoglobin only gets up to 2 per cent in some populations, but these frequencies are still higher than would be expected if the equilibrium were due to mutation balanced by selection against the gene. It thus appears to have a slight selective advantage. Here at the forefront of the advance of the hemoglobin E gene, hemoglobin O has attained these frequencies in the absence of other genes that confer some resistance to malaria. Thus it would seem to be a random mutant that increased slightly during the time between the onset of malaria as a selective force and the arrival of hemoglobin E by gene flow. There is probably some thalassemia in these populations but it has not been investigated. On Amboina to the east, there is a very low frequency of abnormal hemoglobins, but there seems to be as high a frequency of G6PD deficiency as anywhere in Indonesia.

On mainland Southeast Asia the highest frequencies of hemoglobin E are found in eastern Thailand. In Surin Province the Thais seem to have over 50 per cent hemoglobin E, and the Khmers are close to it. These are the only frequencies of over 50 per cent abnormal hemoglobins in any population. From eastern Thailand the frequency of hemoglobin E decreases in all directions, although local malaria conditions have effects on the rate of decrease. In contrast to the distributions of many abnormal hemoglobins and of malaria in other parts of the world, in Southeast Asia it is not the populous delta regions around Bangkok and Saigon that have the most malaria and hence the highest frequencies of abnormal hemoglobins, but the hill areas among the more primitive slash-and-burn agriculturalists. This is due to a great extent to the major vector of malaria, *A. minimus*, which breeds in the small, quick-flowing, clear, sunlit streams in the hills. Recently *A. balabacensis* has been found to be an important vector in Cambodia (242a), but this mosquito is still prevalent in forest environments and not in the greatly altered environment of the rice paddies.

No population studies have been done in Burma, but this country and Laos, Thailand, Cambodia, and Vietnam have comparable malaria endemicities and comparable hemoglobin E frequencies. Malaya, however, does not have much malaria along the coast, except in isolated places, and in these areas hemoglobin E, although present, seems to be lower in frequency. In the interior highlands of Malaya, the vector of malaria is *A. maculatus,* which is not as efficient as *A. minimus* and can be diverted to feeding on cattle. The major plains of Malaya, which are now mostly rice paddies, are also not particularly malarious. However, among the Senoi and some aboriginal Malay groups extremely high frequencies of hemoglobin E are found. These groups also have high frequencies of the G6PD deficiency, so that the two loci are correlated here. The very high hemoglobin E frequencies in these groups are not unexpected because they are slash-and-burn agriculturalists, although the Senoi rely to a greater extent on hunting than do other Malay agriculturalists. But they open up the forest and thus bring about the conditions under which *A. maculatus* thrives. Since the Senoi do not have much livestock, humans are the mosquito's major blood supply and hence malaria is highly endemic (550, 742). However, the Senoi (or Sakai, as they are known in the anthropological literature) together with the Semang Negritos are considered to be the aboriginal inhabitants of Malaya. The high frequencies of hemoglobin E among the Senoi would indicate that they have had malaria and, by implication, agriculture for enough generations for this gene to increase to equilibrium. But the fact that hunters and gatherers in Southeast Asia may have had endemic malaria would provide an alternate explanation. Studies of the Semang Negritos who are still hunters and gatherers and not in close contact with any agriculturalists would help to solve this problem.

Case reports from many countries of Southeast Asia indicate that thalassemia is widespread there, and Flatz et al. (251) have recently shown that this gene is present in most Thai populations. This same study shows that the β-hemoglobin locus has at least three common alleles in many Southeast Asian populations, thus raising the question of possible equilibrium values. To discuss this question, we first have to estimate the fitness values of the genotypes. Although there are many β-thalassemia alleles and they undoubtedly vary in the fitnesses of their genotypes, we will assume the fitness of β-thalassemia homozygotes to be 0.0. Since in many populations in different parts of the world, thalassemia attains a frequency of 20 per cent heterozygotes, we will assume that this is an equilibrium frequency, with thalassemia the only allele present in addition to the normal hemoglobin allele. If the fitness of the normal homozygote is set as 1.0, then the fitness of the thalassemia heterozygote would be 1.125. It is known that persons simultaneously heterozygous for hemoglobin E and β-thalassemia have a severe anemia and are much less fit than hemoglibin E homozygotes. But some E-thalassemia heterozygotes do survive and reproduce, so their fitness will be estimated as 0.2. For hemoglobin E homozygotes, data from Chernoff et al. (164) indicate a moderate anemia.

But according to the data from Flatz et al. (252) hemoglobin E homozyrotes seem to survive and reproduce almost as well as normals. Neither the frequency of the EE genotype among adults nor the number of live-born children of EE women was significantly different from that expected for their data. However, if we take the estimates of survival and reproduction of EE homozygotes in this data (252) at face value and disregard whether or not they are significantly different from normal, then this would seem to give the best estimate of fitness. For Northeast Thailand the EE homozygote survival rate is 85 per cent, and the EE female fertility 77 per cent that of

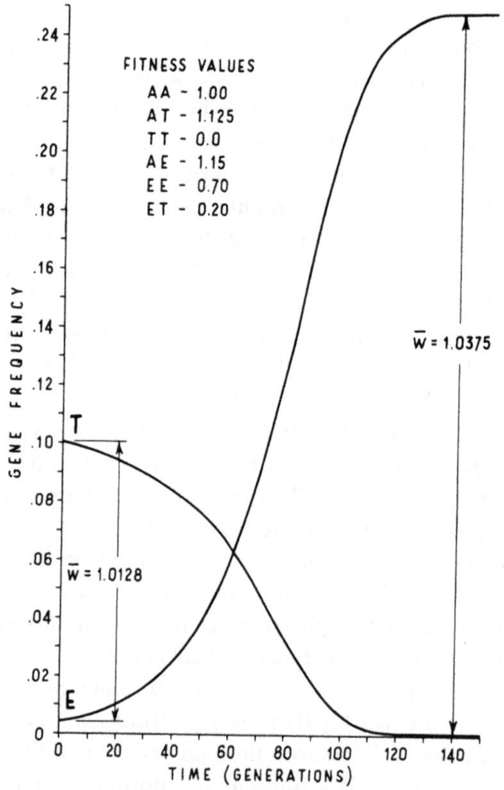

Figure 8. The Replacement of Thalassemia by Hemoglobin E.

normals; hence the fitness of the EE genotype would be about .85 x .77 or .70. Assuming that hemoglobin E can attain a frequency of over 50 per cent carriers, which would be a gene frequency of over .25, then the latter would seem to be a reasonable estimate of the equilibrium frequency; and on this basis the fitness of the hemoglogin E heterozygote would be estimated as 1.15.

Using the method of Bodmer and Parsons (98) which was outlined in Chapter IV, we find k = 1.04, from which we conclude that hemoglobin E will replace thalassemia in a population with endemic malaria. On the other hand, if the equilibrium frequency for thalassemia is estimated as .15 (30 per cent heterozygotes), then the thalassemia heterozygote would have a fitness of 1.21. In this case k = .98, and hemoglobin E would not increase when introduced into the population. If we set the equilibrium frequency of hemoglobin E as .2 (over 40 per cent carriers) and keep the thalassemia heterozygote fitness at 1.125, then k = 1.00. Since this is the exact value which is decisive to the outcome, very small changes in the fitness values will completely alter the course of events—if the fitness values were concentrated around this critical set. Finally, if the fitness of the EE

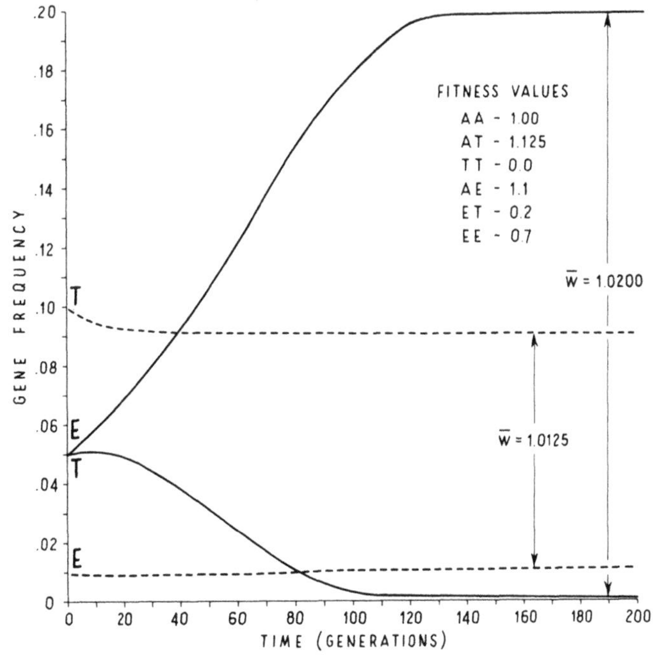

Figure 9. The Interaction of Thalassemia and Hemoglobin E Where the Outcome Is Dependent on the Initial Conditions.

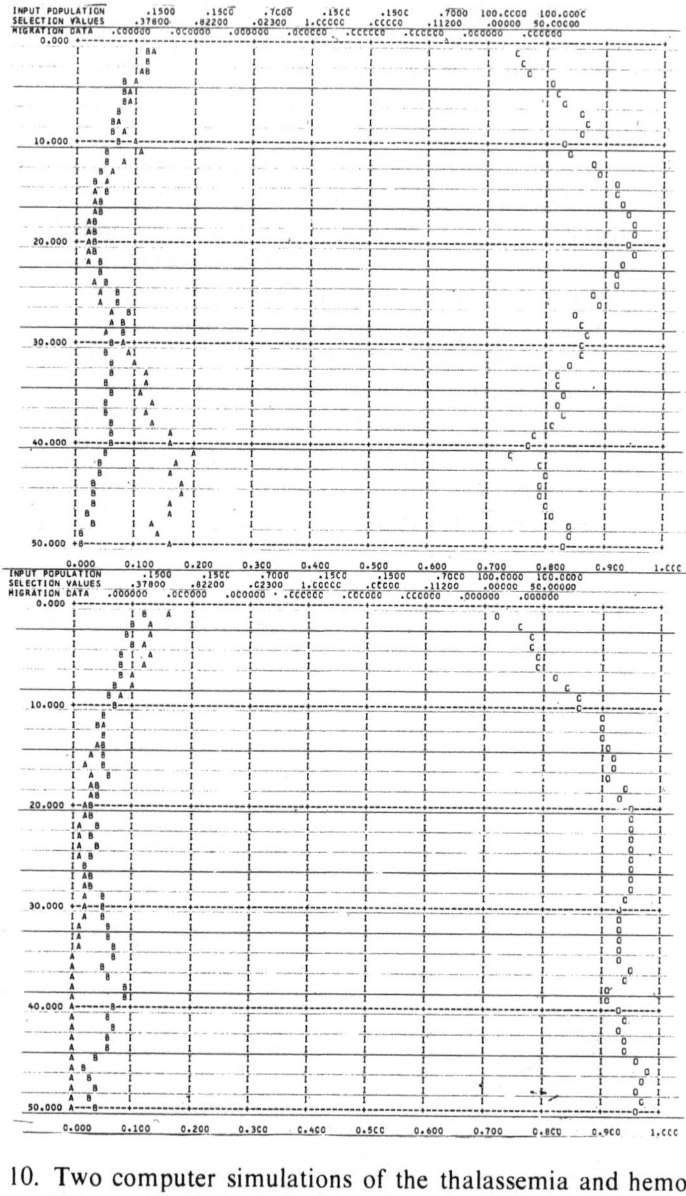

Figure 10. Two computer simulations of the thalassemia and hemoglobin E genes in a breeding population of 200 individuals, when the fitnesses are: AA = 1.0, AT = 1.125, AE, 1.1, TT = 0, EE = .7, and ET = .2. (A is the hemoglobin E gene frequency; B the thalassemia gene frequency; and 0 the hemoglobin A gene frequency.)

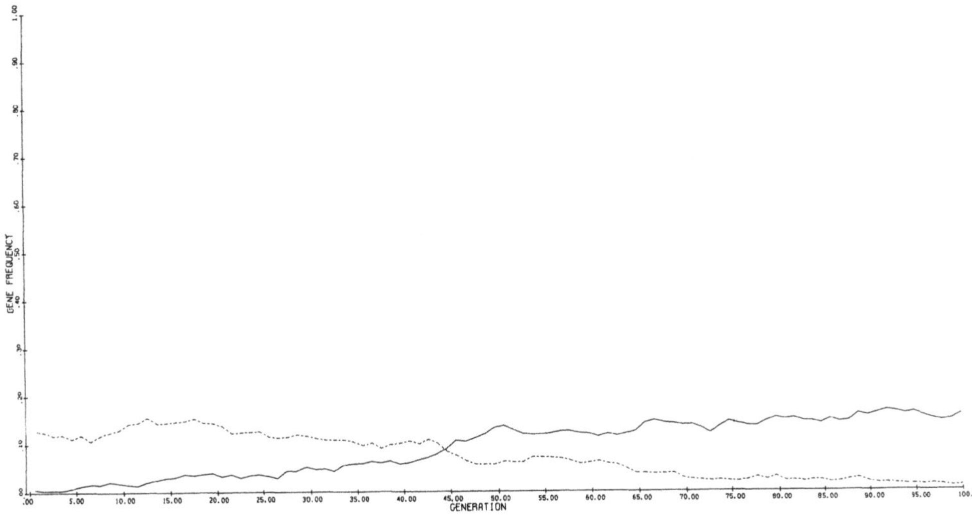

Figure 11. A stochastic model of the replacement of thalassemia by hemoglobin E with gene flow (m = .01) from a population with a hemoglobin E gene frequency of .125, a population of 1000, and fitnesses: W_{AA} = 1.0, W_{AE} = 1.1, W_{EE} = .7, W_{AT} = 1.11, W_{ET} = .2, and W_{TT} = 0. (Thalassemia gene frequency = ----- and hemoglobin E gene frequency = ——.)

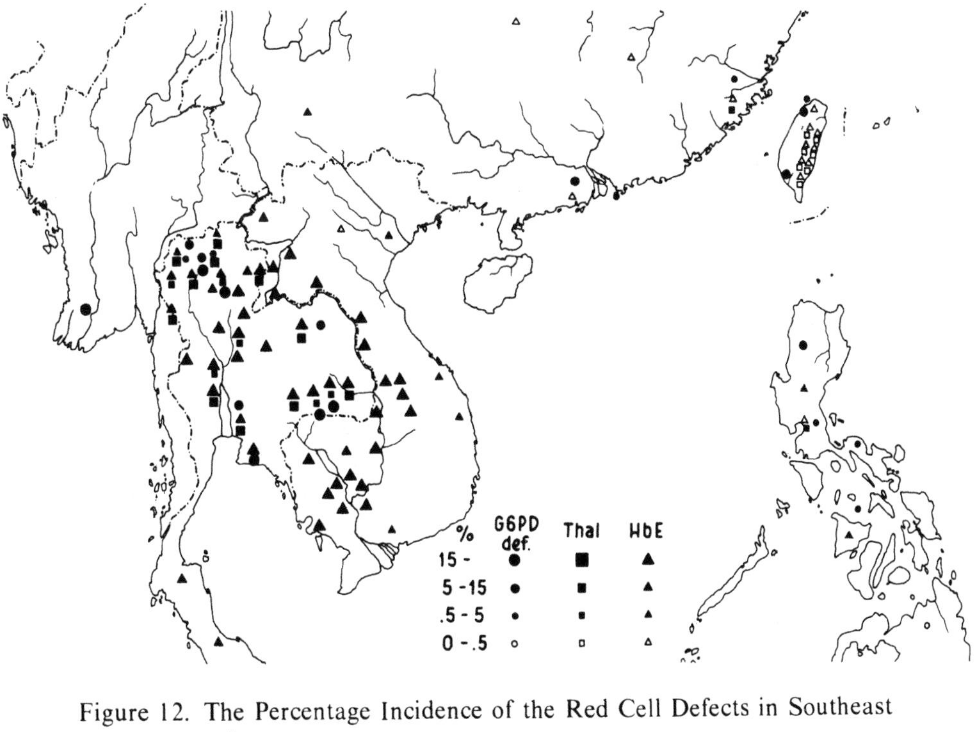

Figure 12. The Percentage Incidence of the Red Cell Defects in Southeast Asia.

homozygote is estimated as .90, then with an equilibrium E frequency of .25, the AE heterozygote would have a fitness of 1.05 and k = .95, with a thalassemia heterozygote fitness of 1.125. So, paradoxically, when the fitness of the EE homozygote is greater, the ability of the hemoglobin E gene to replace the thalassemia gene is less.

Figure 8 is a deterministic computer run based on equation (5) of Chapter IV, showing that hemoglobin E will rapidly replace thalassemia if it has a fitness as high as 1.15 when heterozygous. On the other hand, Figure 9 shows that hemoglobin E will replace thalassemia if both begin with appreciable frequencies, but that it cannot replace thalassemia when introduced at a very small frequency if the fitness of the AE heterozygote is only 1.1.

In order to determine the effects of random gene drift on the outcome of the competition of these two red cell defects, several runs were made with small population sizes. In most cases either one or the other of the red cell defects was eliminated, with about equal frequency. Figure 10 shows two adjacent runs with rather different outcomes. However, most populations in Southeast Asia are much larger than 200, the effective population size used in these runs. To obtain the closest approximation, a population of 1000 was used, and some gene flow from a population with hemoglobin E was introduced (m = .01.). The result is shown on Figure 11 and indicates that hemoglobin E will replace thalassemia. The decreasing hemoglobin E frequencies as one goes out in any direction from eastern Thailand and Cambodia seems to be the result of the spread of a favorable mutant that is replacing thalassemia. But the erratic nature of these clines in Thailand may indicate the operation of gene drift or of small changes in the fitness values which prevent hemoglobin E from replacing thalassemia.

Although much of China has endemic malaria, hemoglobin E has not spread as much to the north as it has out through the Indonesian archipelago (Figure 12). Consequently the populations in the malarious areas of China have thalassemia and the G6PD deficiency in high frequencies. In addition, many rare hemoglobin variants seem to occur in Chinese. The greater number of these rare hemoglobin variants seem to be associated with high frequencies of thalassemia, so that China is like the Mediterranean area and India in this respect. The fact that hemoglobin E has spread south to a greater extent seems reasonable in view of the general direction of gene flow in eastern Asia. The Chinese have "overflowed" to the south for all of history, while there has been little migration in the other direction. And even in prehistoric times a reasonable interpretation of the archeological record indicates continual migration to the south from China (55).

VII

INDIA, TIBET, PAKISTAN, AND CEYLON

IN THE NEIGHBORHOOD of Calcutta, there appears to be a rather marked change in the frequency of hemoglobin E. Assam and East Pakistan have not been investigated in detail; but hemoglobin E is found in East Pakistan (415), and in some isolated tribes of the Northeast Territory such as the Totos it seems to attain very high frequencies (158). A survey of Bengal has found 4 per cent hemoglobin E (157), but to the west in Uttar Pradesh and to the south in Madras and Bihar the frequency of hemoglobin E is practically zero. The high frequencies of hemoglobin S which have been reported from Assam are in recent immigrant populations from Bihar and Orissa. Northern India, from Bihar west to the Punjab, does not have widespread high frequencies of hemoglobin S or any of the other hemoglobin variants that attain high frequencies elsewhere, although occasional populations with high hemoglobin S frequencies have been reported. Malaria is particularly severe along the foothills of the Himalayas, but the indigenous populations have not been studied in detail. However, the findings of an occasional Nepalese with hemoglobin E may indicate that some Nepalese populations in endemic malarious regions have rather high frequencies of this abnormal hemoglobin. On the Ganges Plain malaria is more epidemic than endemic. In the absence of one of the more successful hemoglobin variants such as S or E, hemoglobin D attains frequencies of 4 per cent in these populations, and thalassemia also seems to be prevalent (Figure 13).

In the hilly regions of Peninsular India malaria is holoendemic, and it seems to be more severe among the tribal peoples who practice slash-and-burn agriculture. Bastar has been investigated in detail by Negi (511, 512, 513). In the more urbanized populations, the lower castes—particularly the Mahars—have high frequencies of hemoglobin S both in Bastar and around

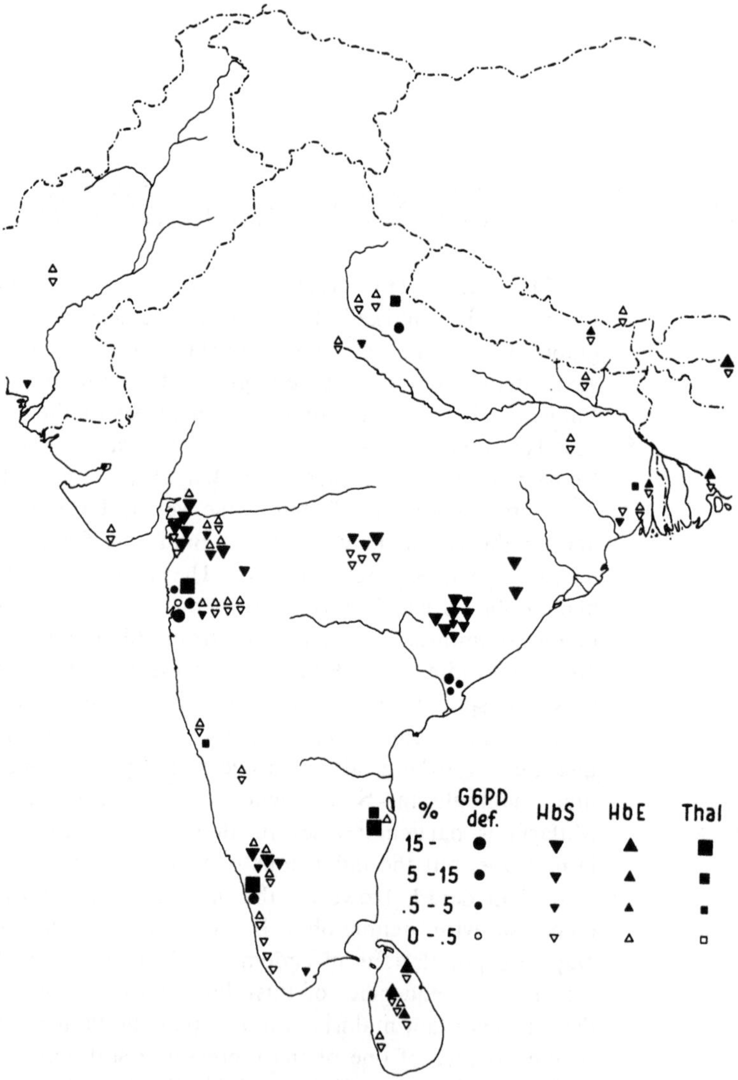

Figure 13. The Percentage Incidence of the Red Cell Defects in India.

Nagpur, while the higher castes have very low frequencies. Although malaria can be severe in these hill regions, its endemicity is still rather erratic. Presumably this great variation in malaria is in part the explanation of the great variability in hemoglobin S frequency among the tribal populations.

In the Nilgiri Hills the Todas, Kotas, and Badagas have low hemoglobin S frequencies, while the Paniyans, Irulas, and Kurumbas have higher frequencies. The latter tribes are quite primitive and are for the most part hunters and gatherers on the forested slopes. In this part of India there does not seem to be a correlation between agriculture and high sickle-cell frequencies, but there is evidence that the association with malaria still holds (122). The Kota are the artisans in this society with many interdependent tribes; they are closely associated with the Toda who are pastoralists. Since the vector of malaria in this area, *A. fluviatilis*, can be easily diverted to feeding on cattle, malaria would be less endemic among pastoralists. In addition, these two tribes, together with the Badaga, live on the top of the Nilgiri Plateau, where there is less malaria than on the forested slopes where the three hunting and gathering tribes live.

The one area of southern India where hemoglobin E has been found is Ceylon. The great majority of Ceylonese populations do not appear to have high frequencies of any hemoglobin variant, but three rather dispersed Vedda villages have very high hemoglobin E frequencies. Malaria is endemic in the hinterland of Ceylon, so that high abnormal hemoglobin frequencies are expectable, but why it should be hemoglobin E is a problem. Assuming that these instances are the same hemoglobin E that is widespread in Southeast Asia, it could be either a separate mutation or gene flow from there. According to Wickremasinghe et al. (743) the presence of hemoglobin E among the Veddas dates back in time to their common anecestry with the Senoi and other primitive peoples of Southeast Asia. But it should be noted that all the Vedda villages tested had mixed considerably with the Tamils and Sinhalese, and the only village that still speaks Vedda, Dambana, has no hemoglobin E. Although a large survey of Ceylonese has revealed no hemoglobin E, there may be more isolated villages in the north with hemoglobin E that could have been the source of this gene in the Vedda; or perhaps contact with Bengal, indicated by the Sinhalese language, could have been the source of this gene. However, malaria may have been common in Paleolithic hunters in Southeast Asia because of the large monkey populations with similar malaria parasites, and this fact makes the presence of hemoglobin E in this area in Paleolithic times a distinct possibility. The other indigenous hunting population in the area, the Andaman Islanders, have not been examined for hemoglobin E. Lehmann (407) tested them for the sickle-cell trait, and they have none, which is expectable. If the Andaman Islanders are found to have hemoglobin E, this would tend to support the position of

Wickremasinghe et al. But since malaria is not endemic in the Andamans, hemoglobin E presumably has not been selected for, and its presence would be unexpected.

From Bombay north through Gujerat, hemoglobin S is found in high frequencies, but only in the tribal peoples or small isolated populations that have endemic malaria. Studies of emigrant Gujerat peoples (567), who come for the most part from urban populations, have found hemoglobin D but no hemoglobin S. This illustrates a point which will arise continually, that small enclaves with very high frequencies of an abnormal hemoglobin can exist within a larger population; hospital or random samples of the total population will not even detect this trait.

Bombay is the only area of India for which the populations have been investigated in any detail for the G6PD deficiency. Although appreciable frequencies of this defect are found in some populations, such as the Parsees, the G6PD-deficiency frequencies for India seem much lower than in comparable areas of the Middle East, Africa, or Southeast Asia.

Few studies have been done in West Pakistan, but it appears to be similar to northern India. Occasional cases of hemoglobin S are found, and hemoglobin D seems to be the most prevalent abnormal hemoglobin. The whole Indian sub-continent, in fact, appears to have many examples of rare abnormal hemoglobins. Hemoglobins D, J, K, L, N, and Q have been found there, although only hemoglobins D in the north and K around Madras appear in appreciable frequencies. In this respect India is like the Mediterranean area, West and Central Africa, and, to a certain extent, China. Every survey in these areas seems to find at least one rare abnormal hemoglobin, while surveys of larger numbers in northern Europe, East Africa, the Pacific, or among American Indians find far fewer cases.

In the absence of one of the more successful hemoglobin variants one would expect to find many different mutants being increased slightly. Particularly in areas of epidemic malaria, where the selective advantage of these abnormal traits would be sporadic both in time and space, one would expect to find many mutants but none in high frequency. Central India from the Punjab to Mysore is this kind of malarious environment, as are parts of Italy, North Africa, the Middle East, and China. On the other hand, the foothill regions of India, West Africa, and Central Africa also have a great variety of abnormal hemoglobins, and in these areas malaria is as endemic as anywhere in the world. One of the hemoglobins that can attain very high frequencies will do so in these areas, and there are many populations with high hemoglobin S frequencies in all of them. But it appears that the introduction of hemoglobin S is rather recent, coming considerably after the beginning of malaria as a selective factor. Hence many different mutants were increased slightly among these populations before the establishment of hemoglobin S, and have not yet been replaced by it.

VIII

THE MIDDLE EAST AND EUROPE

THE GREAT ARIDITY of much of the Middle East makes it an unsuitable environment for endemic malaria, but in the more well-watered oases and river valleys with a suitable mosquito vector of malaria, there is severe endemic malaria. Hence hemoglobin S is found in high frequencies in the oasis populations of Saudi Arabia but not among the Bedouin desert nomads. Hemoglobin S has been reported in Kuwait (729b) and certainly exists in high frequencies in Basra (132), although no surveys have been done here. It is also found through Jordan, Lebanon, and Syria to the Eti-Turks of southeastern Turkey. There is apparently very little hemoglobin S in the rest of Turkey, but extremely high frequencies are found in Macedonia and other areas of northern Greece. In these widespread and ethnically diverse populations, there is a significant correlation between hemoglobin S and endemic malaria. However, there are populations throughout the area who have been subjected to severe malaria but do not have appreciable frequencies of hemoglobin S. Many Jewish groups, particularly those in Kurdistan, have very high frequencies of the G6PD deficiency and some thalassemia, but no hemoglobin S. In the malarious areas of Greece there seems to be a reciprocal relationship between the frequencies of hemoglobin S and β-thalassemia (51) in the indigenous populations, who all also have high G6PD deficiency frequencies.

Since as a general rule hemoglobin S attains higher frequencies than thalassemia, although they both have the same approximate fitness when homozygous, this implies that the fitness of the AS heterozygote is higher than that of the AT heterozygote. Furthermore, this means that hemoglobin S will increase at the expense of thalassemia when introduced into a population at a low frequency. Since the ST heterozygote has a higher fitness than either homozygote, thalassemia will remain in the population at a low frequency for some sets of fitness values. Figure 14 shows this partial replacement and retention of thalassemia when the ST heterozygote has a fitness of .4. This seems rather high. Figure 15 shows the complete replacement of thalassemia by hemoglobin S when the fitness of ST is .2 and the fitnesses of the AS and AT heterozygotes seem more in accord with the data from the Mediterranean area. Thalassemia is found in some areas, such as West Africa, that have high hemoglobin S frequencies but not in other such areas. This may be due to the presence of different thalassemia alleles which have differing severities when combined with hemoglobin S.

The fact that the Kurdish Jews have thalassemia but no hemoglobin S indicates that malaria has been a selective factor among them for a sufficient length of time to increase this gene together with the G6PD deficiency gene. In order to estimate how long this would take, we can use equation (4) of Chapter IV and assume thalassemia as the only abnormal hemoglobin present. If the frequency of the thalassemia gene (.10) is close to equilibrium, then with a homozygote thalassemia fitness of zero and a heterozygote fitness of 1.125, it would take the thalassemia gene only 38 generations to increase from .01 to .09. Since thalassemia and the G6PD deficiency seem to have rather high mutation rates, their presence in the Kurdish Jews could be due to either mutation or gene flow from the outside. On the other hand, hemoglobin S has a much lower mutation rate, so that its absence in the Kurdish Jews and many other populations in the Middle East that have malaria seems to be due to its never having been introduced into these populations.

The frequencies of the G6PD deficiency in the Kurdish Jews, in some oasis populations in Saudi Arabia, and, apparently, in some populations of the Nile Delta are the highest in the world. Some of these frequencies are over 50 percent deficients in males, or a gene frequency of over 50 per cent, implying that the normal genotypes have the lowest fitness. It is possible that the G6PD locus is not a balanced polymorphism among these populations, but this seems unlikely, because total replacement of the normal allele has never occurred. If we assume that these frequencies of over 50 per cent deficients are close to equilibrium, and are not simply the result of random gene drift or selective migration from a small isolate, then as a balanced polymorphism the homozygous and hemizygous deficients would have a greater fitness than homozygous and hemizygous normals, but still a lower fitness than the heterozygote. Strictly speaking only one deficient genotype would

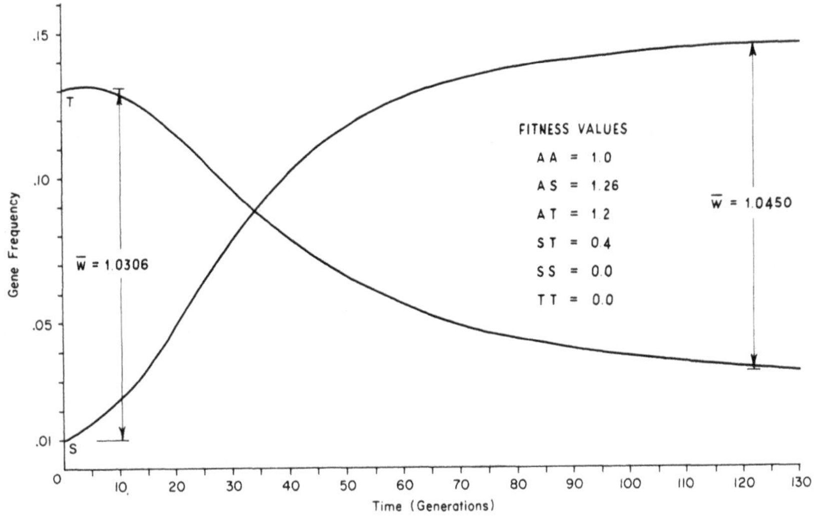

Figure 14. The Partial Replacement of Thalassemia by Hemoglobin S. (From F. B. Livingstone, 1964, *American Journal of Human Genetics*, 16:435-450, by permission.)

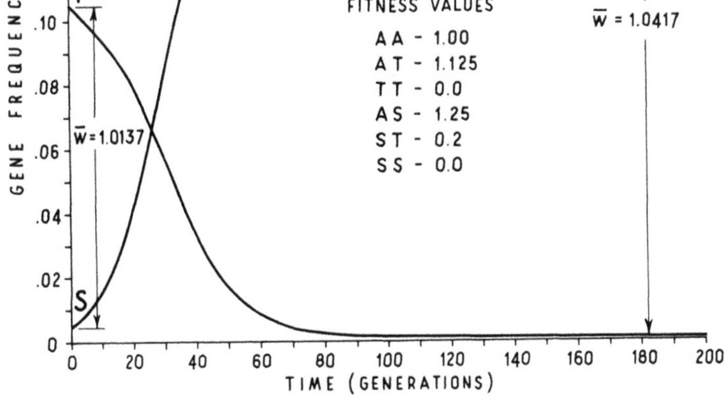

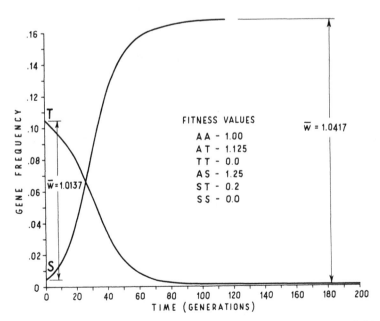

Figure 15. The Complete Replacement of Thalassemia by Hemoglobin S.

have a fitness greater than its normal counterpart, given some sets of fitness values. But since the forces tending to increase one would seem to operate on the other, both types of deficients would most likely be more fit than normals. This is not too unlikely since it would only require a change in fitness value of slightly over 5 per cent, using the maximum estimate of the fitnesses of the homozygous and hemizygous deficients in a non-malarious environment. However, in the Nile Delta the fava bean is eaten as a staple, so that the fitnesses of the deficient genotypes should be decreased. Since malaria can cause a death rate of at least 20 per cent, a 10 per cent change in fitness could occur.

It is possible that selective emigration has altered the equilibrium value, although this has not been demonstrated for the hemoglobin or G6PD loci, or for any others as far as I know. The isolated Jewish groups in Kurdistan are to some extent groups that do not recruit new members but lose a certain number to the outside world or to other more urbanized Jewish communities. Because these migrants as a rule must leave and "go it alone" for some time, they may be assumed to be healthier or have a greater average fitness than those who remain in the group. This may result in less robust genotypes accumulating in the group, which may to a certain extent explain the high frequencies of the G6PD deficiency in Kurdish Jews. But the Nile Delta and Arabian oasis populations do not seem to be so isolated, and although their high frequencies seem to indicate that selection due to malaria can be large enough to result in over 50 per cent G6PD deficients, the Nile Delta at present has rather low malaria parasite rates, 6 per cent near the seacoast and 3–4 per cent in the Upper Delta (301a). However, in the past the rates were higher (49a), and the fact that most of the malaria was due to *P. vivax* may explain the high G6PD-deficiency frequencies and the absence of hemoglobin S in Egypt. The G6PD-deficiency frequencies are correlated with the amount of malaria but seem somewhat high for the endemicity of malaria, particularly with the widespread consumption of fava beans. Since malaria is endemic, everyone would be afflicted sooner or later. Hence all would be subjected to natural selection by the parasite, but they would not be continually reinfected, as occurs elsewhere in Africa and the Middle East where there is severe endemic malaria.

In the populations of the Middle East with high frequencies of hemoglobin S, there are also high frequencies of the G6PD deficiency. Macedonia, southeast Turkey, and the oases of Saudi Arabia all have high frequencies of both. On the other hand, the association between thalassemia and the G6PD deficiency is not so strong. Although the frequency of the G6PD deficiency varies significantly in Greece and Cyprus, thalassemia does not vary so much and does not seem to be so closely correlated with malaria. In the Troodos Mountains of Cyprus there is no malaria, the G6PD-deficiency frequency is zero, and the thalassemia frequency is 9 per cent; while along the seacoast there is endemic malaria, the G6PD deficiency frequency is 11 percent, and a very rough estimate of thalassemia based on red cell morphology and some electrophoresis has found 7 per cent. Other data for thalassemia based on osmotic resistance indicate higher frequencies both in the mountains and on the seacoast, but the higher frequency still is found in the mountains. In five areas of Greece, Stamatoyannopoulos and Fessas (648) have shown that the G6PD deficiency is closely correlated with the endemicity of malaria, while the thalassemia is more loosely correlated with it. In addition, on the island of Malta, Vella (706) has found thalassemia everywhere, with high frequencies in some villages, even though malaria is not known to have been endemic throughout the island. Vella used osmotic resistance as the criterion for thalassemia, which tends to over-estimate the frequency, but most of his positives were undoubtedly thalassemics.

The close correlation of the G6PD deficiency and malaria in the Mediterranean area contrasts with the findings from New Guinea and the Pacific. There would seem to be a relationship to the prolific cultivation of the fava bean in all the areas of the Mediterranean where the correlation is close. There is close correlation on Sardinia and the Italian mainland as well. The disease favism would be a powerful selective factor against hemizygotes and homozygotes for the G6PD deficiency, but presumably would not affect the heterozygotes very much. With this great selective factor introduced into the situation, one would expect much more rapid gene frequency change toward equilibrium and hence expect the frequencies themselves to be closer to the equilibrium values. Of course, there is gene flow between the highland and lowland populations in both regions, and perhaps more gene flow in the Mediterranean area, but more intense selection would be more effective in counterbalancing this gene flow.

If we assume that the advantage of the heterozygote due to malaria is the same in Mediterranean and Kurdish Jewish populations, then we can estimate how much the fitness of the homozygote and hemizygote deficients have changed. Using equation (10) of Chapter IV and assuming the fitnesses of the normal hemizygote and homozygote to be 1.0, and the equilibrium frequency in males to be .25, as it seems to be in coastal Sardinia, we get an expression of W_{12}, the heterozygote fitness, in terms of the fitnesses of the hemizygote and homozygote deficients, or:

$$W_{12} = \frac{W_{2-}(1.5 - .5\, W_{22})}{(W_{2-} + 1)(.75\, W_{2-} - .25)}$$

If we assume W_{2-} and W_{22} to be 0.5, which in view of the seriousness of favism may seem reasonable, then in Sardinia W_{12} would have to be 3.3. This is enormous. Although not impossible, it is yet to be demonstrated. Since there seems to be no differential survival among normal and hemizygous males in Sardinia, W_{2-} *and* W_{1-} are probably much closer in value; so that a fitness of .9 for W_{2-} and also for W_{22} seems to be closer to actuality. Using these values, we find that W_{12} =1.17, which is still quite large.

Using this value of W_{12} and assuming an equilibrium gene frequency of .6, as it seems to be among the Kurdish Jews or some Arabian oasis populations, by the same equation (10) of Chapter IV we find the fitnesses of W_{2-} and W_{22} to be 1.02. As expected, the fitnesses of the deficient genotypes are greater than that of the normal genotypes, but not very much greater. A 12 per cent change due to favism in the fitness of the deficient genotypes seems to be a very conservative estimate. These values are close to the lower limit of the selection coefficient which was discussed in Chapter IV. In any case the upper limit of 50 per cent mortality seems to be much more dubious. To determine how long the increase to equilibrium would take with the fitness estimates for the Kurdish Jews, several runs were made on the computer, using a population of 1000. Starting with a G6PD deficiency frequency of .01, the results were invariably the same and an example is shown on Figure 16. The time in generations is comparable to the previous estimate for the increase in the thalassemia gene.

For the Pacific populations with the G6PD deficiency, it was shown that a small amount of gene flow from a population with a high G6PD-deficiency frequency would counterbalance the effects of selection against this deficiency. Because of the consumption of the fava bean in the Mediterranean area there is more selection against the G6PD deficiency, but there is also more gene flow between the highland and lowland villages of Greece or Sardinia than between the distant island groups of the Pacific. In order to determine how much G6PD deficiency one might expect in the non-malarious areas of the Mediterranean, several runs were made, varying selection against the G6PD deficiency, varying migration, and varying population size. For a wide range of these variables, the stable frequency seemed to be between 5 and 10 per cent G6PD deficiency, and in no case was the frequency much above 10 per cent. A sample run with the fitness, migration, and population values that seem most reasonable is shown in Figure 17. In these models most of the migrants have been assumed to be males, making the amount of gene flow of a sex-linked gene less than if females had been included. Most peasant villages are quite endogamous and residence is usually patrilocal, so that most ideal migration would presumably be females. But for long-distance migration outside the local society, the migrants would more likely be males, and this is the source of migration between breeding populations.

If we estimate m, the amount of gene flow, as .05; S, the selection against the thalassemia homozygote, as 1.0; and Q, the frequency of the thalassemia gene in the population contributing the gene flow, as .1, then using equation (13) of Chapter IV, we find that the equilibrium frequency of

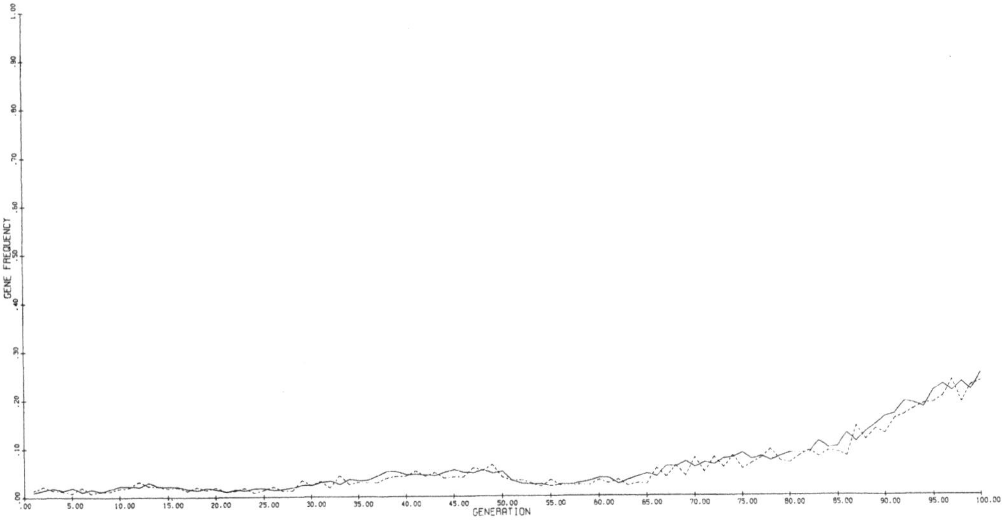

(a)

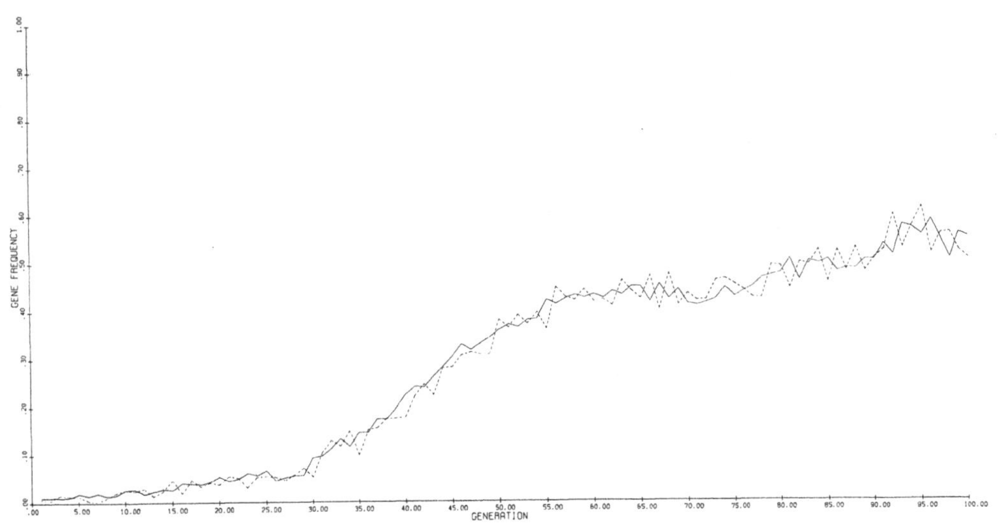

(b)

Figure 16. The approach to equilibrium of the G6PD deficiency with no gene flow, a population of 1000, and fitnesses: (a) $W_{AA} = W_{A-} = 1.0$, $W_{BB} = .945$, $W_{AB} = 1.11$, and $W_{B-} = .95$, (b) $W_{AA} = W_{A-} = 1.0$, $W_{BB} = W_{B-} = 1.02$, and $W_{AB} = 1.17$. (B Gene Frequency in Males = ----, B Gene Frequency in Females = ——).

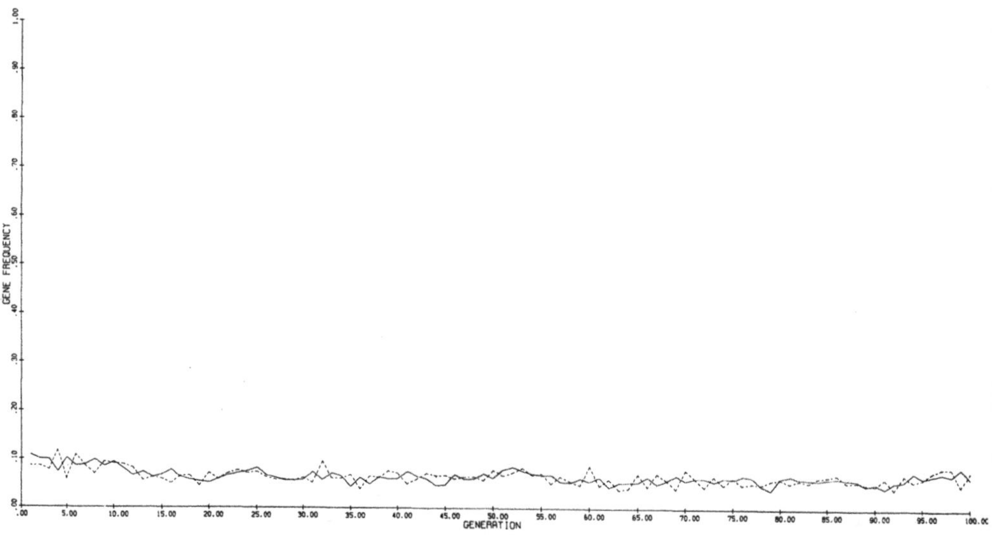

Figure 17. The maintenance of the G6PD deficiency in a population of 1000 by gene flow with m = .05 and 90% of the migrants males from a population with a G6PD-deficiency gene frequency of .20 and fitnesses: $W_{AA} = W_{AB} = W_{A-} = 1.0$, and $W_{BB} = W_{B-} = .8$. (G6PD-deficiency gene (B) frequency in males = ---- and G6PD-deficiency gene frequency in females = ——).

the thalassemia gene in non-malarious populations would be .05 or 10 per cent heterozygotes. This is slightly greater than the expected value for the G6PD deficiency under similar conditions, which may explain the greater correlation of the G6PD deficiency with malaria in the Mediterranean. Most of the frequencies of 3-6 per cent thalassemia on Malta, or the 10 per cent thalassemia in the mountains of Greece, would seem to be explained by this balance of selection and migration (Figure 18). But the few villages on Malta and Gozo with 20 per cent thalassemia seem to be too high. We can always have recourse to the founder effect or random gene drift, but malaria has at some times been endemic on Malta (151a). There does seem to be some correlation between Cassar's (151a) account of malaria in Malta and the populations with high frequencies of thalassemia. Mellieha at the head of St. Paul's Bay has the highest frequency of thalassemia and also is in the area mentioned as having endemic malaria. However, the adjacent town of St. Paul's Bay has a much lower thalassemia frequency. Other selective factors may be involved, however, and there are other places in the Mediterranean, such as the mountain villages of Cyprus, that also seem to require other factors for their explanation.

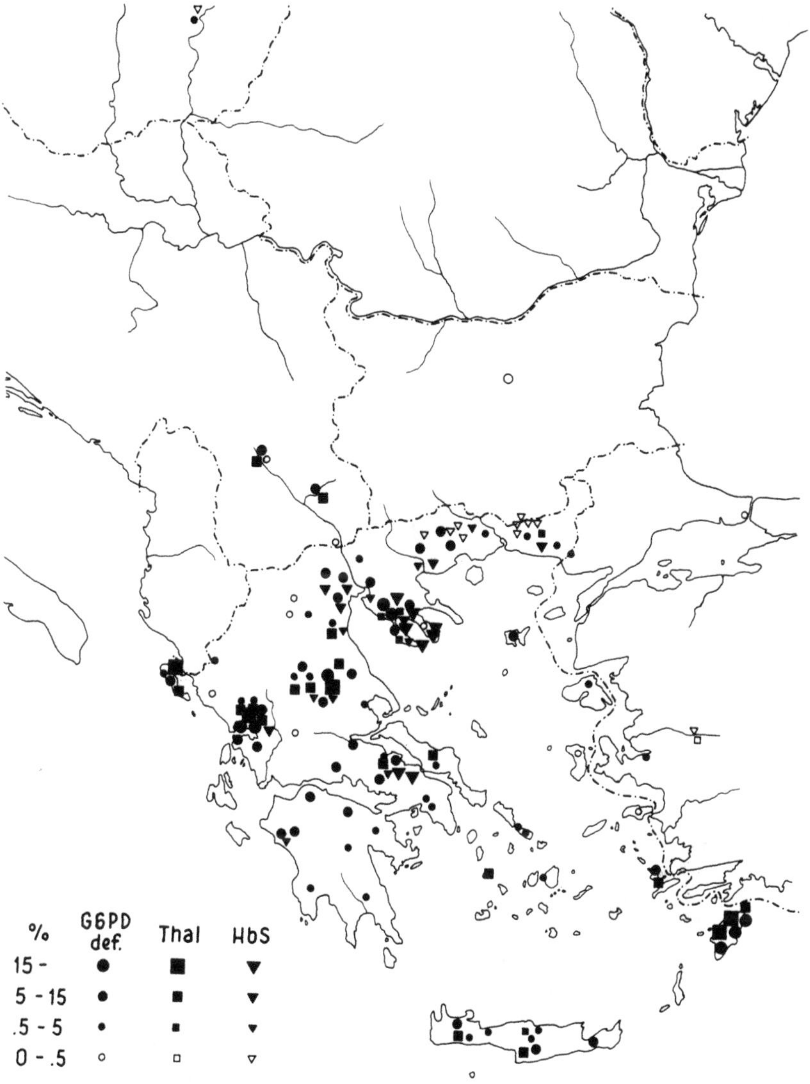

Figure 18. Percentage Incidence of the Red Cell Defects in Greece.

With the exception of thalassemia in Italy, western Mediterranean Europe has not been examined in much detail for abnormal hemoglobins, thalassemia, or the G6PD deficiency. All have been reported from Spain and Portugal, and malaria was endemic in both countries, but few population studies have been done. In both mainland Italy and Sardinia, which has been examined in great detail, the association between malaria and thalassemia is quite convincing (Figure 19). In northern Italy there is a strong correlation between the two in both Verona Province and the Ferrara district at the mouth of the Po River. On Sardinia a similar situation prevails, although a few villages in malarious areas in the north have low thalassemia frequencies. However, Carcassi (149) has shown that their inhabitants are recent immigrants. In southern Italy and in Sicily the data do not indicate so strong an association between malaria and thalassemia, but there seem to be reasons. First, malaria does not seem to have been consistently endemic in South

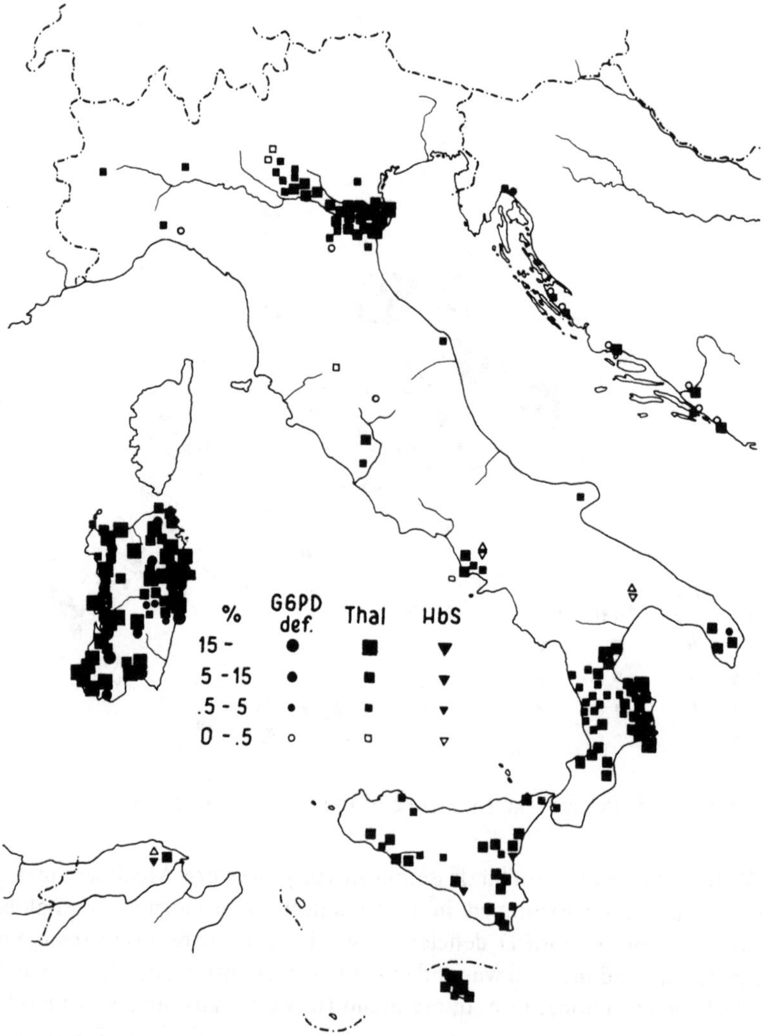

Figure 19. Percentage Incidence of the Red Cell Defects in Italy.

Italy. Second, Brancati's work (112) is the only detailed study in the areas, and it shows that there is a correlation between thalassemia and malaria but that it is not so strong because of the different ethnic groups of recent arrival. In addition, Brancati's work indicates that malaria is not correlated with altitude as strongly in Calabria. Third, the population dynamics of the thalassemia gene are complicated by the presence of hemoglobins S and C, particularly in Sicily (549).

Neither hemoglobin S or C is found in high frequency in Sardinia or northern Italy, which in itself is puzzling, since falciparum malaria is present in both areas. However, in the Po River valley, vivax malaria is the most common type (482). But the absence of hemoglobin S in Sardinia, which has perhaps the most holoendemic malaria in Europe, is a real problem and seems to be due to the absence of gene flow to bring in the hemoglobin S gene. Sardinia is one of the more isolated areas of Mediterranean Europe. To the south in Sicily, the hemoglobin S gene, although present, does not appear to have reached equilibrium in many populations, which seems to argue for its recent arrival. In Sicily there are many different ethnic groups, and some towns are considered to have been established by "Arabs," or peoples from North Africa. Although no investigations have been done among these people, they may well be the gene flow which has brought hemoglobin S to Sicily. Moreover, the villages of the southern coast, which are closer to the source of hemoglobin S, have higher frequencies than the rest of the island.

In Sicily, Sardinia, and much of the rest of the peasant regions of southern Europe, the settlement pattern is conducive to the maintenance of holoendemic malaria and in this way is a partial explanation of the high frequencies of the red cell defects. Differences in these frequencies in Africa seem to have a similar explanation. The two extreme settlement patterns among peasant agriculturalists are, obviously, dispersed single-family (however defined) homesteads and large compact towns or villages. Although malaria can remain endemic in populations with the family homestead pattern, holoendemic malaria seems to be closely associated with large compact settlements. When this type of settlement is found together with a vector that breeds in drains, sewers, and other manmade water sources and readily enters human habitations, the combination produces the most severe malaria.

In Mediterranean Europe, both *A. sacharovi* and *A. labranchiae* enter houses readily, and intense malaria is found everywhere they occur. In much of the area the population lives for most of the year in large towns and moves out—sometimes considerable distances—to their farms. During the harvest or planting seasons they will spend nights near their fields in small shelters. In this situation the large susceptible population in the town is sufficient to maintain the continual transmission of malaria, particularly in the absence of a large livestock population. With single homesteads, however, malaria transmission would be continually interrupted even if the parasite were introduced from the outside. This is particularly true for falciparum malaria, but vivax malaria with its relapsing cycle can apparently maintain itself in a homestead population, as it seems to have done in Holland.

The spontaneous decline of malaria in northern Europe has been explained by Hackett (301) as due to the stabling of domestic animals. Since the vector, *A. maculipennis atroparvus*, is readily deflected from feeding on humans to feeding on animals, the greater availability of this more suitable blood supply interrupted the transmission of human malaria enough to prevent it from remaining endemic. However, with the return of many infected soldiers or other persons from malarious areas, epidemics can occur. In addition to changes in agricultural practices, there was also a large increase in the number of livestock, which contributed to the change in the mosquito's blood preferences. It should be noted that anti-malaria measures and other public health improvements obviously contributed to the continued decline, but it began before such changes were instituted. The principle involved here and in the relationship between malaria endemicity and settlement patterns elsewhere is comparable to Bartlett's (55a) work on the critical size of the city for measles endemicity in the United States. He has shown that Rochester, New York; Akron, Ohio, Providence, Rhode Island; and Winnipeg, Canada, approximate this critical size, below which there are not enough individuals newly susceptible to measles for the disease to remain endemic.

Although northern Europe had endemic malaria up to the nineteenth century, abnormal hemoglobins and the G6PD deficiency are apparently quite rare in all populations. There are, of course, many small isolates that have not been examined, but large surveys in England and Germany have not found any abnormal hemoglobin or thalassemia in appreciable frequency. However, they have uncovered a wide variety of hemoglobin variants in very low frequencies. On the basis of these surveys and the Japanese data, it would appear that hemoglobin variants are found in a frequency of between 1 in 1000 and 1 in 3000 in any human population regardless of its malaria history. Thalassemia and the G6PD deficiency are found occasionally in northern Europe and here, as elsewhere, seem to be more frequent mutants. For example, thalassemia has been reported from Sweden (642), and this case seems to be a random α-thalassemia mutant. Since thalassemia is quite deleterious when homozygous, this may account for its being detected more often.

Because of the prior presence of endemic malaria in northern Europe, higher frequencies of the red cell defects may well have been expected. But there seem to be satisfactory reasons for this absence. First, it is not known how long endemic malaria existed there, and the disease was surely not endemic everywhere. The major vector, *A. maculipennis atroparvus*, breeds in brackish water and hence is found for the most part only along the seacoast. Malaria may have been endemic as far north as Sweden, but the proportion of the population subjected to continual selection by malaria must have been only a small percentage of the total. In Europe the cities, which contained the greater percentage of the total population, were relatively non-malarious. Second, the malaria was due primarily to *P. vivax*, which is a serious disease but not nearly as apt to be fatal as falciparum malaria.

But since there were some small enclaves that were highly endemic, the possibility remains that high frequencies of some red cell defects will be found. In fact there seems to be a little evidence that such exist in Holland. The lowlands of Northern Holland and Friesland were the last area of northern Europe to have endemic malaria and the disease was more endemic there in the past. There are many case reports of thalassemia among pure Dutch (626a, 612b), and the G6PD deficiency seems to be more prevalent there (527). The report (385) of the G6PD deficiency in a large Dutch kindred indicates that in a village west of Amsterdam the gene has increased from one mutant in 1790 to 125 genes today. This is a larger increase than that of the population, indicating either random gene drift or some selective factor. However, one kindred is a biased sample, and its investigation was due in part to its large size.

Very few studies of any red cell defect have been done in eastern Europe, but thalassemia, favism, and the G6PD deficiency have been reported in many countries. A recent study of a population in northeast Hungary has reported 4 per cent of the G6PD deficiency but no hemoglobin S. Malaria has selected for the G6PD deficiency but, in the absence of gene flow, the rare mutant hemoglobin S has not been able to establish itself. Most reports from eastern Europe are of cases that were identified by clinical symptoms, and these seem more common in Bulgaria than elsewhere. Thalassemia (207), an abnormal hemoglobin (371), and favism (39) have all been reported, and the sex ratio of the cases of favism indicates almost 14 per cent as a rough estimate of the G6PD deficiency. Further east, thalassemia has been reported from Poland (498) and Russia (749) and may be quite frequent in the Caucasus Mountain region (722b) and Azerbaijan (5a).

IX

NORTH AND WEST AFRICA

IN THE USUAL racial classification of African peoples, the populations of North and West Africa would never be combined, but with regard to hemoglobin these populations are quite similar. The Sahara never seems to have been a barrier to gene flow in the time that the abnormal hemoglobins have been present in human populations in appreciable frequencies. Except for the Tibesti peoples and the Shuwa Arabs of northern Nigeria, who seem to be more like the populations of East and Central Africa, the abnormal hemoglobins found in North and West Africa have spread throughout the area without regard to "race." Here, as elsewhere, thalassemia is perhaps the most widespread of the hemoglobin genes, but the populations of North and West Africa are unique in having three abnormal hemoglobins, S, C, and K, in appreciable frequencies in diverse and graphically distant populations.

Throughout North Africa malaria has been endemic, but it is rather sporadic due to the aridity of the climate and the strong influence of local environmental factors on the epidemiology of the disease. Some villages will have intense malaria because of a close association with breeding places of the vector, *A. labranchiae*, while others will be practically malaria-free because of the absence of such breeding places. To the west of Algiers, the North African coast is quite malarious, and the indigenous populations have higher frequencies of abnormal hemoglobins. Other areas, such as west of Oran, were comparatively malaria-free, and the populations have much lower abnormal hemoglobin frequencies. In the extreme western part of North Africa, the Rif Berbers, the Berbers of the Atlas Mountains, and the Moors have low frequencies of abnormal hemoglobins, and there is less malaria either because of desert or high altitudes.

In the populations of North and West Africa that have been subjected to malaria and hence have abnormal hemoglobins, there is great variability as to which abnormal hemoglobin is present. The large Arab and Berber urban populations in Algeria have both hemoglobin S and C in small and approximately equal frequencies. On the other hand, among the Berbers of Petite Kabylie, hemoglobin K is found in 8 per cent, which is the highest frequency of this hemoglobin anywhere, but in Grand Kabylie only thalassemia seems to be present. In the Berbers of Dahra Cherchell, which is to the west of Algiers, hemoglobin C seems to have a rather high frequency. Other hemoglobin variants are found throughout North and West Africa as isolated cases. Since the three hemoglobins found in high frequency in North Africa are also found in West Africa, there has been a natural tendency to interpret these occurrences in North Africa as being due to gene flow from the south. Hemoglobin S has been considered to be a "Negro" characteristic, and hemoglobin C seems to be very ancient in West African populations since its highest frequencies are found there. But if all three hemoglobins came from West Africa, why did some get to the Kabyle Mountains and others to Cherchell? Although this state of affairs may seem rather unexplainable, there does seem to be some order to it.

In the isolated populations of North Africa, such as the Berbers of Grand Kabylie, thalassemia has built up to high frequencies in the absence of other abnormal hemoglobins, just as it has in Sardinia or as it is beginning to increase among the Bassa and Kru peoples of Liberia. Hemoglobin K is widespread in North and West Africa, but it doesn't seem to have reached these peoples with thalassemia. It is found in the Mande peoples of central Liberia, in Portuguese Guinea, the Senegal, and among the Gur peoples of Upper Volta. In the Sahara it attains 5 per cent in some populations and is occasionally found in North Africa in areas other than Petite Kabylie. Assuming that these instances of hemoglobin K are the result of the spread of a single or few mutants would seem to imply that it is an ancient mutant in this part of the world. And at present its high frequencies seem to be in long-resident peripheral populations, which also seems to point to a lengthy history. However, in populations such as those in Nigeria, who have high frequencies of hemoglobin S and intense holoendemic malaria, hemoglobin K does not seem to be able to maintain any appreciable frequency.

The fact that hemoglobin C is also found among some of the more primitive peoples of West Africa has been taken to be evidence that it is a rather ancient mutation here. Along with other hemoglobin variants, it seems to have spread across the Sahara, but it is not present in some primitive populations of West Africa, particularly those of the western Ivory Coast and eastern Liberia. Hemoglobin C is found in higher frequencies than hemoglobin K; since it coexists with hemoglobin S in many populations, the question arises whether there is an equilibrium with both S and C present or whether one is replacing the other. The frequencies of hemoglobin C vary quite considerably in West Africa, and this variation is not associated with variation in malarial endemicity. Allison (27) and Rucknagel and Neel (586) have shown that there is an inverse correlation between the frequencies of hemoglobins S and C in West Africa, but there are still many populations with endemic malaria but low frequencies of both hemoglobins. These populations are located for the most part in coastal Portuguese Guinea and in eastern Liberia and the western Ivory Coast. These are the most isolated areas of West Africa, and it seems reasonable to assume that hemoglobin C has not diffused to them. Hemoglobin S is also not found among these populations for the same apparent reason (442). These areas contain the last remnants of relatively unbroken tropical rain forest in West Africa, which is an indication of their low population densities; and they were among the last places to show the effects of man's occupation. Since malaria only attains its intense endemicity where man has changed the environment, it would seem reasonable to assume that the populations in these areas were among the last to experience endemic malaria. Although it seems that neither hemoglobin S nor C has diffused to the populations in these areas, conditions suitable for the maintenance and increase of these hemoglobins are also relatively recent, which would help to account for their low frequencies. Thalassemia is present in eastern Liberia but not in very high frequency. Since this seems to be the first hemoglobin defect to be selected for in other areas when malaria becomes endemic, its presence here seems to indicate that these populations are adapting to malaria but have not been doing it for a very long time.

Returning to the question of possible equilibrium gene frequencies for the abnormal hemoglobins S and C, we must first estimate the fitnesses of the various genotypes. We will assume SS = 0, CC = .5 or .6, and SC = .2, since SC disease is more serious than homozgosity for hemoglobin C, but not as serious as sickle-cell anemia. If the fitness of the normal homozygote is taken to be 1.0, then in order to estimate the fitnesses of the heterozygotes for the normal and either one of the abnormal alleles, we must assume various equilibrium frequencies when only one abnormal allele is present in the population. There are many hemoglobin S frequencies of greater than 30 per cent in many parts of the world, including West Africa, we assume that 33 per cent AS heterozygotes, or a gene frequency of .167, is the equilibrium. The fitness of the AS heterozygote, then, would be 1.25 according to equation (8) of Chapter IV.

The estimation of the AC heterozygote fitness is more difficult since this hemoglobin is not found alone in any population but always with hemoglobin S, which would tend to decrease its frequency. Hemoglobin C is not found in as high frequencies as hemoglobin S, so if we assume its equilibrium gene frequency is .142 and the fitness of the CC homozygote is .5, then the fitness of the AC heterozygote would be 1.1. Given these fitness values, we can determine what would happen if both abnormal hemoglobins were present in a population. The outcome is shown in Figure 20. With these fitnesses hemoglobin S will totally replace hemoglobin C in about seventy generations. If we reverse the equilibrium frequencies so that hemoglobin C when alone has a higher frequency than hemoglobin S, then hemoglobin S will still replace hemoglobin C, but it will take almost three times as long. This is also shown in Figure 20.

The possibility also exists that random gene drift may affect the outcome of these situations. It could not change the equilibrium gene frequency, but it might influence the possibility of the population attaining this equilibrium. For an AS fitness of 1.25 and an AC fitness of 1.1, replacement was even more rapid than the deterministic model; and starting with an S gene frequency of .01, it occurred within thirty generations. Before the outcome was subject to drift, the AC fitness had to be increased to 1.17, with the other fitnesses remaining as in Figure 20. Figure 21 shows one sample run for which hemoglobins S and C have the same equilibrium. This may be true for some populations in West Africa but is not likely to be a widespread phenomenon there.

The preceding analysis made one critical assumption that may restrict its applicability to North and West African populations (Figure 22). This assumption is the constancy of fitness values. Obviously, if the fitnesses of the two superior heterozygotes varied considerably from population to population, then different equilibria would exist, and some of these could favor hemoglobin C. However, for much of West Africa the fitnesses could vary but still not affect the outcome, as Figure 20 indicates.

Throughout West Africa south of the Sahara, endemic falciparum malaria is present even in the Sudan areas just south of the desert. It would thus seem that the AS heterozygote has a very high fitness everywhere. In the Sahara Desert itself and some of its southern approaches, falciparum malaria tends to be replaced by other kinds of malaria, notably that due to *P. malariae*. Hemoglobin S has been shown to confer some resistance to falciparum malaria, but there is little evidence that it considerably increases resistance to the other malaria parasites. Thalassemia is found in the Po River valley of northern Italy, in China, and perhaps in Holland, where the malaria is due mostly to *P. vivax*, which would indicate that this hemoglobin abnormality can confer a resistance to other malarias. On the other hand, hemoglobin S is found in high frequencies only in populations with endemic

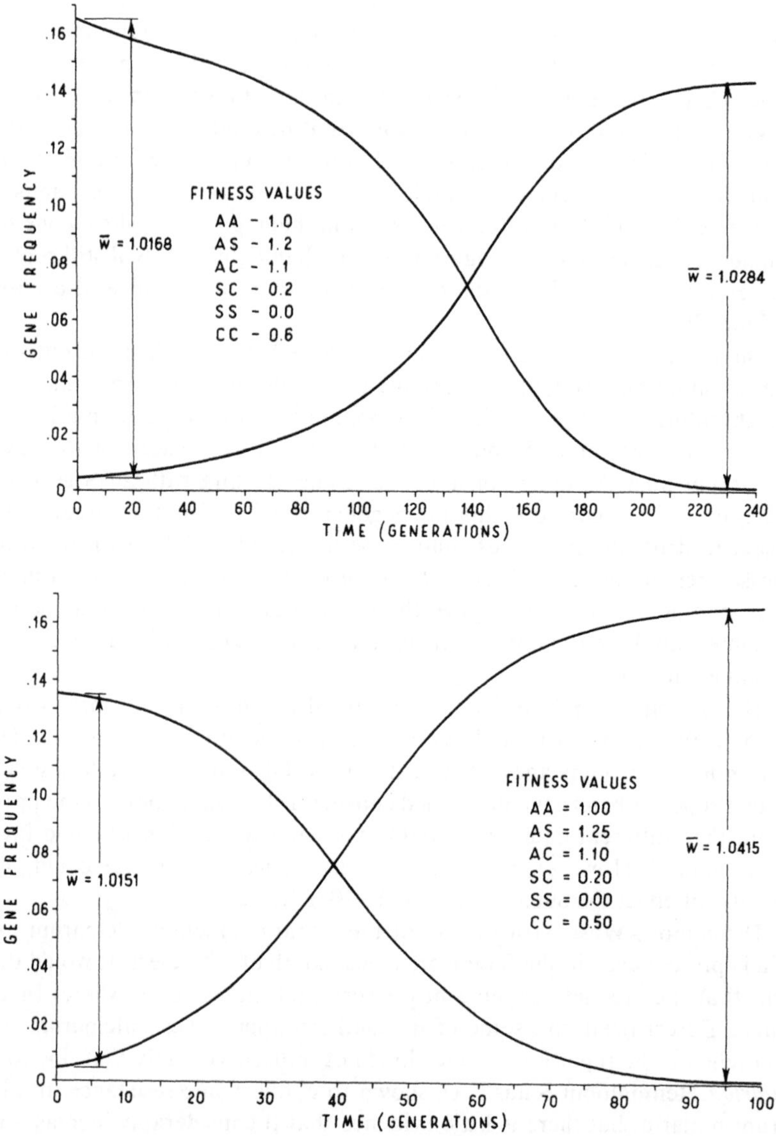

Figure 20. The Replacement of Hemoglobin C by Hemoglobin S with Two Different Sets of Fitness Values.

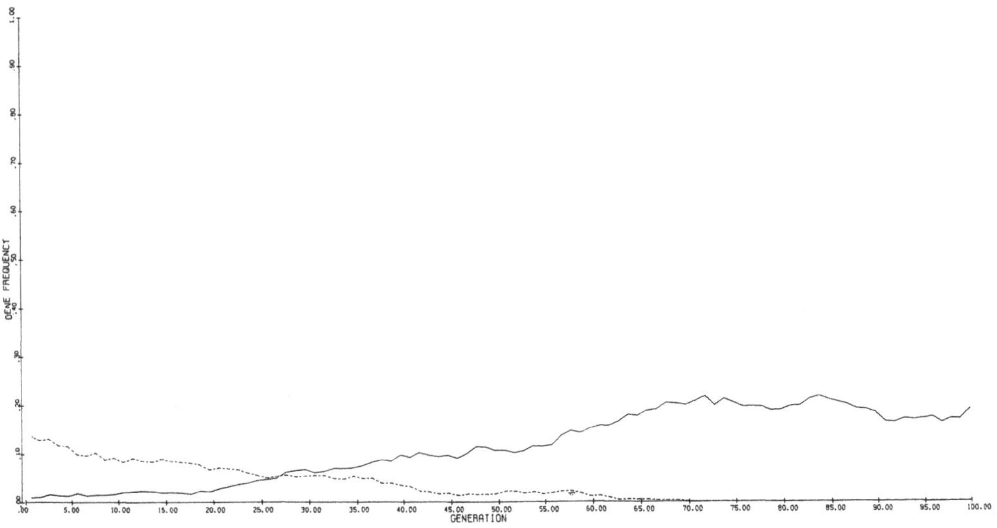

Figure 21. A stochastic model of the replacement of hemoglobin C by hemoglobin S with no gene flow, a population of 1000, and fitnesses: $W_{AA} = 1.0$, $W_{AS} = 1.2$, $W_{SS} = 0$, $W_{AC} = 1.125$, $W_{SC} = .25$, and $W_{CC} = .75$. (Hemoglobin C gene frequency = – – – and hemoglobin S gene frequency = ——).

falciparum malaria. If the physiological explanation for the resistance of hemoglobin S carriers to falciparum malaria lies in a unique interaction of the properties of red cells with hemoglobin S and the falciparum malaria parasite, as postulated by Miller et al. (477b), then it seems reasonable to think that their resistance is confined to this one species of human malaria parasite. For thalassemia, however, there seems to be no such unique interaction, and it would seem that the resistance of thalassemia carriers is simply due to the abnormalities of either their red cell morphology or metabolism.

For hemoglobin C the situation may be similar to thalassemia. The red cell morphology of the hemoglobin C trait is similar to that of thalassemia, deviating from normal in much the same way. In the Sahara Desert, as falciparum malaria is replaced by quartan malaria due to *P. malariae,* the fitness of the AC heterozygote may increase while the fitness of the AS heterozygote is decreased. In addition to the decrease in fitness of the AS heterozygote due to the lessening of falciparum malaria endemicity, the AS heterozygote is also afflicted with hyposthenuria, perhaps further decreasing this genotype's fitness in the desert environment (see Rucknagel and Neel [586] for an extensive discussion of this problem).

L. falciparum is considered to be the latest of the malaria parasites to

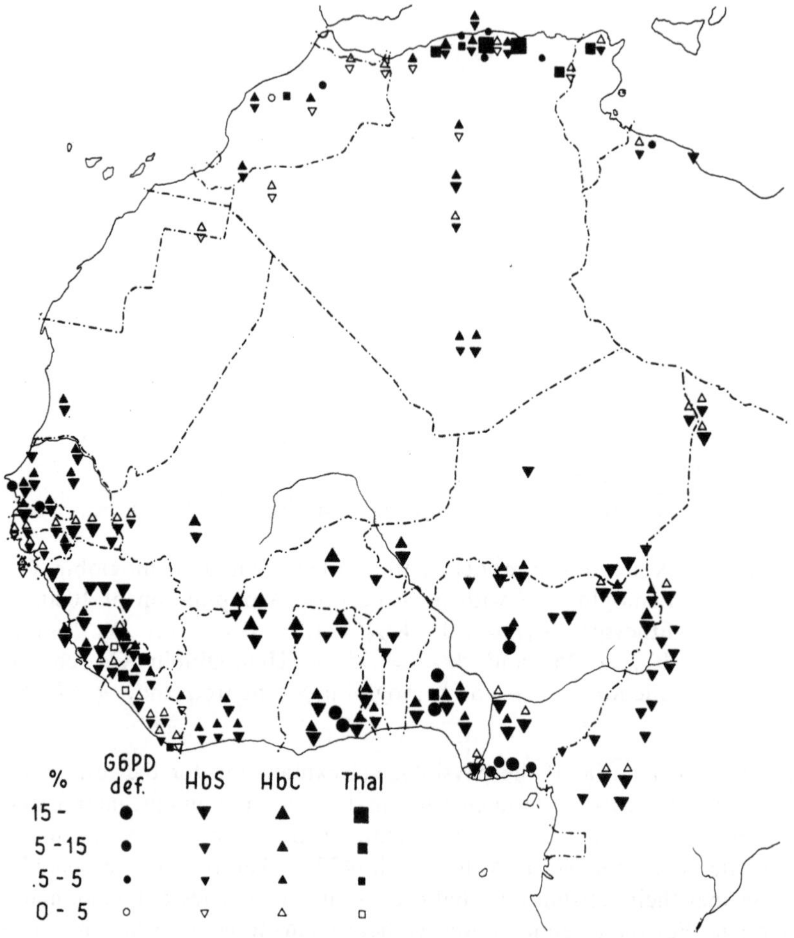

Figure 22. Percentage Incidence of the Red Cell Defects in North and West Africa.

infect man, and *P. malariae* is thought to be the most ancient (271). Since the savanna and Sudan regions of West Africa have the highest frequencies of *P. malariae* in the world, this parasite would seem to be a long-time resident in West Africa. If hemoglobin C confers a resistance to quartan malaria, then it may have been selected for earlier in West Africa than hemoglobin S. It built up to high frequencies in many populations and began to diffuse, but then came into competition with hemoglobin S—a late arrival in the area. Hemoglobin C has been able to maintain itself in areas such as Upper Volta or the Sahara, where *P. malariae* is still found in high frequencies. It has also diffused across the Sahara to the Berbers because of its smaller disadvantage when homozygous as compared to hemoglobin S, but in many populations the latter has overtaken it. And if falciparum malaria were to remain holoendemic among these people, hemoglobin S would replace C. However, since in the absence of its selective advantage, hemoglobin S decreases in frequency much faster than hemoglobin C, the latter will remain longer in the population. This has also undoubtedly happened in the past when a population moved or malaria spontaneously declined. Hence in non-malarious populations or those with an erratic or epidemic malaria situation, hemoglobin C can probably maintain itself better.

In North Africa there is some association beween "Negroid" populations and high frequencies of hemoglobins S and C. Although this association may indicate the direction from which these abnormal hemoglobins came to North Africa, there are other possible reasons for it. The Haratin, who are the Negroid population in the Saharan oases, are the former slaves of the Touareg and are primarily agriculturalists. This occupation and its oasis environment are much more malarious than those of the desert-dwelling nomads. Hence one would expect higher frequencies of abnormal hemoglobins among the Haratin, whatever their "race." Even along the Mediterranean coast in Libya, the most malarious area is the Misurata oasis, which also has a rather high frequency of hemoglobin S. It may have "Negroid" inhabitants, who have a higher hemoglobin S frequency than the other inhabitants; but if the population is panmictic, one would not expect any association between "Negroid" characteristics and abnormal hemoglobin frequency. In any case, abnormal hemoglobins are more associated with malaria in North Africa than with "Negroid" characteristics.

In West Africa very low frequencies of hemoglobin S are found in enclaves along the western coast. In some places, such as the Gambia, high frequencies are found among some populations; but adjacent populations belonging to the same tribe, with similar malaria patterns, sometimes have very low frequencies of this gene. The clines in the frequency of hemoglobin S in Liberia and Portuguese Guinea seem to represent the "wave of advance of an advantageous gene" since malaria is endemic everywhere in these areas of West Africa. Hemoglobin C is also quite low in these populations. But while hemoglobin C is confined to West and North Africa, hemoglobin S is found in even higher frequencies in East and Central Africa. The fact that hemoglobin S is perhaps more frequent in eastern West Africa (Nigeria) than elsewhere in this area seems to indicate that it has diffused into West Africa from the east, or perhaps from the northeast across the desert. Although the first hemoglobin S genes probably got into West Africa by gene flow from across the Sahara, once there, the gene could build up to very high frequencies because of the great selective advantage it possessed in this area. Now, with the very high frequencies of hemoglobin S in West Africa, the net gene flow for hemoglobin S is in the other direction.

The high frequencies of hemoglobin S in the Tibesti Mountains seem to indicate that malaria is present there, but many of the frequencies in the Sahara can be interpreted as the result of gene flow from the south. For example, there are 5 per cent hemoglobin S carriers among the Touareg in Agades (52). Assuming 1 per cent gene flow from the south where the populations have a hemoglobin S gene frequency of .1 (20 per cent heterozygotes), then according to equation (13) of Chapter IV we would expect about 5 per cent hemoglobin S carriers in the Touareg population. So, despite the fact that the hemoglobin S gene may have originally come into West Africa from this direction, it now seems to be "eddying" back.

Investigations on the frequency of the G6PD deficiency in West and North Africa are nowhere near as extensive as those on the abnormal hemoglobins. The few data do not seem to present any surprising results, since there does seem to be a general correlation between the frequency of G6PD deficiency and the intensity of malaria. However, in West Africa, as in East and Central Africa, there are both very intense malaria and high frequencies of abnormal hemoglobins; but the frequency of the G6PD deficiency, although appreciable, is not as high as in some Mediterranean and Near Eastern populations. The highest frequencies of abnormal hemoglobins are found in the areas of most endemic malaria, but the same does not seem to be true for the G6PD deficiency. This is a problem.

X

CENTRAL AND EAST AFRICA

FROM CENTRAL Nigeria eastward throughout sub-Saharan Africa and in Madagascar, hemoglobin S is the only abnormal variant found in high frequencies (Figure 23). Other hemoglobin variants are reported from the Congo Republic (Kinshasa) (697, 699), Uganda (20), and Angola (600), but none attain appreciable frequencies. Thalassemia has also been reported from the Congo Republic (Kinshasa) (699), and a "high fetal" condition from Uganda (348), but these also occur in low frequencies. These reports seem to indicate that hemoglobin S has been present in these populations for a long time, and in that time has driven out all other hemoglobin variants. The ability of hemoglobin S to replace other hemoglobin variants is due to the great fitness of the AS heterozygote. Since the SS homozygote is lethal, the fitness of the AS heterozygote has to be much greater than heterozygotes for abnormal hemoglobins that are not recessive lethals in order for the hemoglobin S gene to attain the same frequency. In addition, the hemoglobin S gene seems to reach higher frequencies than any other variant except hemoglobin E; so that the AS heterozygote must be the most fit of any hemoglobin genotype. Since the fitness of the heterozygote is the most important factor in determining whether a gene will increase when introduced into a population at a low frequency, the ability of the hemoglobin S gene to increase in the face of opposition becomes expectable.

Because of the widespread presence of hemoglobin S

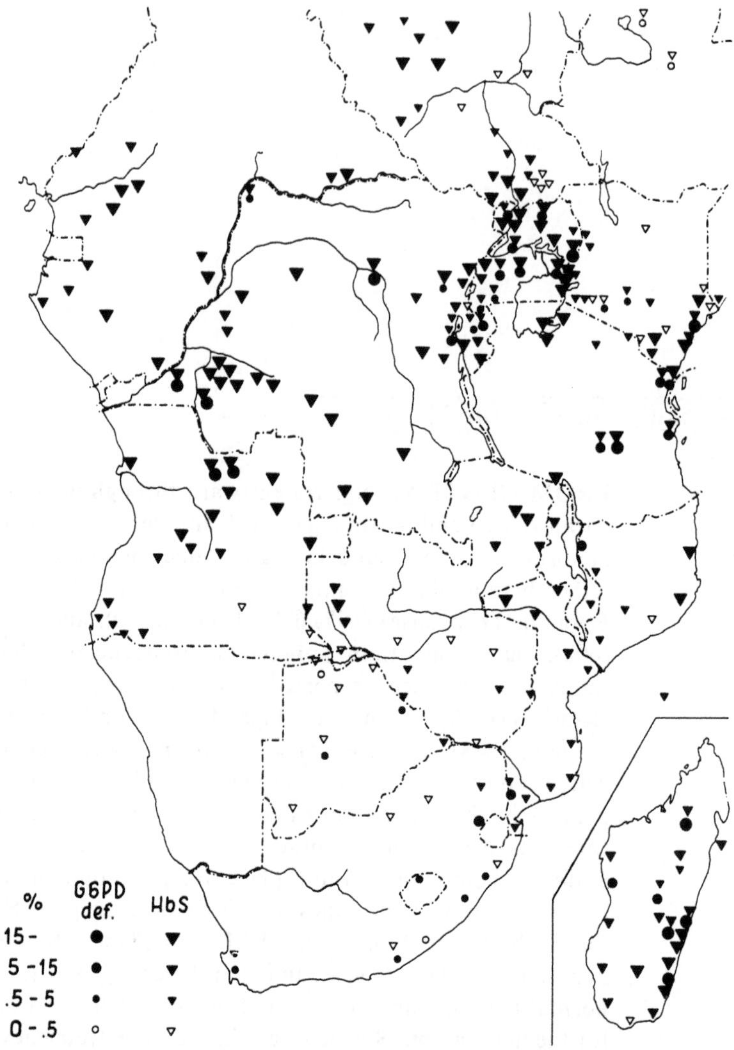

Figure 23. Percentage Incidence of the Red Cell Defects in Central and East Africa.

in central Africa, one is tempted to associate this abnormal hemoglobin with the expansion of the Bantu peoples. The Bantu homeland was most likely somewhere near Lake Chad, and the great similarity of language from Nigeria to Kenya to Zululand indicates that these people began expanding out from Nigeria sometime in the first millenium B.C. All the particulars of the Bantu expansion coincide quite well with the distribution of hemoglobin S and the absence of any other hemoglobin. Originally the Bantu people were undoubtedly much fewer in number, and have expanded rapidly since their geographic expansion began, which is a demographic situation that would favor the spread of a single hemoglobin variant. The expansion of the Bantu was most probably associated with an efficient adaptation of an agricultural economy to the tropical forest, including the growing of tropical root crops and perhaps ironworking (442). This is the type of culture that opens up the forest and is today associated with endemic malaria, but it seems to me to be questionable as to whether the early Bantu had endemic malaria. The population at the beginning was quite small and widely dispersed, and would have had little effect on the vegetation. Among the other primates of central Africa, malaria parasites resembling the *L. falciparum, P. malariae,* and *P. ovale* of man are found; these primates may have been reservoirs of infection and the parasites would have been zoonoses. But with the rapidly expanding human population it would be difficult for malaria to remain endemic, and the very high fertility rate may have reduced the selection for the hemoglobin S heterozygote (445). Hence, although the diffusion of hemoglobin S by the expansion of the Bantu seems plausible, it presents problems.

Since hemoglobin S has presumably been present in East and Central Africa for almost 2000 years, this gene should be close to equilibrium in most populations. It then seems perplexing to find so many low frequencies of hemoglobin S in central Africa, and particularly in the northwestern part where the Bantu originated. The Cameroons and Gabon even today contain more forest than other parts of Central Africa, and is the area where most of the western groups of Pygmies are found. These Pygmies, the Babinga, have a low frequency of hemoglobin S, which is expected since they are hunters. However, Ravisse (570) has found that at present they suffer seriously from malaria. Despite the fact that malaria is ubiquitous in Central Africa in the areas of tropical forest, there do seem to be reasons for believing it to be less severe than elsewhere. In most of Africa south of the Sahara the presence of holoendemic malaria everywhere is due to the two anthropophilic vectors, *A. gambiae* and *A. funestus,* which live in the grass roofs of the mud huts and breed in a great variety of places. Their breeding habits are somewhat complementary; so that during the season when *A. gambiae* is in eclipse, *A. funestus* will be prevalent and vice-versa. But in the forests of the southern Cameroons, these vectors are not present in large numbers (3, 400), and *A. mouchetti* is the major vector of human malaria.

Among the tribes with low hemoglobin S frequencies, the Mpongwe inhabit the coast which, in the absence of *A. melas,* a brackish water vector, is not as malarious as the interior. The low frequency among the Fang was found in the Mitzic District, which has many mountainous areas where malaria is of little public health importance (38). The low frequencies of both hemoglobin S and the G6PD deficiency among the Bwaka, however, do not seem to have a ready explanation, although the fact that this tribe does not speak Bantu may be involved. Around Kinshasa and the mouth of the Congo River, there has been a large, dense human population for many centuries, with a settlement pattern of medium-sized villages. This is the optimum habitat for holoendemic malaria, and throughout the area high frequencies of both hemoglobin S and the G6PD deficiency are found.

In the adjacent area of northern Angola, high frequencies of hemoglobin S and the G6PD deficiency are also found, and these extend south through Angola as far as the highlands around Nova Lisboa, where lower frequencies of hemoglobin S are found. Further south among the primitive peoples of southern Angola, much lower frequencies of hemoglobin S are found. Some of these tribes speak Bushman languages, but low frequencies are also found in Bantu speakers. On the fringe of the Kalahari Desert in southeastern Angola, no hemoglobin S has been found among the Bushmen, which seems expected. In adjacent Bechuanaland neither the Bushmen nor the Mpukshu Bantu have hemoglobin S. However, in recent years most of the population in northern Bechuanaland in the Okavango River Valley seems to have been subjected to intense malaria (639b).

Hemoglobin S has not been found in any Bushman or Hottentot group, and the Bantu of South Africa also have extremely low frequencies. But the Bantu do have the G6PD deficiency in appreciable frequencies, increasing as one proceeds north from Xhosaland. Hemoglobin S also seems to have a north-south cline, but the increase or gradient is not so pronounced. In the Transvaal and Mozambique the frequency of hemoglobin S is only 2–4 per cent. Although hemoglobin S is found in diverse, widespread populations in South Africa, it never seems to have built up to high frequencies there despite the presence of malaria. Similarly, in Rhodesia the frequency of hemoglobin S is very low, and malaria is present, although more epidemic than endemic. In comparison with the populations of Central Africa, those in South Africa have a much lower incidence of endemic malaria.

Part of the reason for this difference in malaria infestation is obviously climatic, but it also seems to be partly due to cultural differences between the Southern and Central African Bantu. In South Africa and Rhodesia the Bantu peoples tended to have a greater reliance on domestic animals, particularly cattle, although most Bantu peoples practice both animal husbandry and agriculture. In the south the basic settlement pattern was one of scattered individual homesteads, which would be closely associated with the cattle. On the other hand, in Central Africa the villages are much larger and tend to be situated close to the local water supply. This settlement pattern is ideal for the transmission of malaria, while the South African one is not. With large numbers of cattle it is even questionable whether malaria could have remained endemic in a population with the homestead pattern.

Since, according to Hackett (301), it was the close association with livestock and the increase in livestock in the nineteenth century that led to the spontaneous decline in malaria in Europe, a similar series of events could have happened among the southern Bantu. It would depend on whether the vector of human malaria could be diverted to feeding on cattle. While *A. gambiae* is not known to be easily diverted, recently Draper and Smith (217) have shown that with an increase in cattle in the Pare area of Tanzania, human malaria declined drastically because the vector, *A. gambiae*, began feeding on cattle. This vector has also been shown to prefer cattle blood on Madagascar (293). Hence, even in tribes such as the Tonga in Rhodesia who live in villages, because their huts are built around the cattle kraal, this would tend to lessen the transmission of human malaria and may explain the low hemoglobin S frequency.

From northern Mozambique to the central Sudan, the frequencies of hemoglobin S and the G6PD deficiency vary enormously. In fact the range of the world's frequencies for hemoglobin S (0–40 per cent heterozygotes) are found in East Africa, and often great differences are found in tribes living next to one another. But for the most part the hemoglobin S and G6PD-deficiency frequencies seem to be close to equilibrium. The great range is due to the fact that the equilibrium frequencies vary greatly in East Africa. In the dry grassland and semi-desert regions of Tanzania and Kenya, the hemoglobin S frequencies among the pastoralists are almost zero, and their G6PD deficiency frequencies are also very low. This seems to be a further example of the lesser selection against the G6PD-deficiency genotypes, which enables this gene to maintain itself in populations for which it has no selective advantage. Allison (22) first showed that just about all populations in East Africa are close to equilibrium for the hemoglobin S gene, as one would expect on the basis of the amount of malaria present. More recently, Marti et al. (464) have shown that in southern Tanzania among closely related Bantu groups, those in the highlands with less malaria have lower frequencies of both hemoglobin S and the G6PD deficiency. However, there do appear to be some exceptions.

On the coast of Kenya and Tanzania, Foy et al. (260, 257) found that among the sub-tribes of the Nyika there appeared to be significant variation in the frequency of hemoglobin S that did not seem to be related to the intensity of malaria. Generally on the coast of Kenya there is a remarkable association between malaria and hemoglobin S. All of the Nyika sub-tribes have at least 10 per cent hemoglobin S and malaria, while the related Teita tribe in the Teita Hills a short distance inland have zero per cent and no malaria. Among the Nyika sub-tribes the Duruma have about 10 per cent, while the other sub-tribes that have been adequately sampled have 20 per cent or more. Although all the Nyika sub-tribes live in similar environments and there is considerable gene flow between them, the Duruma are further inland

and do rely more on pastoralism than the others (558). As elsewhere in East Africa, this reliance on pastoralism with its consequent close association of the people with large herds of cattle may account for the lower hemoglobin S frequency.

Most of the interior of East Africa around Lake Victoria has intense endemic malaria, particularly along the shores of the lake. The Sukuma and allied tribes here have some of the highest hemoglobin S frequencies in the world, while the neighboring Gusii and Kipsigi, who live some distance from the lake and have much less malaria, have very low frequencies. The only tribes whose hemoglobin S frequencies are somewhat difficult to interpret are the Kavirondo Bantu. Their neighbors, the Luo, who are closer to the lake where there is more malaria, have very high frequencies of both hemoglobin S and the G6PD deficiency. The Kavirondo Bantu, though, vary in their hemoglobin S frequencies from 5–20 per cent. Generally the tribes closer to Lake Victoria have higher frequencies. As one proceeds from Lake Victoria up toward the Nandi Escarpment, malaria diminishes with altitude as does the frequency of hemoglobin S. However, in the north near the Uganda border the hemoglobin S frequencies seem to be higher. According to Wagner (725), the Vugusu, the Kavirondo Bantu of this area, lived in sizable walled towns, while the Logoli further to the south lived in scattered homesteads. Here, as in South Africa, there seems to be an association between hemoglobin S frequency and settlement pattern. One further factor which complicates the interpretation of hemoglobin S frequencies in the Kavirondo region is the instability of the epidemiology of malaria here. With the cutting down of the forest in the highlands, malaria has been gradually increasing the altitude at which it can remain endemic (270, 467).

On the western side of Lake Victoria in Uganda the situation is much the same. Near the lake, high frequencies of both hemoglobin S and the G6PD deficiency are found, but in the mountains to the south or the savanna to the north, there are lower frequencies of both genes and of malaria. In Rwanda and southern Uganda the Bantu peoples have rather low hemoglobin S frequencies, but at present there is some malaria here (350, 477). However, due to the increase in agriculture, malaria has been increasing the altitude at which it remains endemic (477). Among the Pygmies or Twa of this region the frequency of hemoglobin S is very low, as one would expect in hunters in mountain forests; and the frequency is also lower among the pastoralist Tutsi than among the agricultural Hutu, which would also be expected on the basis of malaria endemicity.

Just as there does not seem to be a strict concordance between hemoglobin S frequencies and malaria in the mountains of Central Africa because of the unstable altitude limit of endemic malaria, there also, for the same reason, does not seem to be a strict correlation between the two in northern Uganda at the border of endemic malaria in the savanna. A striking cline in the frequency of hemoglobin S seems to exist in many of the large tribes of northern Uganda. But many of the frequencies for the Sudanic, Nilotic, and Nilo-Hamite groups in this area are given by "tribe," and these examinations were done in Kampala on a migrant population. However, there is little doubt that these tribes contain many breeding isolates among which the frequency of hemoglobin S varies significantly. One study of the Lutomi "Kraal" of the Karamojong has found an astounding frequency of 87 per cent hemoglobin S (406). According to the Gullivers (297), the settlement among the Karamojong cluster of tribes tends to be endogamous, so that this frequency probably pertains to a breeding isolate which is very inbred. Most surveys of the Karamojong find very low frequencies of hemoglobin S—including that by Jelliffe et al. (349), which also reported serious endemic malaria. Most of the malaria was due to *P. malariae*, but *L. falciparum* was also present in appreciable frequency.

The Acholi and Lugbara tribes of northern Uganda also vary significantly in their frequencies of hemoglobin S. The Acholi have 27 per cent in Uganda, 15 per cent in northern Uganda, and 11 per cent in the southern Sudan. The Lugbara studied in Kampala have 20 per cent or more of hemoglobin S, but in the Aringa district of the West Nile Province, the most northern area inhabited by the Lugbara, Jelliffe et al. (352) found 2 per cent hemoglobin S but intense endemic malaria. Again, much of the malaria was due to *P. malariae*, but *L. falciparum* was also endemic. Malaria thus seems to have spread farther north into the dry savanna than high frequencies of hemoglobin S. Since hemoglobin S seems to have been present in East Africa long enough for it to have reached equilibrium, the most reasonable interpretation for these non-equilibrium frequencies is the recent spread of falciparum malaria to these populations.

In the southern Sudan, malaria occurs for the most part along the Nile River among the more sedentary, agricultural tribes, and the frequencies of hemoglobin S reflect this. Even among tribes such as the Mandari, who are divided into two sections, the frequency of hemoglobin S is correlated with the amount of malaria. One section of this tribe lives along the Nile and has 17 per cent hemoglobin S; while the other, which is separated from the Nile by an arid unhabited area and is centered around Tali Post, has 7 per cent and less malaria. East of the Nile among the northern Nilo-Hamites the frequencies of hemoglobin S are very low. Although these tribes have lost many of their cattle and much of their pastoral culture in the last 100 years, their previous pastoral life accords with these low frequencies.

Farther north among the pastoral Dinka, Nuer, and Shilluk, the frequency of hemoglobin S is essentially zero. Although malaria occurs among these tribes, it is not endemic, and their history would seem to indicate that it was less frequent in the past. North of the Nilotic peoples and farther out into the desert, there are appreciable frequencies of hemoglobin S among both the Arabic and non-Arabic tribes. Some of these tribes, such as the Habbania, have 20 per cent hemoglobin S but presumably less malaria than the Nilotes farther south; this is a perplexing problem and a real challenge to the malaria hypothesis. It seems to indicate that hemoglobin S has been introduced into this region from the Middle East or the Arabian peninsula. Since the Nilotic tribes are presumably the indigenous inhabitants and have extreme animosity toward strangers, it may well be that the complete absence of gene flow into their populations from the outside has prevented the hemoglobin S gene from becoming established. On the other hand, there may be differences in malaria among these groups, but they have not been reported to my knowledge. The fact that the Shuwa Arabs in Nigeria seem to have higher frequencies of hemoglobin S than the surrounding indigenous peoples may be another indication that the Arabs brought hemoglobin S to this part of the world, which would favor the first possibility.

Among the Arab and other immigrant populations of Khartoum, there seem to be high frequencies of both thalassemia and the G6PD deficiency, but little hemoglobin S. Even such groups as the Armenians, who are not known to have appreciable frequencies of any red cell defects, seem to be like other populations in Khartoum. Malaria is not known to be endemic in Khartoum, but some areas in the Sudan, such as the Gezira, have become malarious in recent years because of irrigation projects.

The populations that have been examined in Ethiopia are all in the highlands, which are not malarious. In southwestern Ethiopia there are many small tribes and kingdoms which have been in existence for millenia and among whom malaria is endemic. The related groups across the border in the Sudan seem to have either hemoglobin S or thalassemia. An examination of these aboriginal groups in southern Ethiopia would probably contribute greatly to solving the problems of the distribution of hemoglobin S in East Africa. The few tests that have been done on Somalis indicate no hemoglobin S in the rest of the Horn of East Africa, which would be expected since malaria is not endemic among them (437).

The final area of East Africa to be considered is Madagascar, which in terms of abnormal hemoglobins is indeed part of the continent. The only abnormal hemoglobin found there is S, and it varies significantly among the tribes of Madagascar. Although it has been claimed to be a genetic "marker" —whatever that is—of African ancestry, its distribution in Madagascar is much more highly correlated with malaria. In the highlands of central Madagascar the inhabitants, the Merina, are said to be less Negroid. They do have less hemoglobin S, but they are also pastoralists with less malaria. On Madagascar, it has been shown that the major vector of human malaria, *A. gambiae*, is the same species as in East Africa but can be diverted to feeding on cattle (293). In addition to the altitude, this seems to be a further reason for the low malaria and hemoglobin S among the Merina. They also have a low G6PD deficiency frequency, which accords with the malaria hypothesis.

On the west coast of Madagascar the Sakalava, together with the inland Bara, are considered to be the most African of the Madagascan tribes. Both these tribes apparently differ internally in their frequencies of hemoglobin S, with the extremes for the island found within both tribes. This internal variation is associated with the endemicity of malaria (362). In the far south of Madagascar, the country is almost desert with very little malaria, and the lowest hemoglobin S frequencies are found here. On the other hand, the small, steep-sided valleys of the east coast are the most malarious part of Madagascar, and the tribes here have the highest hemoglobin S frequencies. As one proceeds toward the highlands from the east coast, the frequency of hemoglobin S diminishes as does the endemicity of malaria. The east coast tribes have never been considered to be particularly African, but more Arab, so that these hemoglobin S frequencies do not accord with the race-mixture hypothesis. However, it may indicate that the Arabs brought the gene to Madagascar. Since the Makoa of the west coast of Madagascar have a very low hemoglobin S frequency and are apparently the same tribe as the Makua of Mozambique, the gene does not seem to have been brought to Madagascar by them. The data for the G6PD deficiency are not as complete as the hemoglobin data, but the known frequencies also accord with the malaria hypothesis.

XI

THE AMERICAS

CONSIDERED AS A whole, the aboriginal populations of the New World have very few abnormal hemoglobins and very little G6PD deficiency. What little of both red cell defects is found among them can reasonably be attributed to recent gene flow from immigrant populations or to very recent mutation. The general picture in the Americas is thus compatible with the hypothesis of the recent introduction of malaria into the New World. The pre-Columbian existence in the New World of many diseases—including malaria—is among the most hotly debated questions in anthropology, parasitology, and medical science. Recently Bruce-Chwatt (118a) has proposed that *P. vivax* and *P. malariae* were present in the New World in pre-Columbian times but not *L. falciparum*. He infers that the first two parasites were carried to the Americas by Bronze Age seafaring peoples from the Middle East or Europe. For this hypothesis he cites three kinds of evidence—linguistic, botanical, and historical.. However, I think that the genetic theory of evolution as applied to both man and his parasites is equally relevant and indicates the opposite conclusion, not only for malaria but also for another controversial disease, syphilis. For malaria, Dunn (224a) has come to the same conclusion; and for syphilis, Hackett (300), Hudson (328), and Weisman (738a) have discussed the issue and come to somewhat different conclusions.

One of the major arguments for the pre-Columbian existence of syphilis in the New World is the rapid spread of this disease in Europe shortly after contact with the Americas. In addition, the disease seemed to spread from Spain to the rest of the continent. But the fact that the American Indian suffered from syphilis so disastrously after contact seems to militate against this conclusion. Several bone lesions on pre-Columbian skeletal material from the Americas have been advanced as evidence for the presence of syphilis, but such lesions are extremely rare (738a). Moreover bone lesions are not syphilis, which is a specific parasite, and they could have been caused by another parasite now extinct. Many other diseases have changed their pathology and perhaps become extinct, for example, the English "sweating sickness" (306). According to evolutionary theory such change should be a relatively frequent phenomenon, and since parasites can evolve much faster than most organisms, it should perhaps be more common among them. It is curious that this possibility is not considered in many discussions of the evolution of parasites or people, but that hypotheses are based instead on the assumption that the morphology and epidemiology of parasites have remained unchanged for hundreds, thousands, and even millions of years.

At the time of contact with the New World by the Spaniards and Portuguese, there was also increased contact and communication with Africa south of the Sahara. Shortly after Columbus' first voyage, a Moroccan army invaded Gao and was defeated, with the remnants retreating back across the Sahara (525). Yaws, which is caused by a treponema indistinguishable morphologically from that causing syphilis, is at present endemic throughout humid tropical Africa. Close contact in the warm humid climate is a sufficiently efficient mechanism of transmission to keep the disease endemic, given the population density and settlement patterns of the indigenous cultures. In the humid tropics, syphilis is rare, but on the southern border of the Sahara, yaws is replaced by syphilis. Here congenital syphilis is endemic. In the typical village of the dry savanna or sudan the entire population is infected (514), and Miner (478a) comments that the inhabitants of Timbuctoo considered the disease inevitable. But in temperate climates these treponemas cannot be transmitted by contact at a sufficient rate to remain endemic. One way for the parasite to adapt to this new environment is to change its mode of transmission. In the case of syphilis, the "close contact" becomes restricted to sexual contact.

Hoare (322) has been shown that another group of African parasites, the trypanosomes, have undergone a similar evolution. The trypanosomes in tropical Africa are quite varied as to their modes of transmission, but most depend on the tsetse fly as the invertebrate host. In the desert, surra, a disease found mostly in camels, is caused by a trypanosome, which is indistinguishable from one found in Central Africa, but is transmitted by the bite of horseflies. In this case the horsefly acts as a simple mechanical agent to carry the parasite from one animal to another, while most trypanosomes undergo a part of their life cycle in the tsetse fly. Finally there is a trypanosome found in horses in temperate climates that is transmitted by sexual contact. These three stages in the adaptation of a tropical parasite to a temperate climate are also found in the treponemas causing yaws and syphilis. The widespread epidemic of syphilis throughout the world at the time of Columbus could have been due to the recent adaptation and spread of the new parasite through the non-immune populations in both the New and Old World. This reconstruction of the evolution of the treponemas is similar theoretically to Hudson (323), but the specific conclusions differ.

Yaws can remain endemic in a relatively small population and thus may have been with the human species during the long prehistoric period when man as a hunter was very sparsely distributed over the face of the earth (300). But malaria requires a larger population or several different host populations to remain endemic. Thus, *Homo erectus*, our ancestor of 500,000 years ago, when the population was between 100,000 and 1,000,000 in the 10,000,000 square miles of Africa, would have been a very poor host for malaria. It seems to me almost a certainty that malaria could not have remained endemic in this population without other hosts. The human malaria parasites could only have been zoonoses at that time and have since become totally human parasites. However, recent investigations have shown that many parasite species and strains are not restricted to humans (170, 183a, 242a).

The human malaria parasites closely resemble the malaria parasites of many monkeys and apes, and those human malaria parasites that are not restricted to the human species are found in other higher primates. Man's close antigenic similarity to his primate cousins has made the transference of a malaria parasite from one to the other a relatively easy matter. The monkeys and apes thus seem to be the obvious source of the malaria parasites that have become endemic in the human species since it became the dominant mammalian species in most of the world. This transference would undoubtedly have occurred when the human species was increasing rapidly, and the former host species of the parasite was becoming extinct in that locality.

The intimate association between the human malaria parasites and those of the monkeys and apes makes an examination of the primate malaria parasites relevant to the problem of the pre-Columbian existence of human malaria in the New World. Among both the apes and Old World monkeys there is a great variety of malaria parasites. This seems to indicate a long evolutionary history of the host-parasite association. In contrast, there is only one common malaria parasite among New World monkeys, *P. brasilianum*, and it is morphologically indistinguishable from the human malaria parasite, *P. malariae*. *P. brasilianum* can also be transmitted readily to man and has been transmitted among humans for several generations (183a). This single parasite among New World monkeys could thus easily be a recent acquisition from humans. Of course, malaria could still have been pre-Columbian in the New World and yet be recent enough for no evolutionary divergence to have occurred among the strains in the New World monkeys. It could not have come across Bering Straits with the Indians and between the original peopling and the time of Columbus there seems to have been no large contact with the Old World that could have carried malaria parasites. When coupled with the almost complete absence of abnormal hemoglobins and the G6PD deficiency in the American Indians, these evolutionary arguments point to an absence of malaria in pre-Columbian America.

In North America the Alaskan Indians and Eskimos and the northern Plains Indians do not have any abnormal hemoglobins in appreciable frequencies, although a hemoglobin D has been found among the latter. The Alaskan Indians and Eskimos do have an hereditary methemoglobinemia (615), but this is due to an enzyme deficiency and not an abnormal hemoglobin (613. It is found in southwestern Alaska in rather high frequencies for a deleterious genetic condition with apparently no selective advantage, and the marked clustering of cases seems to indicate the spread of a single mutant to both the Indian and Eskimo groups. This seems to be a good example of the founder effect.

In southern United States there are reports of hemoglobin S in various tribes. These instances can reasonably be attributed to gene flow from American Negro populations. As would be expected on the basis of this hypothesis, the Seminoles seem to have the highest frequency of hemoglobin S among the Indian tribes. The Seminoles were known to be a haven for runaway slaves; and in addition, there was malaria in Florida.

There are many triracial isolates in southeastern United States. One of these, the Lumbees of Robeson County, North Carolina, has been considered to be more Indian than the others, and they do have a very low frequency of hemoglobin S (2 per cent). However, they have as much hemoglobin C as S, and as much as many Negro populations. Another triracial isolate in Halifax and Warren counties, North Carolina, also has a low hemoglobin S frequency and a very high hemoglobin C frequency in both its divisions. The fact that both the Lumbees and this isolate have more hemoglobin C than expected on the basis of Negro admixture seems to have two possible explanations. One can invoke the founder effect and presume that these groups originated from very few ancestors. Or there may have been selection favoring the hemoglobin C gene in the past in this area. The Negroes of North Carolina seem to have a rather high hemoglobin C frequency, particularly when compared with their hemoglobin S frequency, which may indicate the same selection. However, there is also the possibility that the first Negroes in North Carolina came from West Africa where the frequency of hemoglobin C is high; so that the early mixture resulted in a disproportionate amount of this hemoglobin in the triracial isolates. Malaria was present in many parts of the South in the past century, and in the inland piedmont regions it was mostly due to *P. vivax*. Since hemoglobin S seems to confer a marked resistance to falciparum malaria while hemoglobin C carriers are apparently resistant to all species of malaria, the latter may have increased at the expense of the former in the interior of North Carolina. Of course, since hemoglobin C is not selected against as much as hemoglobin S, if the Negroes of North Carolina and the ancestors of these triracial isolates came from West Africa which had high frequencies of hemoglobin C, it would leave the population at a slower rate than hemoglobin S in the absence of malaria.

A third triracial isolate studied for abnormal hemoglobins and the G6PD deficiency is the Wesort or Brandywine isolate of Prince George and Charles counties, Maryland. These studies also raise questions as to the population dynamics of the hemoglobin genes. The Wesorts have the highest frequency of hemoglobin S (20 per cent) known in the United States. The isolate has probably been in existence for over 200 years but was augmented about 100 years ago from the outside. The area of Maryland where it is located was probably malarious until recently. However, the Negroes in the same area do not have an increased hemoglobin S frequency. Although this high frequency of hemoglobin S does not seem to be due to selection, it is still a possibility. D. L. Rucknagel has informed me that the Wesorts live in small villages of clusters of families, while the usual settlement pattern for the other inhabitants of the area is isolated homesteads. In addition, R. H. Post has proposed that, as a free Negro population in the days of slavery, the Wesorts probably lived on the poorer land which was perhaps swampy and hence very malarious. With their settlement pattern and local environment, malaria could have been much more endemic among the Wesorts than anyone else and the entire population would have been exposed to it.

If selection is not the explanation of the high hemoglobin S frequency among the Wesorts, then one can always resort to the founder effect or gene drift. In this case, there is some evidence that tends to support this. There are only six "core" surnames in the group, and another ten surnames were introduced into it in 1870 (308a), so that there were relatively few ancestors. The Wesorts also have extraordinarily high frequencies of albinism and dentinogenesis imperfecta, which are deleterious conditions due to the presence of a single gene. Since these are not balanced polymorphisms, the hemoglobin S gene may also not be balanced in this population, and its high frequency may be due instead to the same forces that are increasing the frequencies of these deleterious genes. The problem then becomes one of explaining how these deleterious genes can attain appreciable frequencies in these small isolates. The Wesorts are not unique in this respect: the Amish in different areas have high frequencies of hemophilia or the Ellis-vanCrevelt syndrome, and other religious or biracial isolates are also known to be characterized by some such gene.

In an expanding population, a deleterious gene that is present in one or a few ancestors does not have to reproduce at the same rate as the population, but will still be quite frequent in future generations because of this rapid expansion. This seems to be a part of the explanation of the high frequencies of deleterious genes in these circumscribed but expanding isolates. In addition, these are mostly rural populations which are losing members to the cities and could for this reason be subject to selective migration. If the members who leave the population are not a random sample of the genotypes for a particular locus in the population, then some genes may accumulate in the isolate if they tend not to be in the migrants. Among the Wesorts the members with albinism and dentinogenesis imperfecta genes would probably tend not to migrate since these genes when manifest result in observable conditions that would be unsightly to the majority of the U. S. population. Thus, psychologically there would be a tendency for these genotypes to remain in their natal group. The fact that rural areas of many countries tend to have higher frequencies of mental deficients seems to be a result of the same process. For the hemoglobin S gene, it is more difficult to conceive of circumstances wherein the gene would tend to remain home, but the possibility seems to be present.

Although the American Negro is constantly referred to as a single population, the abnormal hemoglobin and G6PD deficiency frequencies, like the other genes that have been studied in detail, indicate that American Negro populations are rather heterogeneous. Some of this heterogeneity is due to varying amounts of gene flow from other populations, particularly American whites, but some of it defies such an explanation. The frequencies of hemoglobin C seem to be much the same, although samples from North Carolina and Mississippi seem to indicate slightly higher frequencies, but the Negro frequencies of hemoglobin S are much more varied.

The Gullah Negroes of South Carolina have much more hemoglobin S (16 per cent) than others, but about the same hemoglobin C (3 per cent). A subdivision of this population on James Island, however, has an even higher hemoglobin S frequency (20 per cent) and very little hemoglobin C (.7 per cent). This was one of the most malarious parts of the United States (169) and much of this malaria could have been due to *L. falciparum*, with the result that the James Island population seems to be the only one in the United States in which hemoglobin S has eliminated hemoglobin C as it has in West Africa and among the Black Caribs of British Honduras. This population has also had less admixture than other American Negro populations, but a comparable population in Evans and Bullock counties, Georgia, has a much lower hemoglobin S frequency (9 per cent). These differences seem to be more related to malaria differences than to admixture, and Cooper et al. (186) have also shown that different loci yield very different estimates of the amount of admixture in the Georgia Negroes.

The Negroes of the northern United States also have lower frequencies of hemoglobin S, but this appears to be due to greater white admixture. Using equation (14) of Chapter IV, we can estimate how the hemoglobin S frequency should have changed in American Negro populations. Assuming $m = .02$ from the White population, $s = 1.0$, and $Q = 0$, then if the American Negro arrived with a hemoglobin S gene frequency of .12, in 10.7 generations the frequency would be .045, which it is on the average today. If the population started instead with a hemoglobin S frequency of .1, then in 9.3 generations it would be .045. Although many simplifying assumptions were necessary to apply the model, it seems to be a reasonable approximation to the hemoglobin S change in the American Negro.

In Mexico and Central America the great majority of the population is of Indian origin. Although there is malaria in many places, there is comparative absence of abnormal hemoglobins and the G6PD deficiency. This is compatible with the idea of malaria being introduced by European contact. But if malaria has been endemic in Central American since then, in the last twenty or more generations one would expect to see the beginning of an increase in either the G6PD deficiency or thalassemia, or perhaps in hemoglobin S if it had been introduced by gene flow. In some populations in Oaxaca, Mexico, hemoglobin S and the G6PD deficiency are found and are the result of gene flow from Africa. But even here the frequencies are quite low, even lower than the American Negro average.

In Central America the highest frequencies of hemoglobin S are found among the Black Carib and in some mixed villages in Panama. The Black Carib speak Carib but are primarily of African ancestry. They are the descendants of shipwrecked slaves who were assimilated into the Carib tribe on St. Vincent Island in the Lesser Antilles and later were deported to Roatan Island off the coast of Honduras, from where they have spread up and down the east coast of Central America. The populations in British Honduras have holoendemic malaria and high frequencies of hemoglobin S. An older study (472) in Honduras has found a lower frequency (8 per cent compared with 20 per cent), indicating that the Black Carib themselves may vary considerably in the frequency of hemoglobin S. On the other hand, the Black Carib have a hemoglobin C frequency that is as low as the average American Negro frequency and lower than those of most Negro populations in the West Indies. This low frequency of hemoglobin C seems to indicate that the selective forces that are maintaining hemoglobin S are not maintaining this other abnormal hemoglobin. Here among the Black Carib of British

Honduras, hemoglobin S is replacing or driving out hemoglobin C just as it is doing in West Africa under similar malarial conditions. However, some of the ancestors of the Black Carib were "Mocoes" from central Nigeria (250). Since there is very little hemoglobin C in this part of Africa, the Black Carib may well have started with very little of this gene.

On Curacao and other Caribbean islands where hemoglobin S does not have a marked selective advantage, hemoglobin C persists to a much greater extent. This may also be due to different areas of origin for the Africans on the different islands, since it would be unrealistic to assume that all populations of African origin in the New World came here with the same hemoglobin frequencies. Most of the Africans imported to the West Indies came in the seventeenth century, particularly the Black Carib and the ancestors of the Bush Negroes of Surinam. The great majority imported to the United States came in the eighteenth century. In the early days of the slave trade the major area of origin was the Gold Coast, or what is now Ghana. Thus, proportionally the Negro populations of the West Indies should have more hemoglobin C, and the fact that the isolated district of Curacao has a very high hemoglobin C frequency (9 per cent) and has lost most of its hemoglobin S (7 per cent) seems to support this interpretation.

Another early renegade Negro population, the Maroons of Jamaica, also have a very low hemoglobin S frequency (4 per cent). The Maroons have probably had little gene flow from other Negro populations in the last 200 years since they were recognized as independent by the British and entered into an agreement with them to return runaway slaves for a reward. They have been in a non-malarious environment for most of this time, and their low hemoglobin S frequency reflects this. The Maroons have not been studied for hemoglobin C, which may be high. The fact that hemoglobin C, like the G6PD deficiency, does not disappear from a population as fast as hemoglobin S in the absence of malaria is illustrated in Figure 24. Although this may explain in part why the Curacao populations have high hemoglobin C frequencies, much of the difference must be due to different origins, since the Lesser Antilles' populations are more like the American Negroes.

South America is similar to Central America in its hemoglobin and G6PD deficiency frequencies. The Indian populations as a rule have practically none, while the urban populations, which contain African admixture in varying amounts, have both. The only Indian groups reported to have these red cell defects are in the Guianas. Cabannes et al. (144) have found hemoglobin S and thalassemia in the Indian tribes of French Guiana, and the Indians of Surinam have been reported to have a very low hemoglobin S frequency (0.5 per cent) (364) and a much higher G6PD deficiency frequency (3-17 per cent) (459a). The hemoglobin S frequencies in the Indians of French Guiana are low (1-10 per cent), and the tribes with this gene are

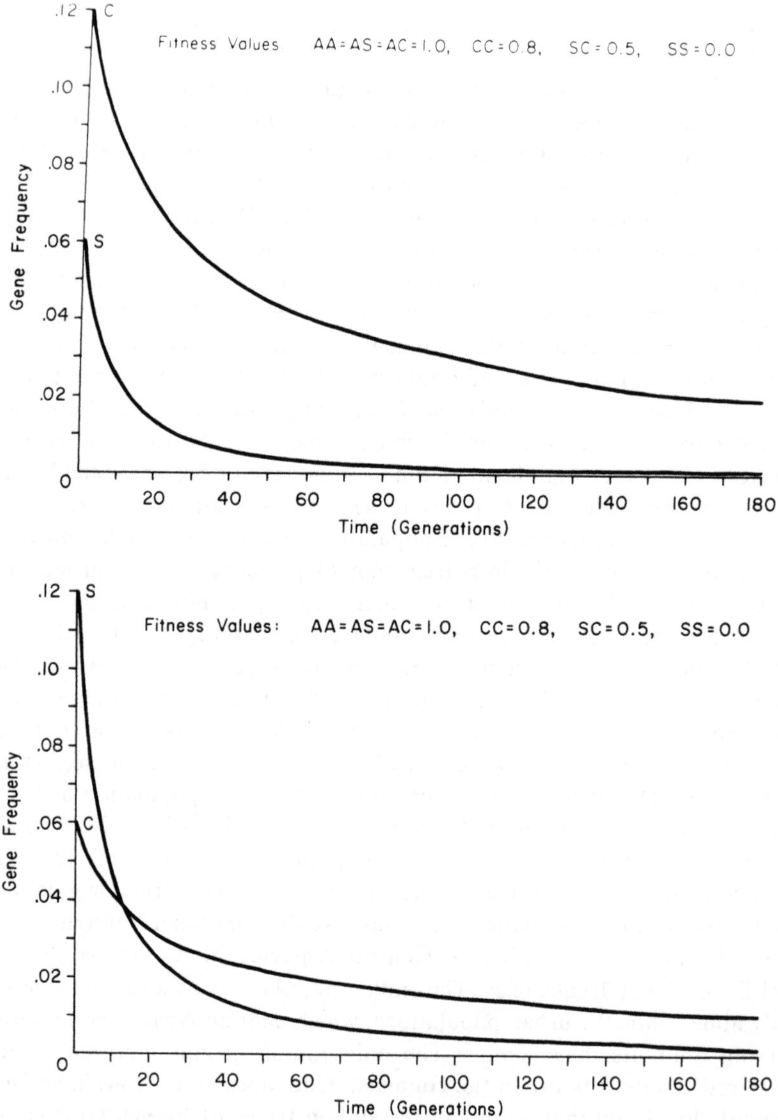

Figure 24. The Decrease in Hemoglobins S and C in the Absence of Malaria. (From F. B. Livingstone, 1964, *American Journal of Human Genetics,* 16:435-450, by permission.)

found along the coast. These frequencies are undoubtedly due to admixture with Africans, and there seems to be a correlation between degree of admixture and hemoglobin S frequency.

All of the Indian tribes of Dutch and French Guiana now have very intense malaria. If malaria were introduced to these Indians after European contact, then the present high endemicity of malaria is quite recent. And as in other parts of the world, the first genes that are usually selected for by malaria are thalassemia and the G6PD deficiency, since they have higher mutation rates. Thus the high thalassemia frequency among the Oyampi, who are in the interior of French Guiana, and the high G6PD deficiency among the Oyana, who are in the interior of Surinam, would seem to be responses to the recent selection by malaria. The Oyana are inland from the Djuka or Bush Negroes, and their G6PD deficiency may be the result of admixture. However, their blood groups (607a) do not indicate any admixture.

While most Negro or mixed groups have hemoglobin frequencies somewhat lower than those of West Africa, the Bush Negroes (who are called Djukas in Surinam and Bonis in French Guiana) like the Black Carib have high frequencies of hemoglobin S. These Negroes escaped to the "bush" about the time of the transfer of Surinam to the Dutch in 1674, but have been augmented by fugitive slaves since then. Their frequencies of hemoglobins S and C vary but on the average are similar to those of the Black Carib. But with 15–20 per cent hemoglobin S and 5 per cent hemoglobin C, they do seem to have slightly less S and more C than the Black Carib. The Negroes transported to the New World by the Dutch were almost all from the Gold Coast, which may explain the high frequency of hemoglobin C. But in any case their hemoglobin C frequency is lower than in Curacao and much lower than the average for the Gold Coast or Ghana today; so that hemoglobin S also seems to have replaced hemoglobin C among the Bush Negroes in the malarious interior of French and Dutch Guiana.

Other populations in South America have abnormal hemoglobin, thalassemia, and G6PD deficiency frequencies that are expectable in terms of their origins. In the northern countries some populations are found with as high as 15 per cent hemoglobin S; these are usually reported to be Negro. Further south the populations have less Negro admixture, less malaria, and less hemoglobin S. In Brazil, the Negro and other populations vary greatly in their hemoglobin S frequencies. In northeast Brazil the frequencies seem to be higher, and there is more malaria. The Negroes of Rio Grande do Sul show a rather low hemoglobin C frequency, particularly when compared to other American Negro populations and when considered in conjunction with their hemoglobin S frequency. However, many more of the slaves imported to Brazil were from Angola, the Congo, and Nigeria than those coming to either North or Central America (361, 592). This would explain their lower hemoglobin C frequency and also their rather high hemoglobin S frequency. Bahia is one part of Brazil that obtained many slaves from West Africa, and the higher hemoglobin C frequency found there and in Minas Gerais seem to reflect this difference of origin.

Finally, the absence of abnormal hemoglobins in Peruvian Indians and also in Tibetans seems to indicate that there have been no adaptations to altitude in human hemoglobin genes (but see 586a). There is also an endemic blood parasite in Peru which causes Oroya fever or Carrion's disease. It is due to a bacteria, *Bartonella bacilliformis*, and is transmitted by sandflies. Although the investigations of abnormal hemoglobins and the G6PD deficiency in Peru have not covered the endemic area, there is no evidence for any hemoglobin adaptations to this disease.

XII

CONCLUSIONS

THE MOST significant conclusion of this examination of the world's frequencies of the abnormal hemoglobin and G6PD-deficiency genes is the great value of the malaria hypothesis for interpreting or explaining these frequencies. There were astonishingly few frequencies that did not seem to be explained directly by this hypothesis. That is, the frequency of the red cell defect did not seem to be in equilibrium for the amount of malaria present now or in the recent past. Of course, one must consider the other factors of evolution, and wherever the frequencies did not seem to be close to equilibrium, gene flow or gene drift seemed to be a plausible explanation. Many of the frequencies that do not appear to be close to equilibrium are found in small, inbred, and isolated populations such as the Wesorts of Maryland or the Kurdish Jews of Northern Iraq. And many of the other non-equilibrium frequencies such as those in the American Negro can be explained on the basis of recent gene flow.

As was stated previously, the logic of an explanation of the frequencies of the red cell defects begins with the question: Why do high frequencies of these deleterious genes exist? Since they are found in many large diverse populations in high frequencies, the only plausible answer to the question is a greater fitness of the heterozygotes for these genes. Furthermore, given the geographical distribution of these high frequencies, malaria seems to be the only selective factor that can account for the greater fitness of the heterozygotes. The implication of this theory is, therefore, that whereever a high frequency of a red cell defect is found, there should be endemic malaria. It does not necessarily follow, however, that wherever there is endemic malaria there should be a high frequency of any particular hemoglobin or G6PD-deficiency variant. If a population with a high frequency of one of the red cell defects were found and it had no history of malaria, this would be concrete evidence that other selective forces besides malaria are involved. The Wesorts come as close to this siuation as any population, but there are still doubts about the history of this isolate and its exposure to malaria.

The fact that no such population has been discovered emphasizes the striking correlation between the distributions of malaria and the red cell defects. But even if such a population were found, it would not "disprove" the malaria hypothesis. There are still the thousands of frequencies in this book that are explained by this hypothesis, and it seems very doubtful that any other selective factor could explain them all. Such a discovery will thus not make us discard the malaria hypothesis but only make us add to the theoretical explanation of the frequencies of the red cell defects. This may well happen for thalassemia. The slight correlation between this defect and malaria in many parts of the Mediterranean area almost seems to require some other factor.

Although the malaria hypothesis has not been disproved, it could also be said that it has not been proved. Proof would consist of a definitive experiment or investigation, one outcome of which would support the malaria hypothesis and another which would not. Much of the experimental or parasite data for hemoglobin S can be considered as such definitive attempts. Some investigations have pointed one way and others the opposite, so that as a whole the evidence still appears equivocal to many. One major reason for the absence of definite proof is that the difference between the outcome predicted by the malaria hypothesis and that expected in the absence of such an association between the red cell defects and malaria is within the range of experimental error or chance variation.

Since the selection against hemoglobins C and E and the G6PD deficiency is much less than that against hemoglobin S, the selective advantage of their respective heterozygotes is also much less. Hence for these genes the difference between the two outcomes of any definitive experiment will be far less than that for hemoglobin S. Considering the difficulties encountered for hemoglobin S, I think that for many of the red cell defects a definitive experiment may never be possible.

Perhaps the techniques of culturing malaria parasites will be perfected to such an extent that conclusive experiments can be devised. Another possibility lies in the development of techniques to determine the hemoglobin and G6PD content of the individual cell. Kruatrachue et al. (389a) have shown that the red blood cells with a deficiency of G6PD have fewer malaria parasites, but not significantly fewer. However, despite these promising possibilities, it is still most likely that the malaria hypothesis will never be proved to everyone's satisfaction. Still, given our present knowledge of the forces of gene frequency change, the malaria hypothesis is the only explanation that has ever been seriously advanced for the high frequencies of the red cell defects, and seems to be the only possible explanation. It seems to me that a "wait and see" attitude with regard to this hypothesis only inhibits further progress, since it will be the basis of any future advances in this field.

BIBLIOGRAPHY

1. ABBOTT, P. H. (1950) The sickle-cell trait among the Zande tribe of the Southern Sudan. *East African Medical Journal*, 27:162–163.
2. ADAM, A. (1962) A survey of some genetical characters in Ethiopian tribes. I. Glutathione stability and glucose-6-phosphate dehydrogenase activity in red blood cells. *American Journal of Physical Anthropology*, 20:172–173.
3. ADAM, J. P. (1956) Note faunistique et biologique sur les Anophèles de la region de Yaoundé et la transmission du paludisme en zone forestiére du Sud Cameroun. *Bulletin de la Société de Pathologie Exotique*, 49:210–220.

3a. ADAMS, J. Q., WHITACRE, F. E., and DIGGS, L. W. (1953) Pregnancy and sickle cell disease. *Obstetrics and Gynecology*, 2:335–352.

4. ADAMSON, P. B. (1951) Haematological and biochemical findings in Hausa males. *Journal of Tropical Medicine and Hygiene*, 54:73–77.
5. AGER, J. A. M. and LEHMANN, H. (1957) Haemoglobin L: a new haemoglobin found in a Punjabi Hindu. *British Medical Journal*, 2:142–143.

5a. AKHUNDOVA, A. M. (1965) Talassemia v Azerbaidzhanskoi SSR. *Problemy Gematologii i Perelivaniya Krovi*, 10:10–18.

6. AKSOY, M. (1955) Sickle-cell trait in South Turkey. *Lancet*, 1:589.
7. AKSOY, M. (1960) The hemoglobin E syndromes. I. Hemoglobin E in Eti-Turks. *Blood*, 15:606–609.
8. AKSOY, M. (1961) Brief note: Hemoglobin S in Eti-Turks and the Allewits in Lebanon. *Blood*, 17:657–659.
9. AKSOY, M. (1962) Haemoglobins S and E in Turkish people. *Nature*, 193: 786–787.
10. AKSOY, M. (1964) The thalassaemia syndromes. III. A severe form of thalassaemia minor with slightly elevated foetal haemoglobin. Study of two families. *Blut*, 10:329–332.
11. AKSOY, M., BIRD, G. W. G., LEHMANN, H., MOURANT, A. E., THEIN, H., and WICKREMASINGHE, R. L. (1955) Haemoglobin E in Asia. *Journal of Physiology*, 130:56P–57P.
12. AKSOY, M., ÇETINGIL, A. I., KOCABALKAN, N., ŞESTAKOF, D., ALADAĞ, T., SECER, F., and BOSTANCI, N. (1963) Thalassemia-hemoglobin E disease

in Turkey, with hypersplenism in one case. *American Journal of Medicine*, 34:851–855.

13. AKSOY, M., IKIN, E. W., MOURANT, A. E., and LEHMANN, H. (1958) Blood groups, haemoglobins, and thalassaemia in Turks in Southern Turkey and Eti-Turks. *British Medical Journal*, 2:937–939.
14. AKSOY, M. and LEHMANN, H. (1957) The first observation of sickle-cell-haemoglobin E disease. *Nature*, 179:1248–1249.
15. ALBAHARY, C., DREYFUS, J. C., LABIE, D., SCHAPIRA, G., and TRAIN, L. (1958) Hémoglobines anormales au Sud-Vietnam (Hémoglobinose C homozygote. Trait E. Hémoglobine nouvelle). *Revue d'Hématologie*, 13:163–170.
16. ALEXANDRIDES, C. (1963) Sur la fréquence des hémoglobinopathies méditerranéenes en Grèce. *Proceedings of the 9th Congress of the European Society of Haematology* (Lisbon, 1963). S. Karger, New York. Pp. 477–495.
17. AL-KHEDAIRY, N. and AL-ABOOSI, A. J. (1964) Haemoglobin C anaemia in an Iraqi child. *Journal of the Faculty of Medicine, Baghdad*, 6:166–167.
18. ALLAN, N., BEALE, D., IRVINE, D., and LEHMANN, H. (1965) Three haemoglobins K: Woolwich, an abnormal, Cameroon and Ibadan, two unusual variants of human haemoglobin A. *Nature*, 208:658–661.
19. ALLARD, R. (1955) A propos de la conservation génétique du sickle cell trait. *Annales de la Société Belge de Médecine Tropicale*, 35:649–660.
20. ALLBROOK, D., BARNICOT, N. A., DANCE, N., LAWLER, S. D., MARSHALL, R., and MUNGAI, J. (1965) Blood groups, haemoglobin and serum factors of the Karamojo. *Human Biology*, 37:217–237.
21. ALLISON, A. C. (1953) The sickle-cell trait in the Mediterranean area. *Man*, 53:31.
22. ALLISON, A. C. (1954) The distribution of the sickle-cell trait in East Africa and elsewhere, and its apparent relationship to the incidence of subtertian malaria. *Transactions of the Royal Society of Tropical Medicine and Hygiene*, 48:312–318.
23. ALLISON, A. C. (1954) Protection afforded by sickle-cell trait against subtertian malarial infection. *British Medical Journal*, 1:290–294.
24. ALLISON, A. C. (1956) The sickle-cell and haemoglobin C genes in some African populations. *Annals of Human Genetics*, 21:67–89.
25. ALLISON, A. C. (1957) Malaria in carriers of the sickle-cell trait and in newborn children. *Experimental Parasitology*, 6:418–447.
26. ALLISON, A. C. (1960) Glucose-6-phosphate dehydrogenase deficiency in red blood cells of East Africans. *Nature*, 186:531–532.
27. ALLISON, A. C. (1964) Polymorphism and natural selection in human populations. *Cold Spring Harbor Symposia on Quantitative Biology*, 29: 137–149.
28. ALLISON, A. C. (1965) Population genetics of abnormal haemoglobins and glucose-6-phosphate dehydrogenase deficiency. In J. H. P. Jonxis (Ed.), *Abnormal Haemoglobins in Africa*, F. A. Davis Co., Philadelphia. Pp. 365–391.
29. ALLISON, A. C., ASKONAS, B. A., BARNICOT, N. A., BLUMBERG, B. S., and KRIMBAS, C. (1963) Deficiency of erythrocyte glucose-6-phosphate dehydrogenase in Greek populations. *Annals of Human Genetics*, 26: 237–242.
30. ALLISON, A. C., CHARLES, L. J., and MCGREGOR, I. A. (1961) Erythrocyte

glucose-6-phosphate dehydrogenase deficiency in West Africa. *Nature*, 190:1198–1199.

31. ALLISON, A. C. and CLYDE, D. F. (1961) Malaria in African children with deficient erythrocyte glucose-6-phosphate dehydrogenase. *British Medical Journal*, 1:1346–1349.
32. ALLISON, A. C. and SMITH, S. M. (1954) Notes on sickle-cell polymorphism. *Annals of Human Genetics*, 19:39–57.
33. DE ALMEIDA, A. (1965) *Bushmen and Other Non-Bantu Peoples of Angola.* Institute for the Study of Man in Africa, Johannesburg. Publication No. 1.
34. ALTMAN, A. (1945) The sickle-cell trait in the South African Bantu. *South African Medical Journal*, 19:457.
35. ALVAR LORÍA, Q. B. P. (1963) Estudios sobre algunas características hematológicas hereditarias en la población Mexicana. III. Deficiencia en la glucosa-6-fosfato deshidrogenasa eritrocítica en 7 grupos Indígenas y algunos mestizos. *Gaceta Médica de México*, 93:299–303.
36. ALVING, A. S., KELLERMEYER, R. W., TARLOV, A., SCHRIER, S., and CARSON, P. E. (1958) Biochemical and genetic aspects of primaquine-sensitive hemolytic anemia. *Annals of Internal Medicine*, 49:240–248.

36a. ANDERSON, J. E. (1966) Anemia and hemoglobin E trait in the Republic of Viet Nam. *Military Medicine*, 131:148–149.

37. ANDIE, R., BESSIS, M., DREYFUS, B., JACOB, S., and MALASSENET, R. (1958) Association d'un syndrome thalassémique et d'un hémoglobine anormale à l'électrophorèsé non encore identifiée, chez un français d'origine Picarde. *Revue d'Hématologie*, 13:31–46.
38. ANDRÉ, L. J. and ANDRÉ-GADRAS, E. (1957) Étude des rapports entre la sicklémie et la lèpre. *Médecine Tropicale*, 17:596–599.
39. ANDRÉEV, I., VAPTZAROV, I., and ANGUELOV, A. (1959) Le favisme en Bulgarie. *Folia Medica(Sofia)*, 1:211–215.
40. ANDREWS, A. C. (1949) The bean and Indo-European totemism. *American Anthropologist*, 51:274–292.

40a. ANONYMOUS (1953) Statement concerning a system of nomenclature for the varieties of human hemoglobin. *Blood*, 8:386–387.

41. ANONYMOUS (1965) Nomenclature of hemoglobins. *Blood*, 25:126–127.
42. ARENDS, T. (1961) Absence of abnormal haemoglobins in Colombian Tunebo Indians. *Nature*, 190:93–94.
43. ARENDS, T. (1963) Estado actual del estudio de las hemoglobinas anormales en Venezuela. *Sangre*, 8:1–14.
44. ARENDS, T. (1963) Frecuencia de hemoglobinas anormales en poblaciones humanas sudamericanas. *Acta Cientifica Venezolana*, 14 Suppl. 1:46–57.
45. ARENDS, T. (1964) Search for abnormal hemoglobins in South American Indians living in malarious zones. *Proceedings of the 7th International Congresses on Tropical Medicine and Malaria*, 4:179–182.
46. ARENDS, T. and GALLANGO, M. L. (1965) Haemoglobin types and blood serum factors in British Guiana Indians. *British Journal of Haematology*, 11:350–359.

46a. ATWATER, J. and REGAN, J. (1964) Hemoglobin O_{Arab} trait in three generations of an American Negro family. *Abstracts of the 10th Congress of the International Society of Haematology* (Stockholm, 1964), L:5.

47. AUNG, THAN BATU (1965) Letter to D. L. Rucknagel.
48. AWNY, A. Y., KAMEL, K., and HOERMAN, K. C. (1965) ABO blood groups

and hemoglobin variants among Nubians, Egypt, U.A.R. *American Journal of Physical Anthropology,* 23:81–82.

48a. Azevedo, E., Morrow, A. C., Kirkman, H. N., and Motulsky, A. G. (1965) Glucose-6-phosphate dehydrogenase mutations in Asiatic Indians. *Abstracts of the Annual Meeting of the American Society of Human Genetics* (Seattle). P. 5.

48b. Baglioni, C. (1962) The fusion of 2 peptide chains in hemoglobin Lepore and its interpretation as a genetic deletion. *Proceedings of the National Academy of Sciences,* 48:1880–1886.

49. Banton, A. H. (1951) A genetic study of Mediterranean anaemia in Cyprus. *American Journal of Human Genetics,* 3:47–64.

49a. Barber, M. A. and Rice, J. B. (1937) A survey of malaria in Egypt. *American Journal of Tropical Medicine,* 17:413–436.

50. Barkhan, P., Stevenson, M. E., Pinker, G., Dance, N., and Shooter, E. M. (1964) Haemoglobin Lepore trait. An analysis of the abnormal haemoglobin. *British Journal of Haematology,* 10:437–441.

51. Barnicot, N. A., Allison, A. C., Blumberg, B. S., Deliyannis, G., Krimbas, C., and Ballas, A. (1963) Haemoglobin types in Greek populations. *Annals of Human Genetics,* 26:229–236.

52. Barnicot, N. A., Ikin, E. W., and Mourant, A. E. (1954) Les groupes sanguins ABO, MNS, et Rh des Touaregs de l'Air. *L'Anthropologie,* 58:231–240.

53. Barnicot, N. A., Krimbas, C., McConnell, R. B., and Beaven, G. H. (1965) A genetical survey of Sphakiá, Crete. *Human Biology,* 37: 274–298.

54. Barnola, J., Tovar-Escobar, G., and Potenza, L. (1953) Enfermedad por células falciformes. *Archivos Venezolanos de Puericultura y Pediatria,* 16:293–376.

55. Barth, F. (1952) The southern Mongoloid migration. *Man,* 52:2.

55a. Bartlett, M. S. (1960) The critical community size for measles in the United States. *Journal of the Royal Statistical Society,* Series A, 123:37–44.

56. Batabyal, J. N. and Wilson, J. M. G. (1958) Sickle-cell anaemia in Assam. *Journal of the Indian Medical Association,* 30:8–11.

57. Baup, H. (1964) Fréquence de l'hémoglobine E au Laos. *Médecine Tropicale,* 24:51–60.

57a. Baur, E. W. and Motulsky, A. G. (1965) Hemoglobin Tacoma—a β chain variant associated with increased Hb. A_2. *Humangenetik,* 1:621–634.

58. Baxi, A. J., Balakrishnan, V., and Sanghvi, L. D. (1961) Deficiency of glucose-6-phosphate dehydrogenase-observations on a sample from Bombay. *Current Science,* 30:16–17.

59. Baxi, A. J., Balakrishnan, V., Undevia, J. V., and Sanghvi, L. D. (1963) Glucose-6-phosphate dehydrogenase deficiency in the Parsee community, Bombay. *Indian Journal of Medical Science,* 17:493–500.

60. Bayrakci, C., Josephson, A., Singer, L., Heller, P., and Coleman, R. D. (1964) A new fast hemoglobin. *Abstracts of the 10th Congress of the International Society of Haematology* (Stockholm, 1964), L:6.

60a. Beacham, W. D. and Beacham, D. W. (1950) Sickle-cell disease and pregnancy. *American Journal of Obstetrics and Gynecology,* 60:1217–1226.

61. Beale, D. and Lehmann, H. (1965) Abnormal haemoglobins and the genetic code. *Nature,* 207:259–261.

62. BEAVEN, G. H., STEVENS, B. L., ELLIS, M. J., WHITE, J. C., BERNSTOCK, L., MASTERS, P., and STAPLETON, T. (1964) Studies on foetal haemoglobin. IV. Thalassaemia-like conditions in British families. *British Journal of Haematology,* 10:1–14.

63. BECQUET, R., GASTEAU, T., and HAPPI, C. (1959) Recherches sur la drépanocytose en pays Bamiléké (Cameroun). *Bulletin de la Société de Pathologie Exotique,* 52:836–843.

64. BECK, J. S. P. and HERTZ, C. S. (1935) Standardizing a sickle-cell method, and evidence of sickle-cell trait. *American Journal of Clinical Pathology,* 5:325–332.

64a. BECKMAN, L., CHRISTODOULOU, C., FESSAS, PH., LOUKOPOULOS, D., KALTSOYA, A. and NILSSON, L-O. (1966) A Swedish haemoglobin variant. *Acta Genetica et Statistica Medica,* 16:362–370.

65. BECKMAN, L. and TAKMAN, J. (1965) On the anthropology of a Swedish Gypsy population. *Hereditas,* 53:272–280.

66. BEEKMAN, E. M. (1949) Klinische en haematologische studies over de sikkelcelziekte. Unpublished thesis, University of Leiden.

67. BEET, E. A. (1946) Sickle cell disease in the Balovale district of Northern Rhodesia. *East African Medical Journal,* 23:75–86.

68. BEET, E. A. (1947) Sickle cell disease in Northern Rhodesia. *East African Medical Journal,* 24:212–222.

69. BEET, E. A. (1949) The genetics of the sickle-cell trait in a Bantu tribe. *Annals of Eugenics,* 14:279–284.

70. BENOIST, J. (1962) Anthropologie physique de la population de l'Île de la Tortue (Haiti). Contribution a l'étude de l'origine des Noirs des Antilles Françaises. *Bulletins et Mémoires de la Société d'Anthropologie de Paris,* 11e Série, 3:315–335.

71. VAN DER BERGHE, L. J. and JANSSEN, P. (1950) Maladie à sickle cells en Afrique noire. *Annales de la Société Belge de Médecine Tropicale,* 30:1553–1566.

72. BERNINI, L., LATTE, B., SINISCALCO, M., PIOMELLI, S., SPADA, U., ADINOLFI, M., and MOLLISON, P. L. (1964) Survival of ^{51}Cr-labelled red cells in subjects with thalassaemia-trait or G6PD deficiency or both abnormalities. *British Journal of Haematology,* 10:171–180.

73. BERNSTEIN, R. E. (1963) Glucose-6-phosphate dehydrogenase deficiency in the Rhodesian Bantu. *South African Journal of Medical Sciences,* 28:111–112.

74. BERNSTEIN, R. E. (1963) Occurrence and clinical implications of red-cell glucose-6-phosphate dehydrogenase deficiency in South African racial groups. *South African Medical Journal,* 37:447–451.

74a. BERTRAUD, E., BAUDIN, L., CLERC, M., and VACHER, P. (1965) A propos de 220 recherches systématiques des hémoglobines anormales à Abidjan. *Médecine Tropicale,* 25:577–582.

75. BEST, W. R. (1959) Absence of erythrocyte G6PDD in certain Peruvian Indians. *Journal of Laboratory and Clinical Medicine,* 54:791.

76. BEST, W. R., LAYRISSE, M., and BERMEJO, R. (1962) Blood group antigens in Aymara and Quechua speaking tribes from near Puno, Peru. *American Journal of Physical Anthropology,* 20:321–329.

77. BETKE, K. and KLEIHAUER, E. (1958) Fetaler und bleibender Blutfarbstoff in Erythrozyten und Erythroblasten von menschlichen Feten und Neugeborenen. *Blut,* 4:241.

78. BETKE, K. and KLEIHAUER, E. (1962) Hämoglobinanomalien in der deutschen Bevölkerung. *Schweizerische Medizinische Wochenschrift,* 92: 1316–1318.

79. BEUTLER, E. (1957) The glutathione instability of drug-sensitive red cells. A new method for the in Vitro detection of drug sensitivity. *Journal of Laboratory and Clinical Medicine,* 49:84–95.

80. BEUTLER, E. (1959) The hemolytic effect of primaquine and related compounds: a review. *Blood,* 14:103–139.

81. BEUTLER, E., DERN, R. J., and FLANAGAN, C. L. (1955) Effect of sickle-cell trait on resistance to malaria. *British Medical Journal,* 1:1189–1191.

82. BEUTLER, E., YEH, M. K. Y., and NECHELES, T. (1959) Incidence of the erythrocytic defect associated with drug sensitivity among Oriental subjects. *Nature,* 183:684–685.

83. BEZON, A. (1955) Proportion de sicklémiques observée en pays Kabré (Togo). *Mêdecine Tropicale,* 15:419–422.

84. BEZON, A. (1955) A propos d'une éventuelle résistance des sicklémiques á l'endémie palustre á "Pl. falciparum". *Mêdecine Tropicale,* 15: 422–427.

85. BHATIA, M. M., THIN, J., DEBRAY, H., and CABANES, J. (1955) Étude anthropologique et génétique de la population du Nord de l'Inde. *Bulletins et Mêmoires de la Sociêtê d'Anthropologie de Paris,* 10e Série, 6:199–213.

86. BHATTACHARJEE, P. N. (1956) A genetic survey in the Rārhi Brahmin and the Muslim of West Bengal: A_1-A_2-B-O, M-N, Rh blood groups, ABH secretion, sickle cell, P.T.C. taste, middle phalangeal hair, and colour blindness. *Bulletin of the Department of Anthropology of the Government of India,* 5:18–26.

87. BIANCO, I., MODIANO, G., BOTTINI, E., and LUCCI, R. (1963) Alteration in the α-chain of haemoglobin $L_{Ferrara}$. *Nature,* 198:395–396.

87a. BIDEAU, J. and COURMES, E. (1965) Enquête sur la fréquence des hémoglobines anormales observées chez les Guadeloupéens. *Journal de Médecine de Bordeaux et du Sud-Ouest,* 142:961–966.

87b. BINI, L., TANNOIA, N., PESCE, M., and FATONE, A. (1966) Frequency and meaning of some red blood cells and haemoglobin abnormalities in a sample of the population from Apulia (South Eastern Italy). *Blut,* 13:305–315.

88. BIRD, G. W. G., IKIN, E. W., MOURANT, A. E., and LEHMANN, H. (1962) The blood groups and haemoglobin of the Malayalis. In T. N. Madan and G. Sarana (eds.), *Essays in Memory of D. N. Majumdar.* Asia Publishing House, New York. Pp. 221–226.

89. BIRD, G. W. G., JAYARAM, T. K., IKIN, E. W., MOURANT, A. E., and LEHMAN, H. (1957) The blood groups and haemoglobin of the Gorkhas of Nepal. *American Journal of Physical Anthropology,* 15:163–169.

90. BIRD, G. W. G. and LEHMANN, H. (1956) Haemoglobin D in India. *British Medical Journal,* 1:514.

90a. BLACKWELL, R. Q., BLACKWELL, B-N., HUANG, J. T-H., CHIEN, L-C., SAMAHARN, A., THEPHUSDIN, C., and BORVORNSIN, C. (1965) Hemoglobin J_{Korat} in Thais. *Science,* 150:1614–1615.

91. BLACKWELL, R. Q., BLACKWELL, B-N., HUANG, J. T-H., and THEPHUSDIN, C. (1965) Haemoglobin J and E in a Thai kindred. *Nature,* 207:767–768.

91a. BLACKWELL, R. Q., DE LA FUENTE, V., FLORENTINO, R. F., ALEJO, L. G., HUANG, J. T-H., and CHIEN, L.-C. (1965) Preliminary report on abnormal hemoglobins in Filipinos. *Journal of the Philippine Medical Association,* 41:703–706.

92. BLACKWELL, R. Q. and HUANG, J. T-H. (1963) Abnormal hemoglobin studies in Taiwan aborigines. *Science,* 139:771–772.

93. BLACKWELL, R. Q., HUANG, J. T-H., and CHIEN, L-C. (1964) Distribution of abnormal hemoglobins among normal Chinese residents of Taiwan. U.S. Naval Medical Research Unit No. 2, *Research Report MR005. 09-1601.7.9.*

94. BLACKWELL, R. Q., HUANG, J. T-H., and CHIEN, L-C. (1965) Haemoglobin E in Vietnamese. *Nature,* 207:768.

94a. BLACKWELL, R. Q., HUANG, J. T-H., and CHIEN, L-C. (1965) Abnormal hemoglobin characteristics of Taiwan Aborigines. *Human Biology,* 37:343–356.

94b. BLANKSMA, L. A. and BREEN, M. (1966) Diagnosis of sickle cell diseases by Microzone electrophoresis system. *The Analyzer,* 7, No. 3, 11–13.

95. BLAQUIÈRE, N. J. (1958) Étude systématique de la répartition de la sicklémie et étude clinique de la sicklanémie en Guinée française. Unpublished thesis, Université de Bordeaux.

96. BLOCH, M. and GAVIDIA, R. (1958) Hemoglobinas anormales. Estudio de una muestra de la población Salvadoreña. *Archivos del Colegio Médico de El Salvador,* 11:89–94.

97. BLUMBERG, B. S., ALLISON, A. C., and GARRY, B. (1959) The haptoglobins and haemoglobins of Alaskan Eskimos and Indians. *Annals of Human Genetics,* 23:349–356.

98. BODMER, W. F. and PARSONS, P. A. (1960) The initial progress of new genes with various genetic systems. *Heredity,* 15:283–299.

99. BOLTON, J. P., HARRISON, B. D. W. and LEHMANN, H. (1964) Abnormal haemoglobins in a small group of tribesmen from Northwest Pakistan. *Man,* 64:134.

99a. BONNÉ, B. (1966) Genes and phenotypes in the Samaritan isolate. *American Journal of Physical Anthropology,* 24:1–19.

99b. BOOKCHIN, R. M., NAGEL, R. L., RANNEY, H. M., and JACOBS, A. S. (1966) Hemoglobin C_{Harlem}: A sickling variant containing amino acid substitutions in two residues of the β-polypeptide chain. *Biochemical and Biophysical Research Communications,* 23:122–127.

100. BORIES, S. (1959) Étude des groupes sanguins ABO, MN, des types Rh, des antigenes Kell et Duffy et de la sicklémie chez les Tahitiens. *Sang,* 30:237–244.

101. BOTURÃO, E. (1952) Incidência de drepanocitóse na Santa Casa de Santos. *Seara Médica,* 6:447–449.

102. BOTURÃO, E. and BOTURÃO, E. (1947) Doença por hematias foiciformes (sickle-cell disease). Incidência na Santa Casa de Santos-observações clínicas e haematológicas. *O Hospital (Rio de Janeiro),* 32:709–728.

102a. BOWMAN, J. E., BREWER, G. J., FRISCHER, H., CARTER, J. L., EISENSTEIN, R. B., and BAYRAKCI, C. (1965) A re-evaluation of the relationship between glucose-6-phosphate dehydrogenase deficiency and the behavorial manifestations of schizophrenia. *Journal of Laboratory and Clinical Medicine,* 65:222–227.

103. BOWMAN, J. E. and WALKER, D. G. (1961) Virtual absence of glutathione instability of the erythrocytes among Armenians in Iran. *Nature,* 191:221–222.

104. Boyer, S. H., Porter, I. H., and Weilbacher, R. G. (1962) Electrophoretic heterogeneity of glucose-6-phosphate dehydrogenase and its relationship to enzymic deficiency in man. *Proceedings of the National Academy of Sciences*, 48:1868–1876.

105. Boyer, S. H., Rucknagel, D. L., Weatherall, D. J., and Watson-Williams, E. J. (1963) Further evidence for linkage between the β and δ loci governing human hemoglobin and the population dynamics of linked genes. *American Journal of Human Genetics*, 15:438–448.

106. Boyo, A. E. (1963) Starch gel electrophoresis of the haemoglobin of Nigerian schoolchildren—a preliminary investigation of the incidence of thalassaemia. *West African Medical Journal*, 12:75–81.

107. Boyo, A. E. and Hendrickse, R. G. (1959) New fast abnormal haemoglobin in newborn Nigerians. *Nature*, 184:997–998.

108. Bradley, T. B., Brawner, J. N., and Conley, C. L. (1961) Further observations on an inherited anomaly characterized by persistence of fetal hemoglobin. *Bulletin of the Johns Hopkins Hospital*, 108:242–257.

109. Brain, P. (1953) The sickle-cell trait. A study of its distribution and effects in some Bantu tribes of South Central Africa. Unpublished thesis, University of Capetown.

110. Brain, P. (1953) The sickle-cell trait: a possible mode of introduction into Africa. *Man*, 53:233.

111. Brain, P. and Lehmann, H. (1955) Incidence of haemoglobin C in the "Coloured" population of Capetown. *Nature*, 175:262–263.

112. Brancati, C. (1962) Diffusione e frequenza della microcitemia e delle anemie microcitemiche in Calabria. *Atti delle Giornate di Studio su "Il Problema Sociale della Microcitemia e del Morbo di Cooley."* Istituto Italiano di Medicina Sociale, Roma. 1:64–77.

113. Brancati, C. and Puccetti, G. (1964) Microcitemie ed emoglobine abnormi in Calabria. *Il Progresso Medico*, 20:635–644.

114. Brandau, G. M. (1932) Sickle-cell anemia. Report of a case. *Archives of Internal Medicine*, 50:635–644.

115. Braunitzer, G., Hilse, K., Rudloff, V., and Hilschmann, N. (1964) The hemoglobins. *Advances in Protein Chemistry*, 19:1–71.

115a. Bray, R. S. (1958) Studies on malaria in chimpanzees. VI. *Lavarania falciparum*. *American Journal of Tropical Medicine and Hygiene*, 7:20–24.

116. Brew, D. St.J. and Edington, G. M. (1965) Haemoglobins S and C in post mortem material in Ibadan, Nigeria. In J. H. P. Jonxis (Ed.), *Abnormal Haemoglobins in Africa*. F. A. Davis, Philadelphia. Pp. 213–231.

117. Brewer, G. J. (1966) Unpublished observations.

117a. Brewer, G. J., Tarlov, A. R., and Alving, A. S. (1960) Met haemoglobin reduction test: a new, simple, in vitro test for identifying primaquine-sensitivity. *Bulletin of the World Health Organization*, 22:633–640.

118. Bronte-Stewart, B., Budtz-Olsen, O. E., Hickley, J. M., and Brock, J. F. (1960) The health and nutritional status of the Kung Bushmen of Southwest Africa. *South African Journal of Laboratory and Clinical Medicine*, 6:187–216.

118a. Bruce-Chwatt, L. J. (1965) Paleogenesis and paleo-epidemiology of primate malaria. *Bulletin of the World Health Organization*, 32:363–387.

118b. Brumpt, L. C. and Brumpt, V. (1958) Resistance au paludisme et hémoglobines anormales (en particulier hémoglobine E). *Bulletin de la Société de Pathologie Exotique*, 51:217–224.

119. BRUMPT, L., BRUMPT, V., COQUELET, M. L., and DETRAVERSE, P. M. (1958) La détection de l'hémoglobine E (Étude des populations Cambodgiennes). *Revue d'Hématologie*, 13:21–30.

120. BRUMPT, L., DETRAVERSE, P., BRUMPT, V., and COQUELET, M. (1957) L'hémoglobine E des Cambodgiens et ses conséquences. *Comptes Rendus des Séances de l'Académie des Sciences, Paris*, 244:496–499.

120a. BRUNETTI, P., PARMA, A., NENCI, G., MIGLIORINI, E., and BRUNELLI, B. (1965) Incidenza del difetto di G-6PD nell' Italia Centrale. *Haematologica*, 50:203–219.

121. BRYSON, V. and VOGEL, H. J. (1965) *Evolving Genes and Proteins*. Academic Press, New York.

122. BUCHI, E. C. (1955) Is sickling a Weddid trait? *The Anthropologist*, 1:25–29.

123. BUCHI, E. C. (1955) Blood, secretion, and taste among the Pallar, a South Indian community. *The Anthropologist*, 2: No. 1:1–8.

124. BUCHI, E. C. (1955) A genetic survey among the Malapantaram, a hill tribe of Travancore. *The Anthropologist*, 2: No. 2:1–11.

125. BUCHI, E. C. (1959) Blut, Geschmack, und Farbensinn bei den Kurumba (Nilgiri, Südindien). *Archiv für Julius Klaus-Stiftung*, 34:310–316.

125a. BUCKLE, A. E. R., HANNING, L., and HOLMAN, C. A. (1964) Routine haemoglobin electrophoresis in at-risk gravid women. *Journal of Obstetrics and Gynaecology of the British Commonwealth*, 71:923–926.

126. BUDTZ-OLSEN, O. E. (1958) Haptoglobins and haemoglobins in Australian Aborigines, with a simple method for the estimation of haptoglobins. *Medical Journal of Australia*, 2:689–693.

127. BUDTZ-OLSEN, O. E. and BURGERS, A. C. J. (1955) The sickle-cell trait in the South African Bantu. *South African Medical Journal*, 29:109–110.

128. BUDTZ-OLSEN, O. and KIDSON, C. (1961) Absence of red cell enzyme deficiency in Australian Aborigines. *Nature*, 192:765.

129. BUETTNER-JANUSCH, J. (1965) Unpublished observations.

130. BUETTNER-JANUSCH, J., BOVE, J. R., and YOUNG, N. (1964) Genetic traits and problems of biological parenthood in two Peruvian Indian tribes. *American Journal of Physical Anthropology*, 22:149–154.

131. BUETTNER-JANUSCH, J. and BUETTNER-JANUSCH, V. (1964) Hemoglobins, haptoglobins, and transferrins in the peoples of Madagascar. *American Journal of Physical Anthropology*, 22:163–169.

132. BUNI, S. (1964) Sickle cell disease in Basra (Iraq). *Journal of the Iraqi Medical Professions*, 12:25–29.

133. BURKA, E. R. and MARKS, P. A. (1963) Ribosomes active in protein synthesis in human reticulocytes: a defect in thalassaemia major. *Nature*, 199:706–707.

134. BURKE, J., DEBOCK, G., and DEWULF, O. (1958) La drépanocytémie simple et l'anémie drépanocytaire au Kwango (Congo belge). *Académie royale des Sciences coloniales, Bruxelles, Mémoires in-8°*, Nouvelle Série, Tome VII, fasc. 3.

134a. BUXTON, P. A. (1927) Researches in Polynesia and Melanesia. *Memoir No. 1, London School of Hygiene and Tropical Medicine*.

135. CABANNES, R. (1960) The distribution of abnormal haemoglobins in Algeria, the Hoggar, and High Volta: Anthropological incidences. *Journal of the Royal Anthropological Institute of Great Britain and Ireland*, 90:306–319.

136. Cabannes, R. (1960) La hemoglobina C. Distribución en el Norte y Oeste de Africa. Incidencias antropológicas. *Sangre*, 5:51–66.
137. Cabannes, R. (1962) Étude des types hémoglobiniques rencontrés dans les populations de la partie occidentale du continent Africain. Unpublished thesis, Université de Toulouse.
138. Cabannes, R. J. (1962) Distribuzione, frequenza, ed importanza delle emopatie ereditarie in Algeria. *Atti delle Giornate di Studio su "Il Problema Sociale della Microcitemia e del Morbo di Cooley."* Istituto Italiano di Medicina Sociale, Roma. 1:116–129.
139. Cabannes, R. (1965) Répartition des hémoglobines anormales dans la partie ouest du continent africain. In J. H. P. Jonxis (Ed.), *Abnormal Haemoglobins in Africa*. F. A. Davis, Philadelphia. Pp. 291–317.
140. Cabannes, R., Beurrier, A., and Larrouy, G. (1965) La thalassémie chez les indiens de Guyane Française. *Nouvelle Revue Française d'Hématologie*, 5:617–630.
141. Cabannes, R. and Ruffie, J. (1961) Les hémoglobinoses dans le bassin méditerranéen. *Toulouse Médical*, 62:955–984.
142. Cabannes, R. and Ruffie, J. (1961) Les types hémoglobiniques des populations indigenes du Tibesti. *Comptes Rendus de la Société de Biologie de Paris*, 155:2449–2451.
143. Cabannes, R. and Ruffie, J. (1961) Les types hémoglobiniques dans les populations des massifs montagneux du Sahara central (Hoggar et Tibesti). *L'Anthropologie*, 65:467–483.
144. Cabannes, R., Ruffie, J., Larrouy, G., and Beurrier, A. (1963) Les hémoglobines anormales dans la population Indienne de Guyane Française. *Proceedings of the 9th Congress of the European Society of Haematology* (Lisbon, 1963). S. Karger, New York. Pp. 551–558.
144a. Cabannes, R., Taleb, N., Ghorra, F., and Schmitt-Beurrier, A. (1965) Étude des types hémoglobiniques dans la population du Liban. *Nouvelle Revue Française d'Hématologie*, 5:851–856.
145. Calero, C. M. (1946) Drepanocitemia y anemia drepanocitica en el istmo Panamá. *Archivos del Hospital Santo Tomas*, 1: No. 2:27–35.
146. Cannon, D. S. H. (1958) Malaria and prematurity in the Western Region of Nigeria. *British Medical Journal*, 2:877–878.
147. Capps, F. P. A., Gilles, H. M., Jolly, H., and Worlledge, S. M. (1963) Glucose-6-phosphate dehydrogenase deficiency and neonatal jaundice in Nigeria. *Lancet*, 2:379–383.
148. Carbonell, L. M. and Aleman, C. A. (1951) Investigaciónes de la drepanocitemia entre los indios de la Sierra de Perijá. *Gaceta Médica de Caracas*, 59:2–9.
149. Carcassi, U. (1962) Frequenza della microcitemia e del morbo di Cooley in Sardegna. *Atti delle Giornate di Studio su "Il Problema Sociale della Microcitemia e del Morbo Cooley."* Istituto Italiano di Medicina Sociale, Roma. 1:78–97.
150. Cardozo, W. W. (1957) Immunologic studies of sickle cell anemia. *Archives of Internal Medicine*, 60:623–653.
150a. Carrell, R. W., Lehmann, H. and Hutchison, H. E. (1966) Haemoglobin Köln (β 98 Valine→Methionine): an unstable protein causing inclusion-body anaemia. *Nature*, 210:915–917.
151. Carson, P. E., Flanagan, C. L., Ickes, C. E., and Alving, A. S. (1956) Enzymatic deficiency in primaquine-sensitive erythrocytes. *Science*, 124:484–485.

151a. CASSAR, P. (1964) *Medical History of Malta.* Wellcome History of Medicine Library, London.

152. CAVALIERI, S. and GAROFALO, E. (1962) La microcitemia nel veronese. Nota II. Frequenza e distribuzione geografica. *Fracastoro,* 55:349–359.

152a. CAVALLI-SFORZA, L. L. (1966) Personal communication.

153. CHABEUF, M. and ZELDINE, G. (1962) Groupes sanguins et drépanocytose dans l'île de Sainte Marie (Madagascar). *Médecine Tropicale,* 22: 261–267.

153a. CHAN, A. C., JONGCO, A., and MENDOZA, R. R. (1965) G-6-P D deficiency as a cause of jaundice in the newborn period (preliminary report). *Philippine Journal of Pediatrics,* 14:405–410.

154. CHAN, T. K., TODD, D., and WONG, C. C. (1964) Erythrocyte glucose-6-phosphate dehydrogenase deficiency in Chinese. *British Medical Journal,* 2:102.

155. CHARLES, L. J. (1960) Observations on the haemolytic effect of primaquine in 100 Ghanaian children. *Annals of Tropical Medicine and Parasitology,* 54:460–470.

156. CHARLTON, R. W. and BOTHWELL, T. H. (1961) Primaquine-sensitivity of red cells in various races in Southern Africa. *British Medical Journal,* 1:941–944.

157. CHATTERJEA, J. B. (1959) Haemoglobinopathy in India. In J. H. P. Jonxis and J. L. Delafresnaye (Eds.), *Abnormal Haemoglobins.* C. C. Thomas. Springfield, Ill. Pp. 322–339.

158. CHAUDHURI, S., CHAKRAVARTTI, M. R., MUKHERJEE, B., SEN, S. N., GHOSH, J., and MAITRA, A. (1964) Study of haematological factors, blood groups, anthropometric measurements and genetics of some of the tribal and caste groups of: 1. South India—Kerala, Nilgiris, and Andhra Pradesh. 2. North Eastern India (Indo-Bhutan border)—Totopara. *Proceedings of the 9th Congress of the International Society of Blood Transfusion* (Mexico, 1962) S. Karger, New York. Pp. 196–205.

159. CHAUDHURI, S., GHOSH, J., and MUKHERJEE, B. (1964) Study of haemoglobin variants and blood groups in Santal tribe of Midnapore District of West Bengal, India. *Abstracts of the 10th Congress of the International Society of Haematology* (Stockholm, 1964), L:11.

160. CHAUDHURI, S., SEN, S. N., MUKHERJEE, B., and GHOSH, J. (1963) Haematological field survey in Anglo-Indian community of Kharagpore, W. Bengal. *Journal of the Association of Physicians of India,* 11:955–960.

161. CHEDIAK, M., CALDERÓN, J. C. and VARGAS, G. P. (1939) Anemia á hématies falciformes. Contribución a su estudio en Cuba. *Archivos de Medicina Interna,* 5:313–370.

162. CHERNOFF, A. I. (1956) On the prevalence of hemoglobin D in the American Negro. *Blood,* 11:907–909.

163. CHERNOFF, A. I. (1959) The distribution of the thalassemia gene: an historical review. *Blood,* 14:899–912.

163a. CHERNOFF, A. I. (1964) Hgb A_4, a naturally occurring hemoglobin possessing only α chains. *Journal of Clinical Investigations,* 43:1266.

164. CHERNOFF, A. I., MINNICH, V., NA-NAKORN, S., TUCHINDA, S., KASHEMSANT, C., and CHERNOFF, R. R. (1956) Studies on hemoglobin E. I. The clinical, hematologic, and genetic characteristics of the hemoglobin E syndromes. *Journal of Laboratory and Clinical Medicine,* 47:455–489.

165. CHERNOFF, A. I. and PETTIT, N. M. (1964) The amino acid composition of hemoglobin. III. A qualitative method for identifying abnormalities of the polypeptide chains of hemoglobin. *Blood,* 24:750–756.

166. CHERNOFF, A. I. and WEICHSELBAUM, T. E. (1958) A microhemolyzing technic for preparing solutions of hemoglobin for paper electrophoretic analysis. *American Journal of Clinical Pathology,* 30:120–125.

167. CHERRIE, A. L. (1963) The sickling phenomenon in a college population. *Journal of the National Medical Association,* 55:142–147.

168. CHILDS, B. and ZINKHAM, W. H. (1959) The genetics of primaquine sensitivity of the erythrocytes. *CIBA Foundation Symposium on Biochemistry of Human Genetics.* Little, Brown, Boston. Pp. 76–95.

169. CHILDS, ST. J. R. (1940) *Malaria and the Colonization of the Carolina Low Country 1526–1696.* The Johns Hopkins Press, Baltimore.

170. CHIN, W., CONTACOS, P. G., COATNEY, G. R., and KIMBALL, H. R. (1965) A naturally acquired quotidian-type malaria in man transferable to monkeys. *Science,* 149:865.

171. CHOREMIS, C., FESSAS, P., KATTAMIS, C., STAMATOYANNOPOULOS, G., ZANNOS-MARIOLEA, L., KARAKLIS, A., and BELIOS, G. (1963) Three inherited red cell abnormalities in a district of Greece. *Lancet,* 1:907–909.

172. CHOREMIS, C., IKIN, E. W., MOURANT, A. E., LEHMAN, H., and ZANNOS, L. (1957) Blood groups of a Greek community with a high sickling frequency. *Lancet,* 2:1333–1334.

172a. CHOREMIS, C., KATTAMIS, CH. A., KYRIAZAKOU, M., and GAVRIILIDOU, E. (1966) Viral hepatitis in G.-6-P.D. deficiency. *Lancet,* 1:269–270.

173. CHOREMIS, C., ZANNOS-MARIOLEA, L., and KATTAMIS, M. D. C. (1962) Frequency of glucose-6-phosphate dehydrogenase deficiency in certain highly malarious areas of Greece. *Lancet,* 1:17–18.

174. CHUNG, A. E. and LANGDON, R. G. (1963) Human erythrocyte glucose-6-phosphate dehydrogenase. *Journal of Biological Chemistry,* 238:2309–2324.

175. CLEGG, J. B., NAUGHTON, M. A., and WEATHERALL, D. J. (1965) An improved method for the characterization of human haemoglobin mutants: identification of $\alpha_2\beta_2^{95glu}$, haemoglobin N (Baltimore). *Nature,* 207:945–947.

176. CLYDE, D. F. and EMANUEL, E. (1965) Malaria distribution in Tanganyika. Part V. The North. *East African Medical Journal,* 42:438–446.

177. COLBOURNE, M. J. and EDINGTON, G. M. (1956) Sickling and malaria in the Gold Coast. *British Medical Journal,* 1:784–787.

178. COLBOURNE, M. J., EDINGTON, G. M., and HUGHES, M. H. (1950) A medical survey in a Gold Coast village. *Transactions of the Royal Society of Tropical Medicine and Hygiene,* 44:271–296.

179. COLBOURNE, M. J., IKIN, E. W., MOURANT, A. E., LEHMANN, H., and THEIN, H. (1958) Haemoglobin E and the Diego blood group antigen in Sarawak and Burma. *Nature,* 181:119–120.

180. COLLET, A. (1958) Recherche des hémoglobines chez les lépreux. *Archives de l'Institut Pasteur de Martinique,* 11:16.

181. COLLIER, W. A. and DE LA PARRA, D. A. (1952) Sickle-cell trait in Surinam Creoles. *Tropical and Geographical Medicine,* 4:223–225.

182. CONARD, R. A., MEYER, L. M., SUTOW, W. M., MOLONEY, W. C., LOWREY, A., HICKING, A., and RIKLON, E. (1963) Medical Survey of Rongelap People Eight Years After Exposure to Fallout. Brookhaven

National Laboratory, U.S. Atomic Energy Commission, *BNL 780 (T-296)*.

183. CONLEY, C. L., WEATHERALL, D. J., RICHARDSON, S. N., SHEPARD, M. K., and CHARACHE, S. (1963) Hereditary persistence of fetal hemoglobin; A study of 79 affected persons in 15 Negro families in Baltimore. *Blood,* 21:261–281.

183a. CONTACOS, P. G. and COATNEY, G. R. (1963) Experimental adaptation of simian malarias to abnormal hosts. *Journal of Parasitology,* 49:912–918.

184. COOLEY, T. B. and LEE, P. (1925) Series of cases of splenomegaly in children with anemia and peculiar bone changes. *Transactions of the American Pediatric Society,* 37:29–30.

185. COOLEY, T. B. and LEE, P. (1926) The sickle cell phenomenon. *American Journal of Diseases of Childhood,* 32:334–340.

186. COOPER, A. J., BLUMBERG, B. S., WORKMAN, P. L., and MCDONOUGH, J. R. (1963) Biochemical polymorphic traits in a U.S. white and Negro population. *American Journal of Human Genetics,* 15:420–428.

187. CORRAL, J. F. and UNANUE, E. R. (1960) Survey sobre hemoglobinas en la raza negra en Cuba. *Revista Cubana de Laboratorio Clinico,* 14:57–59.

188. CORDEIRO FERREIRA, N. (1963) Talassémia—Contribuição para o estudo da sua heterogeneidade bioquímica em Portugal. *Anais do Instituto de Medicina Tropical, Lisboa,* 20:175–312.

188a. COTTER, J. and PRYSTOWSKY, H. (1963) Routine hemoglobin electrophoresis in Negro gravidas. *Obstetrics and Gynecology,* 22:610–611.

189. COULTER, W. W. (1965) Incidence of hemoglobin "C" trait in tuberculous Negroes. *Journal of the Louisiana Medical Society,* 117:242–244.

190. CRESTA, M. (1964) Antropologia morfologica e sierologica dei N'Zakara della Repubblica Centroafricana. *La Ricerca Scientifica,* 34, Rendiconti B. serie 2, 4:131–142.

190a. CROOKSTON, J. H., BEALE, D., IRVINE, D., and LEHMANN, H. (1965) A new haemoglobin, J Toronto (α 5 Alanine → Aspartic Acid). *Nature,* 208: 1059–1061.

191. CROSBY, W. H. (1956) Newsletter—Favism in Sardinia. *Blood,* 11:91–92.

192. CRUZ-HERNANDEZ, M. (1962) La thalassemia maior in Spagna. *Atti delle Giornate di Studio su "Il Problema Sociale della Microcitemia e del Morbo di Cooley."* Istituto Italiano di Medicina Sociale, Roma. 1:200–207.

193. CURTAIN, C. C. (1964) A structural study of abnormal haemoglobins occurring in New Guinea. *Australian Journal of Experimental Biology and Medical Science,* 42:89–97.

194. CURTAIN, C. C., GAJDUSEK, D. C., and ZIGAS, V. (1961) Studies on kuru. II. Serum proteins in natives from the kuru region of New Guinea. *American Journal of Tropical Medicine and Hygiene,* 10:92–109.

195. CURTAIN, C. C., KIDSON, C., GAJDUSEK, D. C., and GORMAN, J. G. (1962) Distribution pattern, population genetics and anthropological significance of thalassemia and abnormal hemoglobins in Melanesia. *American Journal of Physical Anthropology,* 20:475–483.

196. DAS, S. R., MUKHERJEE, D. P., and SASTRY, D. B. (1967) Sickle-cell trait in Koraput District and other parts of India. *Acta Genetica et Statistica Medica,* 17:62–73.

197. DAS, S. R., KUMAR, N., BHATACHARJEE, P. N., and SASTRY, D. B. (1961) Blood groups (ABO, M-N, and Rh), ABH secretion, sickle-cell, P.T.C. taste, and colour blindness in the Mahar of Nagpur. *Journal of the*

Royal Anthropological Institute of Great Britain and Ireland, 91:345–355.

198. DasGupta, C. R., Chatterjea, J. B., Ray, R. N., Ghosh, S. K., and Choudhury, A. B. (1958) Observations on Cooley's anemia (thalassemia). *Proceedings of the 6th International Congress of the International Society of Hematology* (Boston, 1956). Grune and Stratton, New York. Pp. 733–742.

199. Delbrouck, J. (1958) Contribution à la génétique de la sicklémie. Maintein de la fréquence élevée de sicklémie au Congo belge. *Annales de la Société Belge de Médecine Tropicale,* 38:103–133.

200. Deliyannis, G. A. and Tavlarakis, N. (1955) Sickling phenomenon in Northern Greece. *British Medical Journal,* 2:229–301.

201. Deliyannis, G. A. and Tavlarakis, N. (1955) Compatibility of sickling with malaria. *British Medical Journal,* 2:301–303.

201a. Dern, R. J., Glynn, M. F., and Brewer, G. J. (1963) Studies on the correlation of the genetically determined trait, glucose-6-phosphate dehydrogenase deficiency, with behavioral manifestations in schizophrenia. *Journal of Laboratory and Clinical Medicine,* 62:319–329.

202. DeSilva, C. C. (1957) Abnormal haemoglobins and haemoglobinopathies. *Journal of the Lady Ridgeway Hospital for Children* (Colombo, Ceylon), 1:16–32.

203. DeSilva, C. C., Bulugahapitiza, D. T. D., DeSilva, J., Wickremasinghe, R. L., and Jonxis, J. H. P. (1962) Sinhalese family with haemoglobin S. *British Medical Journal,* 1:1519–1521.

204. Dherte, P., Lehmann, H., and Vandepitte, J. (1959) Haemoglobin P in a family in the Belgian Congo. *Nature,* 184:1133–1135.

205. Didier, R. and Diacono, G. (1956) Enquête sur la sicklémie en Tunisie. *Archives de l'Institut Pasteur de Tunis,* 33:61–64.

206. Diggs, L. W., Ahmann, C. F., and Bibb, J. (1933) Incidence and significance of the sickle-cell trait. *Annals of Internal Medicine,* 7:769–777.

207. Dimitrow, St. and Nineu, Sch. (1962) Beitrag zur anämie Cooley. *Proceedings of the 8th Congress of the European Society of Haematology* (Vienna, 1961). S. Karger, New York. Part II, No. 310.

208. Dodin, A. (1965) Déficit en glucose-6-phosphate déshydrogénase. Premières recherches à Madagascar. *Archives de l'Institut Pasteur de Madagascar,* 33:233–240.

209. Doehnert, H. R. (1957) Consideraciones sobre la patologia de la drepanocitosis. *Acta Cientifica Venezolana,* 8:26–60.

210. Dolgopol, V. B. and Stitt, R. H. (1929) Sickle-cell phenomenon in tuberculosis patients. *American Review of Tuberculosis,* 19:454–460.

211. Douglas, R., Jacobs, J., Greenhough, R., and Staveley, J. M. (1964) Blood groups, serum genetic factors, and hemoglobins in New Hebrides Islanders. *Transfusion,* 4:177–184.

212. Douglas, R., Jacobs, J., Hoult, G. E., and Staveley, J. M. (1962) Blood groups, serum genetic factors, and hemoglobins in Western Solomon Islanders. *Transfusion* 2:413–418.

213. Douglas, R., Jacobs, J., Sherliker, J., and Staveley, J. M. (1961) Blood groups, serum genetic factors, and haemoglobins in Gilbert Islanders. *New Zealand Medical Journal,* 60:146–152.

214. Douglas, R., Jacobs, J. Sherliker, J., and Staveley, J. M. (1961) Blood groups, serum genetic factors and haemoglobins in Ellice Islanders. *New Zealand Medical Journal,* 60:259–261.

214a. Douglas, R., McCarthy, D. D., Staveley, J. M., and Jacobs, J. (1966)

Blood group, serum genetic factors, and hemoglobins in Cook Islanders. I. Aitu Island. II. Rarotonga. *Transfusion*, 6:319–326.

215. Douglas, R. and Stavely, J. M. (1959) The blood groups of Cook Islanders. *Journal of the Polynesian Society*, 68:14–20.

216. Doxiadis, S. A., Vales, T., Karaklis, A., and Stavrakakis, D. (1964) Risk of severe jaundice in glucose-6-phosphate dehydrogenase deficiency of the newborn. Differences in population groups. *Lancet*, 2:1210–1212.

217. Draper, C. C. and Smith, A. (1957) Malaria in the Pare area of N.E. Tanganyika. *Transactions of the Royal Society of Tropical Medicine and Hygiene*, 51:137–151.

218. Dresbach, M. (1904) Elliptical human red corpuscles. *Science*, 19:469–470.

219. Dreyfus, J-C., Maleknia, N., and Kaplan, J-C. (1964) Recherches sur le déficit en glucose-6-phosphate déshydrogénase en France. A propos de 200 dosages. *Nouvelle Revue Française d'Hématologie*, 4:791–802.

220. Dreyfuss, F. and Benyesch, M. (1952) Sickle-cell trait in Arabs. *Lancet*, 1:1213.

221. Dreyfuss, F., Ikin, E., Lehmann, H., and Mourant, A. E. (1952) An investigation of blood-groups and a search for sickle-cell trait in Yemenite Jews. *Lancet*, 2:1010.

222. Dreyfuss, F. and Pinkhas, J. (1958) Search for abnormal haemoglobins in Oriental Jews. *Lancet*, 2:1180.

223. Du, S-D. (1952) Favism in West China. *Chinese Medical Journal*, 70:17–26.

224. Dube, B., Kumar, S., and Mangalik, V. S. (1959) Absence of abnormal haemoglobins in 235 subjects in Uttar Pradesh. *Indian Journal of Medical Research*, 47:148–149.

224a. Dunn, F. L. (1965) On the antiquity of malaria in the Western Hemisphere. *Human Biology*, 37:385–393.

225. East African Common Services Organization. (1962) *Annual Report of the East African Institute of Malaria and Vector-Borne Diseases*, July 1961–June 1962 (G. Pringle, Director). Kenya Government Printer, Nairobi.

226. Edington, G. M. (1955) The pathology of sickle-cell disease in West Africa. *Transactions of the Royal Society of Tropical Medicine and Hygiene*, 49:253–267.

227. Edington, G. M. (1959) *Annual Report of the Department of Pathology*, University College, Ibadan, Nigeria.

228. Edington, G. M. and Laing, W. N. (1957) Relationship between haemoglobins C and S and malaria in Ghana. *British Medical Journal*, 2:143–145.

229. Edington, G. M. and Lehmann, H. (1954) A case of sickle cell-haemoglobin C disease and a survey of haemoglobin C incidence in West Africa. *Transactions of the Royal Society of Tropical Medicine and Hygiene*, 48:332–335.

230. Edington, G. M. and Lehmann, H. (1956) The distribution of haemoglobin C in West Africa. *Man*, 56:36.

231. Edington, G. M. and Watson-Williams, E. J. (1965) Sickling, haemoglobin C, glucose-6-phosphate dehydrogenase deficiency and malaria in Western Nigeria. In J. H. P. Jonxis (Ed.), *Abnormal Haemoglobins in Africa*. F. A. Davis, Philadelphia. Pp. 393–401.

231a. Edozien, J. C. (1964) Deficiency of glucose-6-phosphate dehydrogenase (G-6-P D) in Nigeria. *Bulletin of the World Health Organization*, 31:417–421.

232. Edozien, J. C. (1965) Deficiency of glucose-6-phosphate dehydrogenase in Nigeria. In J. H. P. Jonxis (Ed.), *Abnormal Haemoglobins in Africa.* F. A. Davis, Philadelphia. Pp. 197–205.

233. Edozien, J. C., Boyo, A. E., and Morley, D. C. (1960) The relationship of serum gamma globulin concentration to malaria and sickling. *Journal of Clinical Pathology,* 13:118–123.

234. Eisen, B. and Abildgaard, C. C. (1960) Hemoglobin electrophoretic patterns and blood groups of San Blas Indians. *Vox Sanguinis,* 5:560–561.

235. El-Dewi, S. and Fahmi, T. (1958) The sickle-cell trait in Egypt. *Journal of the Egyptian Medical Association,* 41:425–432.

236. Ellis, F. R., Cawley, L. P., and Lasker, G. W. (1963) Blood groups, hemoglobin types, and secretion of group-specific substance at Hacienda Cayaltí, North Peru. *Human Biology,* 35:26–52.

237. English, R. B. (1945) Sicklaemia occurring in Africans in Northern Rhodesia. *South African Medical Journal,* 19:431.

238. Erdohazi, M. and Highman, W. J. (1962) Glucose-6-phosphate dehydrogenase deficiency in Britain. *Lancet,* 2:1274.

239. vanErp, Th. (1954) Detection of sickle cells as anthropological method. *Tropical and Geographical Medicine,* 6:278–279.

240. Esrachowitz, S. R., Friedlander, S., Radloff, G., and Saunders, S. (1952) The sickle cell trait in Cape Coloured persons. *South African Medical Journal,* 26:239–240.

241. Etcheverry, R., Guzmán, C., Hille, A., Nagel, R., and Covarrubias, E. (1963) Types of haptoglobins in Araucanian Indians of Chile. *Nature,* 197:187–188.

242. Evans, R. W. (1944) The sickling phenomenon in the blood of West African natives. *Transactions of the Royal Society of Tropical Medicine and Hygiene,* 37:281–286.

242a. Eyles, D. E., Wharton, R. H., Cheong, W. H., and Warren, McW. (1964) Studies on malaria and *Anopheles balabacensis* in Cambodia. *Bulletin of the World Health Organization,* 30:7–21.

242b. Fairbanks, V. F. and Beutler, E. (1962) A simple method for detection of erythrocyte glucose-6-phosphate dehydrogenase deficiency (G-6-P-D spot test). *Blood,* 20:591–601.

243. Feinbrun, N. (1938) New data on some cultivated plants and weeds of the early Bronze Age in Palestine. *Palestine Journal of Botany,* Series J, 1:238–240.

244. Fessas, Ch., Karaklis, A., Loukopoulos, D., Stamatoyannopoulos, G., and Fessas, Ph., (1965) Haemoglobin Nicosia: an α-chain variant and its combination with β-thalassaemia. *British Journal of Haematology,* 11:323–330.

245. Fessas, Ph., Karaklis, A., and Gnafakis, N. (1961) A further abnormality of foetal haemoglobin. *Acta Haematologica,* 25:62–70.

246. Fessas, Ph., Mastrokalos, N., Fostiropoulos, G., Vella, F., Ager, J. A. M., and Lehmann, H. (1959) New variant of human foetal haemoglobin. *Nature,* 183:30–32.

247. Fessas, Ph. and Stamatoyannopoulos, G. (1964) Hereditary persistence of fetal hemoglobin in Greece: a study and a comparison. *Blood,* 24:223–240.

248. Fessas, Ph., Stamatoyannopoulos, G., and Karaklis, A. (1962) Hemoglobin "Pylos": study of a hemoglobinopathy resembling thalassemia in the heterozygous, homozygous, and double heterozygous state. *Blood,* 19:1–22.

249. FINDLAY, C. M., ROBERTSON, W. M., and ZACHARIAS, F. J. (1946) The incidence of sicklaemia in West Africa. *Transactions of the Royal Society of Tropical Medicine and Hygiene,* 40:83–86.

250. FIRSCHEIN, I. L. (1961) Population dynamics of the sickle-cell trait in the Black Caribs of British Honduras, Central America. *American Journal of Human Genetics,* 13:233–254.

251. FLATZ, G., PIK, C., and SRINGAM, S. (1965) Haemoglobinopathies in Thailand II. Incidence and distribution of elevations of haemoglobin A_2 and haemoglobin F; a survey of 2790 people. *British Journal of Haematology,* 11:227–241.

252. FLATZ, G., PIK, C., and SRINGAM, S. (1965) Haemoglobin E and β-thalassaemia: their distribution in Thailand. *Annals of Human Genetics,* 29:151–170.

253. FLATZ, G., PIK, C., and SUNDHARAGIATI, B. (1964) Malaria and haemoglobin E in Thailand. *Lancet,* 2:385–387.

254. FLATZ, G. and SRINGAM, S. (1964) Glucose-6-phosphate dehydrogenase deficiency in different ethnic groups in Thailand. *Annals of Human Genetics,* 27:315–318.

255. FLATZ, G., SRINGAM, S., and KOMKRIS, V. (1963) Negative balancing factors for the glucose-6-phosphate dehydrogenase polymorphism in Thailand. *Acta Genetica et Statistica Medica,* 13:316–327.

256. FLOCH, H. and DELAJUDIE, P. (1944) Sur la méniscocytémie en Guyane Française. *Publications de l'Institut Pasteur de la Guyane,* No. 92.

257. FOY, H., BRASS, W., MOORE, R. A., TIMMS, G. L., KONDI, A., and OLUOCH, T. (1955) Two surveys to investigate the relation of sickle-cell trait and malaria. *British Medical Journal,* 2:1116–1118.

258. FOY, H. and KONDI, A. (1961) Report on incidence, aetiology, treatment and prophylaxis of the anaemias in the Seychelles: a study in iron-deficiency anaemias and ancylostomiasis in the tropics. *Annals of Tropical Medicine and Parasitology,* 55:25–45.

259. FOY, H., KONDI, A., REBELLO, A., and MARTINS, F. (1952) The distribution of sickle-cell trait and the incidence of sickle-cell anaemia in the Negro tribes of Portuguese East Africa. *East Africa Medical Journal,* 29:247–251.

260. FOY, H., KONDI, A., TIMMS, G. L., BRASS, W., and BUSHRA, F. (1954) The variability of sickle-cell rates in tribes of Kenya and the Southern Sudan. *British Medical Journal,* 1:294–297.

261. FRAZER, G. R., DEFARANAS, B., KATTAMIS, C. A., RACE, R. R., SANGER, R., and STAMATOYANNOPOULOS, G. (1964) G-6-P D, colour vision and X_g blood groups in Greece: linkage and population data. *Annals of Human Genetics,* 27:395–403.

261a. FRAZER, G. R., GRUNWALD, P., and STAMATOYANNOPOULOS, G. (1966) Glucose-6-phosphate dehydrogenase (G6PD) deficiency, abnormal haemoglobins and thalassaemia in Yugoslavia. *Journal of Medical Genetics,* 3:35–41.

262. FRAZER, G. R., STAMATOYANNOPOULOS, G., KATTAMIS, C., LOUKOPOULOS, D., DEFARANAS, B., KITSOS, C., ZANNOS-MARIOLEA, L., CHOREMIS, C., FESSAS, P., and MOTULSKY, A. (1964) Thalassemias, abnormal hemoglobins, and glucose-6-phosphate dehydrogenase deficiency in the Arta area of Greece: diagnostic and genetic aspects of complete village studies. *Annals of the New York Academy of Sciences,* 119:415–435.

262a. Freese, E. and Yoshida, A. (1965) The role of mutations in evolution. In V. Bryson and H. J. Vogel (eds.), *Evolving Genes and Proteins*. Academic Press, New York. Pp. 341–355.
263. Fujiki, N., Ohkawara, Y., Yamamoto, M., Fukuda, K., Nishimura, J., Takenaka, S., Ishimaru, H. and Takanashi, T. (1965) Hematological survey in the isolated villages in Japan. *Israel Journal of Medical Sciences*, 1:712–713.
264. Fullerton, W. T., Hendrickse, J. P. deV., and Watson-Williams, E. J. (1965) Haemoglobin SC disease in pregnancy. A review of 190 cases. In J. H. P. Jonxis (ed.), *Abnormal Haemoglobins in Africa*. F. A. Davis, Philadelphia. Pp. 411–433.
265. Furuhjelm, V. and Vuopio, P. (1961) Glucose-6-phosphate dehydrogenase deficiency. *Lancet*, 2:1366.
265a. Gall, J. (1966) Personal communication.
265b. Gallango, M. L. and Arends, T. (1966) Haemoglobin types and blood serum factors in Colombian Indians. *Acta Genetica et Statistica Medica*, 16:162–168.
266. Gamet, A. (1964) Première étude sur les hémoglobinoses au centre-Cameroun. *Bulletin de la Société de Pathologie Exotique*, 57:1125–1133.
267. Gammack, D. B., Huehns, E. R., Lehmann, H., and Shooter, E. M. (1961) The abnormal polypeptide chains in a number of haemoglobin variants. *Acta Genetica et Statistica Medica*, 11:1–16.
268. Garlick, J. P. (1960) Sickling and malaria in South-west Nigeria. *Transactions of the Royal Society of Tropical Medicine and Hygiene*, 54:146–154.
269. Garlick, J. P. and Barnicot, N. A. (1957) Blood groups and haemoglobin variants in Nigerian (Yoruba) schoolchildren. *Annals of Human Genetics*, 21:420–425.
270. Garnham, P. C. C. (1948) The incidence of malaria at high altitudes. *Journal of the National Malaria Society*, 7:275–284.
271. Garnham, P. C. C. (1963) Distribution of simian malaria parasites in various hosts. *Journal of Parasitology*, 49:905–911.
272. Gavarrino, M. (1956) Contribution a l'étude de la sicklémie à Madagascar. *Bulletin de la Société de Pathologie Exotique*, 49:403.
273. Gedda, L. and Romei, L. (1961) Un focolaio di microcitemia nella provincia di Roma. *Acta Geneticae Medicae et Gemellologiae*, 10:265–269.
274. Gelfand, M. (1960) Sickle cell anaemia in an African infant from Northern Rhodesia. *Central African Journal of Medicine*, 6:401–402.
275. Gelpi, A. P. (1965) Glucose-6-phosphate dehydrogenase deficiency in Saudi Arabia: a survey. *Blood*, 25:486–493.
276. Gentilini, M., Laroche, V., and Degremont, A. (1964) Aspects de la pathologie tropicale parasitaire et infectieuse en République d'Haiti. *Bulletin de la Société de Pathologie Exotique*, 57:565–570.
276a. Gerald, P. S. and Diamond, L. K. (1958) The diagnosis of thalassemia trait by starch block electrophoresis of the hemoglobin. *Blood*, 13:61–69.
277. Gessain, R., Ruffié, J., Kane, Y., Kane, O., Cabannes, R., and Gomila, J. (1965) Note sur la séro-anthropologie de trois populations de Guinée et du Sénégal: Coniagui, Bassari, et Bedik. *Bulletins et Mémoires de la Société d'Anthropologie de Paris*, 11e série, 8:5–18.

278. Giblett, E. R. and Best, W. R. (1961) Haptoglobin and transferrin types in Peruvian Indians. *Nature*, 192:1300–1301.

279. Gibson, F. D. (1958) Malaria parasite survey of some areas in the Southern Cameroons under United Kingdom Administration. *West African Medical Journal*, 7:170–178.

280. Giles, E. (1962) Favism, sex-linkage, and the Indo-European kinship system. *Southwestern Journal of Anthropology*, 18:286–290.

280a. Gilles, H. M. (1964) *Akufo: An Environmental Study of a Nigerian Village*. University of Ibadan Press, Ibadan, Nigeria.

281. Gilles, H. M. and Taylor, B. G. (1961) The existence of the glucose-6-phosphate dehydrogenase deficiency trait in Nigeria and its clinical implications. *Annals of Tropical Medicine and Parasitology*, 55:64–69.

282. Gilles, H. M., Watson-Williams, J., and Taylor, B. G. (1960) Glucose-6-phosphate dehydrogenase deficiency trait in Nigeria. *Nature*, 185:257–258.

283. Githens, J. H. (1961) Prevalence of abnormal hemoglobins in American Indian children. Survey in the Rocky Mountain area. *Journal of Laboratory and Clinical Medicine*, 57:755–758.

284. Göksel, V., and Tartaroglu, N. (1962) Thalassémie et hémoglobines anormales dans la région égéene de l'Anatolie. *Revue Medicale du Moyen Orient*, 19:58–64.

285. Goldstein, M. A., Patpongpaij, N., and Minnich, V. (1964) The incidence of elevated hemoglobin A_2 levels in the American Negro. *Annals of Internal Medicine*, 60:95–99.

286. Gómez, O. L. and Carbonell, L. (1946) Drepanocitos en Venezuela. *Gaceta Médica de Caracas*, 54:48–50.

287. Gorman, J. G. and Kidson, C. (1962) Distribution pattern of an inherited trait, red cell enzyme deficiency, in New Guinea and New Britain. *American Journal of Physical Anthropology*, 20:347–356.

288. Gosden, M. and Reid, J. D. (1948) An account of blood results in Sierra Leone. *Transactions of the Royal Society of Tropical Medicine and Hygiene*, 41:637–640.

289. Graham, G. S. and McCarty, S. H. (1930) Sickle cell (meniscocytic) anemia. *Southern Medical Journal*, 23:598–607.

290. Grelier, L. J. and Roge (1959) Drépancocytose des habitants de la côte sud-est de Madagascar. *Archives de l'Institut Pasteur de Madagascar*, 27:75–78.

291. Griffiths, S. B. (1953) Absence of sickle cell trait in the Bushmen of South-West Africa. *Nature*, 171:577–578.

292. Griffiths, S. B. (1954) The distribution of the sickle-cell trait in Africa. *South African Journal of Medical Sciences*, 19:56–57.

293. Grjebine, A. (1956) Aperçu sommaire du peuplement anophèlien de Madagascar. *Bulletin of the World Health Organization*, 15:593–611.

294. Gross, R. T., Hurwitz, R. E., and Marks, P. A. (1958) An hereditary enzyme defect in erythrocyte metabolism: glucose-6-phosphate dehydrogenase deficiency. *Journal of Clinical Investigations*, 37:1176–1184.

294a. Grozdea, I., Benegmos, J., and Levêque, M. (1966) Hémoglobines anormales chez des malades marocaîns cancéreux. *Acta Haematologica*, 35:53–55.

295. Guevara, I., Guevara, J. M., Guevara, M. E., Gonzalez, B., and Arends, T. (1963) Busqueda de hemoglobinas anormales en el Estado Trujillo. *Acta Científica Venezolana*, 14:153–155.

296. GUEVARA, J. M. and ARENDS, T. (1962) Frecuencia de las hemoglobinas anormales en niños de Venezuela. *Sangre*, 7:386–396.

297. GULLIVER, P. and GULLIVER, P. H. (1953) *The Central Nilo-Hamites*. Ethnographic Survey of Africa, Part VII, International African Institute, London.

298. GUZMAN, L. C., ETCHEVERRY, B. R., MURANDA, R. M., REGONESI, L. C., and DURAN, N. (1964) Hemoglobinas anormales y hemoglobinopatias en Chile. Drepanocitosis. *Proceedings of the 9th Congress of the International Society of Hematology* (Mexico, 1962), 3:71–80.

299. GUZMAN, C. ETCHEVERRY, R., PUGA, F., REGONESI, C., MURANDA, M., DURAN, N., and MUÑOZ, E. (1964) Anemias hemolíticas por defecto enzimatico (Deficiencia de glucosa-6-fosfato dehidrogenasa). *Revista Médica de Chile*, 92:592–600.

300. HACKETT, C. J. (1963) On the origin of the human treponematoses. *Bulletin of the World Health Orgainzation*, 29:7–41.

301. HACKETT, L. W. (1937) *Malaria in Europe*. Oxford University Press, London.

301a. HACKETT, L. W. (1949) Conspectus of malaria incidence in Northern Europe, the Mediterranean Region, and the Near East. In M. F. Boyd (Ed.), *Malariology*. W. Blakiston, Philadelphia. 2:788–799.

302. HAILES, A. M. and ROBERTS, D. F. (1962) Glucose-6-phosphate dehydrogenase deficiency screening in Madeira. *Human Biology*, 34:206–213.

302a. HALDANE, J. B. S. (1948) The theory of a cline. *Journal of Genetics*, 48:277–284.

302b. HALDANE, J. B. S. (1949) Disease and evolution. *La Ricerca Scientifica*, 19: Suppl. 1:3–10.

303. HALL-CRAGGS, M., MARSDEN, P. D., RAPER, A. B., LEHMANN, H., and BEALE, D. (1964) Homozygous sickle-cell anaemia arising from two different haemoglobins S. *British Medical Journal*, 2:87–89.

304. HANADA, M. (1965) Personal communication.

305. HANSEN-PREUSS, O. C. (1936) Experimental studies of the sickling of red blood cells. *Journal of Laboratory and Clinical Medicine*, 22:311–315.

306. HARE, R. (1955) *Pomp and Pestilence*. Philosophical Library, New York.

307. HARRIES, J. R. and CHARTERS, J. D. (1962) Glucose-6-phosphate dehydrogenase deficiency and malaria. *East African Medical Journal*, 39:37–39.

308. HARRIS, R. and GILLES, H. M. (1961) Glucose-6-phosphate dehydrogenase deficiency in the peoples of the Niger Delta. *Annals of Human Genetics*, 25:199–206.

308a. HARTE, T. J. (1959) Trends in mate selection in a tri-racial isolate. *Social Forces*, 37:215–221.

309. HATHORN, M. (1963) Haemoglobin levels in pregnant women in Accra. *Ghana Medical Journal*, 2:55–61.

310. HAYNIE, T. P., DOBSON, H. L., and HETTIG, R. A. (1957) Molecular diseases of hemoglobin. I. Introduction and incidence. *Annals of Internal Medicine*, 46:1031–1038.

311. HEANGSUN, SOK (1958) *L'Hémoglobine E au Cambodge*. École Française d'Extrême-Orient, Paris.

312. HELLER, P. (1965) The molecular basis of the pathogenicity of abnormal hemoglobins—some recent developments. *Blood*, 25:110–125.

313. HELMS, M. W. (1964) Glucose-6-phosphate dehydrogenase enzyme deficiency on the East Coast of Nicaragua. *Papers of the Michigan Academy of Science, Arts, and Letters*, 44:239–244.

314. HENDRICKSE, R. G. (1965) Fast haemoglobins in Nigerian infants. In J. H. P. Jonxis, (Ed.), *Abnormal Haemoglobins in Africa,* F. A. Davis, Philadelphia. Pp. 249–256.

315. HENDRICKSE, R. G., BOYO, A. E., FITZGERALD, P. A., and RANSOME-KUTI, S. (1960) Studies on the haemoglobins of newborn Nigerians. *British Medical Journal,* 1:611–614.

316. HENRY, M. U. (1963) The haemoglobinopathies in Trinidad. *Caribbean Medical Journal,* 25:26–40.

317. HERRERA CABRAL, J. M. (1950) *Revista Medica Dominicana,* 5:265. Quoted in W. A. Collier and D. A. de la Parra. (1952) Sickle-cell trait in Surinam Creoles. *Tropical and Geographical Medicine,* 4:223–225.

318. HERRICK, J. B. (1910) Peculiar, elongated and sickle-shaped red corpuscles in a case of severe anemia. *Archives of Internal Medicine,* 6:517–521.

319. HIERNAUX, J. (1952) La génétique de la sicklémie et l'intérêt anthropologique de sa fréquence en Afrique noire. *Annales du Musée Royal du Congo Belge,* Tervuren (Belgique). Série in 8°, *Sciences de l'homme, Anthropologie,* vol. 2.

320. HIERNAUX, J. (1956) Analyse de la variation des caractères physiques humain en une région de l'Afrique centrale: Ruanda-Urundi et Kivu. *Annales du Musée Royal du Congo Belge,* Tervuren. Série in 8°, *Anthropologie,* vol. 3

321. HIERNAUX, J. (1962) Données génétiques sur six population de la République du Congo (groupes sanguins ABO et Rh, et taux de sicklémie). *Annales de la Société Belge de Médecine Tropicale,* 42:145–174.

321a. HIERNAUX, J. (1966) Personal communication.

322. HOARE, C. A. (1957) The spread of African trypanosomes beyond their natural range. *Zeitschrift für Tropenmedizin und Parasitologie,* 8:157–161.

322a. HOBOLTH, N. (1965) Haemoglobin M_{Arhus}. *Acta Paediatrica Scandinavica,* 54:357–368.

323. HODGKIN, E. P. (1956) The transmission of malaria in Malaya. Institute for Medical Research, Kuala Lumpur, Publication No. 27.

323a. HOERMAN, K. C., KAMEL, K., and AWNY, A. Y. (1961) Haemoglobin E in Egypt. *Nature,* 189:69–70.

323b. HOLLAN, S. R. and SZELÉNYI, J. (1963) Some new data on hemoglobin$_{Kiskunhalas}$. *Proceedings of the 9th Congress of the European Society of Haematology* (Lisbon, 1963) S. Karger, New York. Pp. 538–542.

324. HOROWITZ, A. (1963) Polymorphic characters and genetic affinities of the Jewish community from Urfa. *Israle Journal of Zoology,* 12:219.

325. HORSFALL, W. R. and LEHMANN, H. (1953) Absence of the sickle-cell trait in seventy-two Australian Aboriginals. *Nature,* 172:638.

326. HORSFALL, W. R. and LEHMANN, H. (1956) Absence of abnormal haemoglobins in some Australian Aboriginals. *Nature,* 177:41–42.

327. HORTON, B., PAYNE, R. A., BRIDGES, M. T., and HUISMAN, T. H. J. (1961) Studies on an abnormal minor hemoglobin component (Hb B_2). *Clinica Chemica Acta,* 6:246–253.

328. HUDSON, E. H. (1965) Treponematosis and man's social evolution. *American Anthropologist,* 67:885–901.

329. HUEHNS, E. R., FLYNN, F. V., BUTLER, E. A., and BEAVEN, G. H. (1961) Two new haemoglobin variants in a very young human embryo. *Nature,* 189:496–497.

330. HUEHNS, E. R. and SHOOTER, E. M. (1965) Human haemoglobins. *Journal of Medical Genetics,* 2:48–90.

331. Huisman, T. H. J. and Sydenstricker, V. P. (1962) Difference in gross structure of two electrophoretically identical 'minor' haemoglobin components. *Nature*, 193:489–491.

332. Humphreys, J. (1952) Observations on the sickle cell trait in Nigerian soldiers. *Journal of Tropical Medicine and Hygiene*, 55:173–176.

333. Hunt, J. A. and Ingram, V. M. (1959) Human haemoglobin E, the chemical effect of gene mutation. *Nature*, 184:870–872.

334. Hunt, J. A. and Lehmann, H (1959) Haemoglobin "Barts," a foetal hemoglobin without α chains. *Nature*, 184:872–873.

335. Huntsman, R. G., Hall, M., Lehmann, H., and Sukumaran, P. K. (1963) A second and third abnormal haemoglobin in Norfolk. *British Medical Journal*, 1:720–722.

336. Hutchison, H. E., Pinkerton, P. H. and Waters, P. (1965) Haemoglobinopathies in the West of Scotland. *Scottish Medical Journal*, 10:159–164.

337. Hutchison, H. E., Pinkerton, P. H., Waters, P., Douglas, A. S., Lehmann, H., and Beale, D. (1964) Hereditary Heinz-body anaemia, thrombocytopenia, and haemoglobinopathy(Hb Köln) in a Glasgow family. *British Medical Journal*, 2:1099–1103.

338. Ibbotson, R. N. and Crompton, B. A. (1963) The incidence of β-thalassaemia in Greek and Italian migrants in Australia and its effect in pregnancy. *British Journal of Haematology*, 9:523–531.

339. Ikin, E. W., Mourant, A. E., and Lehmann, H. (1965) The blood groups and haemoglobins of the Assyrians of Iraq. *Man*, 65:99.

339a. Ingram, V. M. (1961) *Hemoglobin and Its Abnormalities*. C. C. Thomas, Springfield, Ill.

339b. Ingram, V. M. (1963) *The Hemoglobins in Genetics and Evolution*. Columbia University Press, New York.

339c. Ingram, V. M. and Stretton, A. O. W. (1959) Genetic basis of the thalassaemia diseases. *Nature*, 184:1903–1909.

340. Iribarren, J. M. G. (1963) Frecuencia de hemoglobinas anormales en niños sanos y enfermos. Unpublished thesis, Instituto Venezolano de Investigaciónes Científicas, Caracas.

340a. Itano, H. A. (1965) The synthesis and structure of normal and abnormal hemoglobins. In J. H. P. Jonxis (Ed.), *Abnormal Haemoglobins in Africa*. F. A. Davis, Philadelphia. Pp. 3–16.

341. Itano, H. A., Bergen, W. R., and Sturgeon, P. (1954) Identification of fourth abnormal human hemoglobin. *Journal of the American Chemical Society*, 76:2278.

342. Itano, H. A. and Pauling, L. (1961) Thalassaemia and the abnormal human haemoglobins. *Nature*, 191:398–399.

342a. Itano, H. A. and Robinson, E. (1959) Formation of normal and doubly abnormal haemoglobins by recombination of haemoglobin I with S and C. *Nature*, 183:1799–1800.

343. Jackson, F. S., Lehmann, H., and Sharih, A. (1960) Thalassaemia in a Tibetan discovered during a haemoglobin survey among the Sherpas. *Nature*, 188:1121–1122.

344. Jacob, G. F. (1955) A survey for haemoglobins C and D in Uganda. *British Medical Journal*, 1:521–522.

345. Jacob, G. F. (1957) A study of the survival rate of cases of sickle-cell anaemia. *British Medical Journal*, 1:738–739.

346. Jacob, G. F. (1957) A study of the relationship between sickling and hookworms. *East African Medical Journal*, 34:597–600.

347. JACOB, G. F., LEHMANN, H., and RAPER, A. B. (1956) Haemoglobin D in Indians of Gujerati origin in Uganda. *East African Medical Journal,* 33:135–138.

348. JACOB, G. F. and RAPER, A. B. (1958) Hereditary persistence of foetal haemoglobin production and its interaction with the sickle-cell trait. *British Journal of Haematology,* 4:138–149.

349. JELLIFFE, D. B., BENNETT, F. J., JELLIFFE, E. F. P., and WHITE, R. H. R. (1964) Ecology of childhood disease in the Karamojong of Uganda. *Archives of Environmental Health,* 9:25–36.

350. JELLIFFE, D. B., BENNETT, F. J., STROUD, C. E., NOVOTNY, M. E., KARRACH, H. A., MUSOKE, L. K., and JELLIFFE, E. F. P. (1961) Field survey of the health of Bachiga children in the Kayonza District, Kigezi, Uganda. *American Journal of Tropical Medicine and Hygiene,* 10:435–445.

351. JELLIFFE, D. B., BENNETT, F. J., STROUD, C. E., WELBOURN, H. F., WILLIAMS, M. C., and Jelliffe, E. F. P. (1963) The health of Acholi children. *Tropical and Geographical Medicine,* 15:411–421.

352. JELLIFFE, D. B., BENNETT, F. J., WHITE, R. H. R., CULLINAN, T. R., and JELLIFFE, E. F. P. (1962) The children of the Lugbara: a study in the techniques of paediatric field survey in tropical Africa. *Tropical and Geographical Medicine,* 14:33–50.

353. JELLIFFE, D. B. and HUMPHREYS, J. (1952) The sickle-cell trait in Western Nigeria. *British Medical Journal,* 1:405.

354. JELLIFFE, D. B., STUART, K. L., and WILLS, V. G. (1954) The sickle-cell trait in Jamaica. *Blood,* 9:144–152.

355. JELLIFFE, E. F. P. and JELLIFFE, D. B. (1963) *Plasmodium malariae* in Ugandan children. I. Prevalence in young children in rural communities. *American Journal of Tropical Medicine and Hygiene,* 12:296–297.

356. JELLIFFE, R. S. (1954) The sickle-cell trait in three Northern Nigerian tribes. *West African Medican Journal,* 3:26–28.

356a. JENKINS, M. E. and CLARK, J. F. (1962) Studies into maternal influences on the well-being of the fetus and newborn. *American Journal of Obstetrics and Gynecology,* 84:57–61.

357. JENKINS, T. (1963) Sickle cell anaemia in Wankie, Southern Rhodesia. *Central African Journal of Medicine,* 9:307–319.

358. JILLY, P. and NKRUMAH, F. K. (1964) A survey of anaemia in children in the Korle Bu Hospital, with special reference to malaria. *Ghana Medical Journal,* 3:118–124.

359. JIM, R. T. S. and YARBRO, M. T. (1960) Survey of haemoglobin types in Hawaii. *Acta Haematologica,* 23:398–400.

360. JOHNSON, F. B. and TOWNSEND, E. W. (1937) Sickle-cell anemia. A report of 30 cases. *Southern Medicine and Surgery,* 99:377–381.

361. JOHNSTON, H. H. (1910) *The Negro in the New World.* Methuen, London.

362. JONCOUR, G. (1956) La lutte contre le paludisme à Madagascar. *Bulletin of the World Health Organization,* 15:711–723.

362a. JONES, R. T. (1966) Personal communication.

363. JONXIS, J. H. P. (1957) Sickle cell gene in Indonesia. *Nature,* 179:876.

364. JONXIS, J. H. P. (1959) The frequency of haemoglobin S and haemoglobin C carriers in Curaçao and Surinam. In J. H. P. Jonxis and J. F. Delafresnaye (Eds.), *Abnormal Haemoglobins.* C. C. Thomas, Springfield, Ill. Pp. 300–306.

365. JONXIS, J. H. P., HUISMAN, T. H. J., DA COSTA, G. J., and METSELAAR, D. (1958) Absence of abnormal haemoglobins in some groups of the Papua population of Dutch New Guinea. *Nature*, 181:1279.

366. JOSEPHS, H. (1928) Clinical aspects of sickle cell anemia. *Bulletin of the Johns Hopkins Hospital*, 43:397–398.

367. JUILLAN, M. (1961) Enquête sur la fréquence des hématies falciformes en Algérie. *Archives de l'Institut Pasteur d'Algérie*, 39:261–270.

367a. JUKES, T. H. (1965) The Genetic Code, II. *American Scientist*, 53:477–487.

368. KALMUS, H. (1957) Defective colour vision, P.T.C. tasting and drepanocytosis in samples from fifteen Brazilian populations. *Annals of Human Genetics*, 21:313–317.

369. KALMUS, H., DEGARAY, A. L., RODARTE, U., and COBO, L. (1964) The frequency of PTC tasting, hard ear wax, colour blindness and other genetical characteristics in urban and rural Mexican populations. *Human Biology*, 36:134–145.

370. KAMEL, K., HOERMAN, K. C., MIALE, A., and AWNY, Y. A. (1960) L'incidence d'hémoglobines congénitalement anormales chez les enfants au Caire, R. A. U.. *Sang*, 31:307–310.

371. KANTCHEV, K. N., TCHOLAKOV, B., BAGLIONI, C., and COLOMBO, B. (1965) Haemoglobin O_{Arab} in Bulgaria. *Nature*, 205:187–188.

372. KARL, A. R. (1957) Estudio electroforético de la hemoglobina de los indígenas "Mazatecos" de la cuenca del Papaloapan. *Ciencia*, 17:85–86.

373. KERSTEN, H. G. and KLEIHAUER, E. (1964) Hämoglobin M Köln, eine neue Hämoglobinvariante. Zugleich ein Beitrag zur Differentdiagnose der Zyanöse. *Die Medizinische Welt*, 2:1607–1611.

374. KIDSON, C. (1961) Erythrocyte glucose-6-phosphate dehydrogenase deficiency in New Guinea and New Britain. *Nature*, 190:1120–1121.

375. KIDSON, C. (1961) Deficiency of glucose-6-phosphate dehydrogenase; some aspects of the trait in people of Papua-New Guinea. *Medical Journal of Australia*, 2:506–509.

376. KIDSON, C. and GAJDUSEK, D. C. (1962) Glucose-6-phosphate dehydrogenase deficiency in Micronesian peoples. *Australian Journal of Science*, 25:61–62.

377. KIDSON, C. and GAJDUSEK, D. C. (1962) Congenital defects of the central nervous system associated with hyperendemic goiter in a neolithic highland society of Netherlands New Guinea. II. Glucose-6-phosphate dehydrogenase in the Mulia population. *Pediatrics*, 29:364–368.

378. KIDSON, C. and GORMAN, J. G. (1962) A challenge to the concept of selection by malaria in glucose-6-phosphate dehydrogenase deficiency. *Nature*, 196:49–51.

379. KILLINGSWORTH, W. P. and WALLACE, S. A. (1936) Sicklemia in the Southwest. *Southern Medical Journal*, 29:941–944.

379a. KIRIMLIDES, ST., POLITIS, E., DROSSOS, CH., SCALOUMBAKAS, N., PAPAIOANNOU, M., and PHILIPPIDIS, PH. (1965) Glucose-6-phosphate dehydrogenase deficiency in Greece. *Helvetica Paediatrica Acta*, 20:490–496.

380. KIRK, R. L., LAI, L. Y. C., VOS, G. H., and VIDYARTHI, L. P. (1962) A genetical study of the Oraons of the Chota Nagpur Plateau (Bihar, India). *American Journal of Physical Anthropology*, 20:375–385.

381. KIRK, R. L., LAI, L. Y. C., VOS, G. H., WICKREMASINGHE, R. L., and

Perera, D. J. B. (1962) The blood and serum groups of selected populations in South India and Ceylon. *American Journal of Physical Anthropology*, 20:485–497.

382. Kirkman, H. N. and Hendrickson, E. M. (1963) Sex-linked electrophoretic difference in glucose-6-phosphate dehydrogenase. *American Journal of Human Genetics*, 15:241–258.

383. Kirkman, H. N., Rosenthal, I. M., Simon, E. R., Carson, P. E., and Brinson, A. G. (1964) "Chicago 1" variant of glucose-6-phosphate dehydrogenase in congenital hemolytic disease. *Journal of Laboratory and Clinical Medicine*, 63:715–725.

384. Kirkman, H. N., Simon, E. R., and Pickard, B. M. (1965) Seattle variant of glucose-6-phosphate dehydrogenase. *Journal of Laboratory and Clinical Medicine*, 66:834–840.

385. Klein Obbink, H. J. (1965) Glucose-6-phosphate dehydrogenase deficiency in a Dutch family. *Acta Genetica et Statistica Medica*, 15:21–32.

386. Knight, R. H. and Robertson, D. H. H. (1963) The prevalence of the erythrocyte glucose-6-phosphate dehydrogenase deficiency among Africans in Uganda. *Transactions of the Royal Society of Tropical Medicine and Hygiene*, 57:95–100.

387. Knox, E. G. and McGregor, I. A. (1965) Glucose-6-phosphate dehydrogenase deficiency in a Gambian village. *Transactions of the Royal Society of Tropical Medicine and Hygiene*, 59:46–58.

387a. Konigsberg, W., Huntsman, R. G., Wadia, F., and Lehmann, H. (1965) Haemoglobin D β Punjab in an East Anglian family. *Journal of the Royal Anthropological Institute*, 95:295–306.

388. Kraus, A. P., Neely, C. L., Carey, F. T., and Kraus, L. M. (1962) Detection of deficient erythrocyte regeneration of reduced triphosphopyridine nucleotide from glucose-6-phosphate. *Annals of Internal Medicine*, 56:765–773.

389. Kruatrachue, M., Charoenlarp, P., Chongsuphajaisiddhi, T., and Harinsuta, C. (1962) Erythrocyte glucose-6-phosphate dehydrogenase and malaria in Thailand. *Lancet*, 2:1183–1186.

389a. Kruatrachue, M., Klongkumnuanhara, K., and Harinasuta, C. (1966) Infection-rates of malarial parasites in red blood-cells with normal and deficient glucose-6-phosphate dehydrogenase. *Lancet*, 1:404–406.

390. Kruatrachue, M., NaNakorn, S., and Charoenlap, P. (1961) Trophozoite induced malaria and hemoglobinopathies. *Proceedings of the 8th Congress of the International Society of Hematology* (Tokyo, 1960) Pan Pacific Press, Tokyo. Pp. 1233–1236.

391. Kruatrachue, M., Na-Nakorn, S., Charoenlarp, P., and Suwanakul, L. (1961) Haemoglobin E and malaria in Southeast Thailand. *Annals of Tropical Medicine and Parasitology*, 55:468–473.

392. Kumar, N. (1957) A genetic survey among the Tentulia Bagdi and the Duley of Hooghly District in West Bengal. *Bulletin of the Department of Anthropology of the Government of India*, 6:81–88.

392. Kumar, N. and Ghosh, A. K. (1967) ABO blood groups and sickle-cell trait investigations in Madhya Pradesh, Ujjain and Dewas Districts. *Acta Genetica et Statistica Medica*, 17:55–61.

392a. Kunkel, H. G. and Wallenius, G. (1955) New hemoglobin in normal adult blood. *Science*, 122:288.

393. LABIE, D., ROSA, J., and PAVIOT, J-J. (1961) Sur l'existence de différentes anomalies de l'hémoglobine dans une population du Sud de l'Inde. *Nouvelle Revue Française d'Hématologie*, 1:562–568.

393a. LABIE, D. and SCHAPIRA, G. (1966) New variant of haemoglobin G. Haemoglobin G_{Paris}. *Nature*, 209:1033–1034.

394. LALOUEL, J. (1955) La sicklémie au Gabon. *Bulletins et Mémoires de la Société d'Anthropologie de Paris*, 10e série, 6:129–132.

394a. LAMBERT, S. M. (1949) Malaria incidence in Australia and South Pacific. In M. F. Boyd (Ed.), *Malariology*. W. Blakiston, Philadelphia. 2:820–830.

395. LAMBOTTE-LEGRAND, J. and LAMBOTTE-LEGRAND, C. (1951) L'anémie à hématies falciformes chez l'enfant indigène du Bas-Congo. *Annales de la Société Belge de Médecine Tropicale*, 31:207–234.

396. LAMBOTTE-LEGRAND, J. and LAMBOTTE-LEGRAND, C. (1958) Notes complémentaires sur la drépanocytose. I. Sicklémie et malaria. *Annales de la Société Belge de Médecine Tropicale*, 38:45–53.

397. LAMBOTTE-LEGRAND, J. and LAMBOTTE-LEGRAND, C. (1958) Notes complémentaires sur la drépanocytose. II. Sicklémie et anémie par ankylostomiase. *Annales de la Société Belge de Médecine Tropicale*, 38:55–56.

398. LAMBOTTE-LEGRAND, J., LAMBOTTE-LEGRAND, C., AGER, J. A. M., and LEHMANN, H. (1960) L'hémoglobinose P. A propos d'un cas d'association des hémoglobines P et S. *Revue d'Hématologie*, 15:10–18.

399. LANGUILLON, J. (1951) L'anémie a hématies falciformes. A propos 6 observations personelles chez les Noirs de la Guadeloupe. *Revue de Médecine et d'Hygiene d'Outre-Mer*, 23:114–126.

400. LANGUILLON, J. (1957) Carte épidémiologique du paludisme au Cameroun. *Bulletin de la Société de Pathologie Exotique*, 50:585–600.

401. LANGUILLON, J. (1957) Note sur la présence d'hémoglobines anormales chez les Bantous du Sud-Cameroun. *Bulletin de la Société de Pathologie Exotique*, 50:726–728.

402. LANGUILLON, J. and DELAS, A. (1957) Note sur la sicklémie et les groupes sanguins chez diverse populations du Cameroun. *Médecine Tropicale*, 17:830–835.

403. LAYRISSE, M., LAYRISSE, Z., and WILBERT, J. (1960) Blood groups antigens among the Paraujano. *American Journal of Physical Anthropology*, 18:131–139.

404. LAYRISSE, M., LAYRISSE, Z., and WILBERT, J. (1963) Blood group antigen studies of four Chibchan tribes. *American Anthropologist*, 65:36–55.

405. LEE, T-C., SHIH, L.-Y., HUANG, P.-C., LIN, C.-C., BLACKWELL, B.-N., BLACKWELL, R. Q., and HSIA, D. Y.-Y. (1963) Glucose-6-phosphate dehydrogenase deficiency in Taiwan. *American Journal of Human Genetics*, 15:126–132.

406. LEHMANN, H. (1951) Sickle-cell anaemia and sickle-cell trait as homo- and heterozygous gene combinations. *Nature*, 167:931–933.

407. LEHMANN, H. (1954) Distribution of the sickle cell gene. *Eugenics Review*, 46:101–121.

407a. LEHMANN, H. (1962) Haemoglobins and haemoglobinopathies. In H. Lehmann and K. Betke (Eds.), *Haemoglobin Colloquium*. Georg Thieme Verlag, Stuttgart. Pp. 1–14.

408. LEHMANN, H. and MACKEY, J. P. (1955) The absence of haemoglobin C in 104 East Africans living in Dar es Salaam. *Man*, 55:200.

409. LEHMANN, H., MARANJIAN, G., and MOURANT, A. E. (1963) Distribution of sickle-cell haemoglobin in Saudi Arabia. *Nature*, 198:492–493.
410. LEHMANN, H., NORTH, A., and STAVELEY, J. M. (1958) Absence of the Diego blood group and abnormal haemoglobins in 92 Maoris. *Nature*, 181:791–792.
411. LEHMANN, H. and NWOKOLO, C. (1959) The River Niger as a barrier in the spread eastwards of haemoglobin C: a survey of haemoglobins in the Ibo. *Nature*, 183:1587–1588.
412. LEHMANN, H. and RAPER, A. B. (1949) Distribution of the sickle-cell trait in Uganda, and its ethnological significance. *Nature*, 164:494–495.
413. LEHMANN, H. and RAPER, A. B. (1956) Maintenance of high sickling rate in an African community. *British Medical Journal*, 2:333–336.
414. LEHMANN, H., SHARIH, A., GILAT, T., and LENZ, R. (1962) A survey of some genetical characters in Ethiopian tribes. II. Hemoglobin examinations. *American Journal of Physical Anthropology*, 20:174.
415. LEHMANN, H., SHARIH, A., and ROBINSON, G. L. (1961) Sickle-cell haemoglobin in a Pathan. *Man*, 61:134.
416. LEHMANN, H. and SINGH, P. B. (1956) Haemoglobin E in Malaya. *Nature*, 178:695–696.
417. LEHMANN, H., STORY, P., and THEIN, H. (1956) Haemoglobin E in Burmese. *British Medical Journal*, 1:544.
418. LEHMANN, H. and SUKUMARAN, P. K. (1956) Examination of 146 South Indian Aboriginals for haemoglobin variants. *Man*, 56:97.
419. LEJEUNE (1952) Premiers résultats d'une enquête sur la fréquence du "sickle cell trait" chez les nourrisons des consultations du Cercle de Feshi. *Rapport de Foréami*, pp. 102–104.
420. LELE, R. D., SOLANKI, B. R., BHAGWAT, R. B., INGLE, V. N., and SHAH, P. M. (1962) Haemoglobinopathies in Aurangabad region. *Journal of the Association of Physicians of India*, 10:263–271.
421. LÉON, RULX (1953) *Les Maladies en Haiti.* Imprimerie de l'Etat, Port-au-Prince.
422. LESSA, A. and DESSAI, M. (1955) Enquêtes sur la drépanocytose. *Proceedings of the 5th International Congress of Blood Transfusion* (Paris). Pp. 507–508.
423. LEVY, J. (1929) Sicklemia. *Annals of Internal Medicine*, 3:47.
424. LI, C. C. (1955) The stability of an equilibrium and the average fitness of a population. *American Naturalist*, 89:281–296.
425. LIACHOWITZ, C., ELDERKIN, J., GUICHIRIT, I., BROWN, H. W., and RANNEY, H. M. (1958) Abnormal hemoglobins in the Negroes of Surinam. *American Journal of Medicine*, 24:19–24.
425a. LIDDELL, J., BROWN, D., BEALE, D., LEHMANN, H., and HUNTSMAN, R. G. (1964) A new haemoglobin $J_{\alpha\ \mathrm{Oxford}}$ found during a survey of an English population. *Nature*, 204:269–270.
426. LIE-INJO LUAN ENG (1957) Sickle cell gene in Indonesia. *Nature*, 179:381.
427. LIE-INJO LUAN ENG (1959) Haemoglobin of newborn infants in Indonesia. *Nature*, 183:1125.
428. LIE-INJO LUAN ENG (1959) Pathological haemoglobins in Indonesia. In J. H. P. Jonxis and J. F. Delafresnaye (Eds.), *Abnormal Haemoglobins.* C. C. Thomas, Springfield, Ill. Pp. 363–383.
429. LIE-INJO LUAN ENG (1962) The significance of "Barts" or Fessas and Papaspyrou hemoglobin. *Eugenics Quarterly*, 9:49–53.
429a. LIE-INJO LUAN ENG (1965) Hereditary ovalocytosis and haemoglobin E-ovalocytosis in Malayan Aborigines. *Nature*, 208:1329.

430. Lie-Injo Luan Eng and Chin, J. (1964) Abnormal haemoglobin and glucose-6-phosphate dehydrogenase deficiency in Malayan Aborigines. *Nature*, 204:291–292.

431. Lie-Injo Luan Eng, Chin, J., and Ti, T. S. (1964) Glucose-6-phosphate dehydrogenase deficiency in Brunei, Sabah, and Sarawak. *Annals of Human Genetics*, 28:173–176.

431a. Lie-Injo Luan Eng, Pillay, R. P., and Virik, H. K. (1966) Haemolysis due to glucose-6-phosphate dehydrogenase deficiency in Malaya. *Transactions of the Royal Society of Tropical Medicine and Hygiene*, 60:262–266.

432. Lie-Injo Luan Eng and Poey-Oey Hoey Giok (1964) Glucose-6-phosphate dehydrogenase deficiency in Indonesia. *Nature*, 204:88–89.

433. Lie-Injo Luan Eng and Ti, T. S. (1961) The fast moving haemoglobin component in healthy newborn babies in Malaya. *Medical Journal of Malaya*, 16:107–114.

434. Lie-Injo Luan Eng and Ti, T. S. (1964) Glucose-6-phosphate dehydrogenase deficiency in Malayans. *Transactions of the Royal Society of Tropical Medicine and Hygiene*, 58:500–502.

435. Linhard, J. (1952) Note complémentaire sur la sicklémie dans la région de Dakar. *Revue d'Hématologie*, 7:561–566.

436. Linhard, J., Baylet, R., and Malvoisin, J. (1964) Premiers résultats sur les déficiences en G6PD dans la région de Dakar. *Bulletin de la Société Médecine d'Afrique Noire en Langue Française*, 9:269–270.

437. Lipparoni, E. (1954) Rilievi sul nomadismo nelle sue correlazioni nosografiche ed epidemiologiche in Somalia. *Archivio Italiano di Scienze Mediche Tropicali e di Parassitologia*, 35:134–154.

438. Lisker, R. (1963) Estudios sobre algunas características hematologicas hereditarias en la población Mexicana. II. Hemoglobinas anormales en 7 grupos indígenas y algunos mestizos. *Gaceta Médica de Mexico*, 93:289–297.

439. Lisker, R., Alvar Loria, Q. B. P., and Reyes, G. R. (1964) Frecuencia de hemoglobinas anormales en Mexico. *Proceedings of the 9th Congress of the International Society of Hematology* (Mexico City, 1962), 3:45–49.

440. Lisker, R., Loria, A., Cordova, M. Soledad (1965) Studies on several genetic hematological traits of the Mexican population. VIII. Hemoglobin S, glucose-6-phosphate dehydrogenase deficiency and other characteristics in a malarial region. *American Journal of Human Genetics*, 17:179–187.

440a. Lisker, R., Zarate, G., and Loria, A. (1966) Studies on several genetic hematologic traits of Mexicans. IX. Abnormal hemoglobins and erythrocytic glucose-6-phosphate dehydrogenase deficiency in several Indian tribes. *Blood*, 27:824–830.

440b. Lister, R. W., Orr, N. W. M., Botting, D., Ikin, E. W., Mourant, A. E., and Lehmann, H. (1966) The blood groups and haemoglobin of the Bedouin of Socotra. *Man* (new series), 1:82–86.

441. Livingstone, F. B. (1957) Sickling and malaria. *British Medical Journal*, 1:762–763.

442. Livingstone, F. B. (1958) Anthropological implications of sickle cell gene distribution in West Africa. *American Anthropologist*, 60:533–562.

443. Livingstone, F. B. (1960) The wave of advance of an advantageous gene: the sickle cell gene in Liberia. *Human Biology*, 32:197–202.

444. LIVINGSTONE, F. B. (1961) Balancing the human hemoglobin polymorphisms. *Human Biology*, 33:205–219.
445. LIVINGSTONE, F. B. (1962) Population genetics and population ecology. *American Anthropologist*, 64:44–53.
446. LIVINGSTONE, F. B. (1964) Aspects of the population dynamics of the abnormal hemoglobin and glucose-6-phosphate dehydrogenase deficiency genes. *American Journal of Human Genetics*, 16:435–450.
447. LIVINGSTONE, F. B. (1966) The origin of the sickle cell gene. *Publications of the Boston University School of African Studies.* (In press)
448. LIVINGSTONE, F. B. (1966) Unpublished data.
449. LIVINGSTONE, F. B., GERSHOWITZ, H., BACON, E., KELLER, F. J., and ROBINSON, A. R. (1960) The blood groups, abnormal hemoglobins, and hemoglobin values of pregnant women in Liberia. *American Journal of Physical Anthropology*, 18:1–4.
450. LONG, W. K. (1965) Personal communication.
451. LONG, W. K., KIRKMAN, H. N., and SUTTON, H. E. (1965) Electrophoretically slow variants of glucose-6-phosphate dehydrogenase from red cells of Negroes. *Journal of Laboratory and Clinical Medicine*, 65:81–87.
451a. LOTTI, F. (1962) Osservazioni sulla microcitemia nel Gargano. *Atti delle Giornate di Studio su "Il Problema Sociale della Microcitemia e del Morbo di Cooley".* Istituto Italiano di Medicina Sociale, Roma. 1:238–243.
452. LUCCI, R. and SOFFRITTI, E. (1959) Presenza di emoglobine abnormi nella popolazione del delta Padano. *Arcispedale de Santa Anna di Ferrara*, 12:419–429.
453. LUTTRELL, V. and LEA, C. (1965) Glucose-6-phosphate dehydrogenase deficiency in East Africans. *East African Medical Journal*, 42:313–315.
454. LUZZATTO, L., ALLAN, N. C., and DE FLORA, A. (1965) Genetic polymorphism of glucose-6-phosphate dehydrogenase. *Biochemical Journal*, 97:19P–20P.
455. MACHADO, L. (1958) Da incidência da drepanocitemia em grupos de indivíduos da Cidade do Salvador. *Medicina, Cirurgia, e Farmâcia*, 270:471–475.
456. MALAMOS, B., FESSAS, PH., and STAMATOYANNOPOULOS, G. (1962) Types of thalassaemia-trait carriers as revealed by a study of their incidence in Greece. *British Journal of Haematology*, 8:5–14.
457. MANDEL, S. P. H. (1963) A note on the initial progress of new genes. *Heredity*, 18:535–538.
458. MARDER, V. J. and CONLEY, C. L. (1959) Electrophoresis of hemoglobin on agar gels. Frequency of hemoglobin D in a Negro population. *Bulletin of the Johns Hopkins Hospital*, 105:77–88.
459. MARGOLIES, M. P. (1951) The incidence of sickling. *American Journal of the Medical Sciences*, 221:270–272.
459a. MARKS, P. A. (1965) Personal communication.
460. MARKS, P. A., BANKS, J., and GROSS, R. T. (1962) Genetic heterogeneity of glucose-6-phosphate dehydrogenase deficiency. *Nature*, 194:454–456.
461. MARKS, P. and BURKA, E. R. (1964) Hemoglobins A and F: formation in thalassemia and other hemolytic anemias. *Science*, 144:552–553.
462. MARKS, P. A. and GROSS, R. T. (1959) Erythrocyte glucose-6-phosphate dehydrogenase deficiency. Evidence of differences between Negroes and Caucasians with respect to this genetically determined trait. *Journal of Clinical Investigations*, 38:2253–2262.

462a. MARTI, H. R. (1964) Les hémoglobines normales et anormales. *Praxis*, 53:646–651.

463. MARTI, H. R. and BÜTLER, R. (1961) Hämoglobin F und hämoglobin A_2—Vermehrung bei der Schweizer Bevölkerung. *Acta Haematologica*, 26:65–74.

464. MARTI, H. R., SCHOEPF, K., and GSELL, O. R. (1965) Frequency of haemoglobin S and glucose-6-phosphate dehydrogenase deficiency in Southern Tanzania. *British Medical Journal*, 1:1476–1477.

464a. MARTINS, J. M., PITOMBEIRA, M. S., and CUNHA, R. V. (1965) Hemoglobinopatias. Estudos feitos no Estado do Ceará. *O Hospital*, 68:701–709.

465. MASUDA, M. and FUJIKI, N. (1961) Recent biochemical studies on the genetic role in red blood cell formation. *Proceedings of the 8th International Congress of the International Society of Hematology* (Tokyo, 1960). Pan Pacific Press, Tokyo. Pp. 1120–1122.

466. MATHUR, K. S., MEHROTRA, T. N., DAYAL, R. S., and YADAR, S. N. S. (1962) Incidence of haemoglobin E and thalassaemia in Uttar Pradesh. *Journal of the Indian Medical Association*, 39:172–177.

467. MATSON, A. T. (1957) The history of malaria in Nandi. *East African Medical Journal*, 34:431–441.

468. MATSON, G. A., SUTTON, H. E., SWANSON, J., and ROBINSON, A. R. (1963) Distribution of haptoglobin, transferrin, and hemoglobin types among Indians of Middle America: Southern Mexico, Guatemala, Honduras, and Nicaragua. *Human Biology*, 35:474–483.

469. MATSON, G. A., SUTTON, H. E., SWANSON, J., and ROBINSON, A. R. (1965) Distribution of haptoglobin, transferrin, and hemoglobin types among Indians of Middle America: In British Honduras, Costa Rica, and Panama. *American Journal of Physical Anthropology*, 23:123–130.

469a. MATSON, G. A., SUTTON, H. E., SWANSON, J., ROBINSON, A. R., and SANTIANA, A. (1966) Distribution of hereditary blood groups among Indians in South America. I. In Ecuador. *American Journal of Physical Anthropology*, 24:51–69.

469a! MATSON, G. A., SUTTON, H. E., SWANSON, J., and ROBINSON, A. (1966) Distribution of hereditary blood groups among Indians of South America. II. In Peru. *American Journal of Physical Anthropology*, 24:325–350.

469b. MATSUNAGA, E., SHINODA, T., and HANDA, Y. (1965) A genetic study on the quantitative variation in erythrocyte glucose-6-phosphate dehydrogenase activity of apparently healthy Japanese. *Japanese Journal of Human Genetics*, 10:1–12.

469c. MAUZE, J. (1946) Contribution à l'étude du paludisme dans la Nouvelles-Hebrides (particulièrement pendant la campagne du Sud-Ouest Pacifique Janvier 1942-Décembre 1943). *Médecine Tropicale*, 6:109–138.

470. MCCORMICK, W. F. (1960) Abnormal hemoglobins. I. Incidence in Memphis and Western Tennessee, with special reference to autopsy material. *American Journal of Clinical Pathology*, 34:220–224.

470a. MCCURDY, P. R., KIRKMAN, H. N., NAIMAN, J. L., JIM, R. T. S., and PICKARD, B. M. (1966) A Chinese variant of glucose-6-phosphate dehydrogenase. *Journal of Laboratory and Clinical Medicine*, 67:374–385.

471. MCFADZEAN, A. J. S. and TODD, D. (1964) The distribution of Cooley's

anaemia in China. *Transactions of the Royal Society of Tropical Medicine and Hygiene,* 58:490–499.

472. McGAVACK, T. H. and GERMAN, W. M. (1944) Sicklemia in the Black Carib Indians. *American Journal of the Medical Sciences,* 208:350–355.

472a. McGUINESS, R. (1966) Cataracts in glucose-6-phosphate dehydrogenase deficiency. *British Medical Journal,* 1:613.

473. MEERA KHAN, P. (1964) Glucose-6-phosphate dehydrogenase deficiency. *Journal of Genetics,* 59:14–18.

474. DEMENDONCA, J. M. (1942) Meniscocitemia—frequência no Brasil. *Brasil-Medico,* 56:382–384.

475. MENÉNDEZ CORRADA, R. (1957) Hemoglobin survey in San Patricio Hospital: filter paper electrophoresis of the hemoglobin of 500 patients. *Boletín de la Asociación Médica de Puerto Rico,* 49:262–267.

476. MERA, B. (1943) Preliminares del estudio de la meniscocitemia en Colombia. *Boletín de la Oficina Sanitaria Pan-Americana,* 22:680–682.

477. MEYERS, H., LIPS, M., and CAUBERGH, H. (1962) L'état actuel du problème du paludisme d'altitude au Ruanda-Urundi. *Annales de la Société Belge de Médecine Tropicale,* 42:771–782.

477a. MILLER, M. J. (1958) Observations on the natural history of malaria in the semi-resistant West African. *Transactions of the Royal Society of Tropical Medicine and Hygiene,* 52:152–168.

477b. MILLER, M. J., NEEL, J. V., and LIVINGSTONE, F. B. (1956) Distribution of parasites in the red cells of sickle-cell trait carriers infected with *Plasmodium falciparum. Transactions of the Royal Society of Tropical Medicine and Hygiene,* 50:294–296.

478. MILNER, P. (1963) Haemoglobin D in Jamaica. *West Indian Medical Journal,* 12:141–142.

478a. MINER, H. (1965) *The Primitive City of Timbuctoo.* Doubleday and Co., Garden City, N. Y.

479. MINNICH, V., CORDONNIER, J. K., WILLIAMS, W. J., and MOORE, C. V. (1962) Alpha, beta, and gamma hemoglobin polypeptide chains during the neonatal period with description of a fetal form of hemoglobin $D_{\alpha \text{ St. Louis}}$. *Blood,* 19:137–167.

480. MINNICH, V., HILL, R. J., KHURI, P. D., and ANDERSON, M. E. (1965) Hemoglobin Hope: a beta chain variant. *Blood,* 25:830–838.

481. MISRA, G. M. (1960) A study of abnormal haemoglobin found in Western Uttar Pradesh. Unpublished thesis, Agra University.

482. MISSIROLI, A. (1933) Tipe epidemico delle febbri malariche nel nord d'Italia. *Rivista di Malariologia,* 12:675–688.

483. MITAL, M. S., PAREKH, J. G., SUKUMARAN, P. K., SHARMA, R. S., and DAVE, P. J. (1962) A focus of sickle cell gene near Bombay. *Acta Haematologica,* 27:257–267.

483a. MIWA, S., TERAMURA, K., IRISAWA, K., and OHYAMA, H. (1965) Glucose-6-phosphate dehydrogenase (G-6-P D) deficiency. II. Incidence of G-6-P D deficiency in Japanese. *Acta Haematologica Japonica,* 28:590–592.

484. MIYAMOTO, K. and KORB, J. H. (1927) Menyscocytosis (latent sickle cell anemia), its incidence in St. Louis. *Southern Medical Journal,* 20:912–916.

484a. MODIANO, G., BENERECETTI-SANTACHIARA, A. S., GONANO, F., ZEI, G., CAPALDO, A., and CAVALLI-SFORZA, L. L. (1965) An analysis of ABO,

MN, Rh, Tf, and G-6-PD types in a sample from the human population of the Lecce Province. *Annals of Human Genetics*, 29:19–31.

485. MODICA, R., LIVADIOTTI, M., and MACALUSO, A. S. (1960) Incidenza della sicklemia pregressa malaria e distribuzione razziale nell' oasi costiera di Tauorga. *Archivio Italiano di Scienze Mediche Tropicali e di Parassitologia*, 41:595–604.

486. MODICA, R. and MACALUSO, A. S. (1960) Inchiesta sulla presenza di emoglobine anormali in Tripolitania. *Bollettino Sanitario della Tripolitania* (Jan.-Mar.) Pp. 20–22.

487. MODICA, R. and MARAINI, G. (1957) Ricerche sulla presenza della falcemia (s.c.t.) in Tripolitania. *Archivio Italiano di Scienze Mediche Tropicali e di Parassitologia*, 38:209–218.

488. MOFFITT, E. M. and MCDOWELL, C. W. (1959) The incidence of abnormal hemoglobins by paper electrophoresis in Sourthern Louisiana. *Bulletin of the Tulane Medical Faculty*, 19:167–180.

489. MONEKOSSO, G. L. (1964) Clinical survey of a Yoruba village. *West African Medical Journal*, 13:47–59.

489a. MONEKOSSO, G. L. and IBIAMA, A. A. (1966) Splenomegaly and sickle-cell trait in a malaria-endemic village. *Lancet*, 1:1347–1348.

490. MONTESTRUC, E., BERDONNEAU, R., BENOIST, J., and COLLET, A. (1959) Hémoglobines anormales et groupes sanguins ABO chez les Martiniquais. *Bulletin de la Société de Pathologie Exotique*, 52:156–158.

491. MOORE, R. A., BRASS, W., and FOY, H. (1954) Sickling and malaria. *British Medical Journal*, 2:630–631.

491a. MORTON, N. E. (1966) Personal communication.

492. MOTULSKY, A. G. (1956) Genetic and haematological significance of haemoglobin H. *Nature*, 178:1055–1056.

493. MOTULSKY, A. G. (1960) Metabolic polymorphisms and the role of infectious diseases in human evolution. *Human Biology*, 32:28–62.

494. MOTULSKY, A. G. (1965) Theoretical and clinical problems of glucose-6-phosphate dehydrogenase deficiency. Its occurrence in Africans and its combination with hemoglobinopathy. In J. H. P. Jonxis (Ed.), *Abnormal Haemoglobins in Africa*. F. A. Davis, Philadelphia. Pp. 143–196a.

494a. MOTULSKY, A. G. and CAMPBELL-KRAUT, J. M. (1961) Population genetics of glucose-6-phosphate dehydrogenase deficiency of the red cell. In B. S. Blumberg (Ed.), *Proceedings of the Conference on Genetic Polymorphisms and Geographic Variations in Disease*. Grune and Stratton, New York. Pp. 159–180.

495. MOTULSKY, A. G., LEE, T-C., and FRAZER, G. R. (1965) Glucose-6-phosphate dehydrogenase (G6PD) deficiency, thalassaemia, and abnormal haemoglobins in Taiwan. *Journal of Medical Genetics*, 2:18–20.

496. MOTULSKY, A. G., STRANSKY, E., and FRAZER, G. R. (1964) Glucose-6-phosphate dehydrogenase (G6PD) deficiency, thalassaemia, and abnormal haemoglobins in the Philippines. *Journal of Medical Genetics*, 1:102–106.

497. MOURA PIRES, F. (1959) Contribuição para o estudo da drepanocitemia nos indígênas da Lunda. *Anais do Instituto de Medicina Tropical, Lisboa*, 16:453–460.

498. MUSIAL, W., KRYKOWSKI, E., KOLCZYCKA, Z., and MURAWSKI, E. (1961)

Thalassemia minor w polskiej rodzinie. *Polskie Archiwum Medycyny Wewnetrznej*, 31:1541–1549.

499. MYERSON, R. M., HARRISON, E., and LOHMULLER, H. W. (1959) Incidence and significance of abnormal hemoglobins. *American Journal of Medicine*, 26:543–546.

499a. NAGEL, R., RANNEY, H. M., JACOBS, A. S., ANDERSON, H. M., and KRITZLER, R. A. (1964) Hemoglobin Columbia: an α chain variant found in a Russian Jewish family: its association with a hemolytic state. *Abstracts of the Annual Meeting of the American Society of Human Genetics*. P. 2.

500. NA-NAKORN, S. (1959) Haemoglobinopathies in Thailand. In J. H. P. Jonxis and J. F. Delafresnaye (Eds.), *Abnormal Haemoglobins*. C. C. Thomas, Springfield, Ill. Pp. 357–367.

501. NA-NAKORN, S., MINNICH, V., and CHERNOFF, A. I. (1956) Studies of hemoglobin E. II. The incidence of hemoglobin E in Thailand. *Journal of Laboratory and Clinical Medicine*, 47:490–498.

502. NANCE, W. E. (1963) Genetic control of hemoglobin synthesis. *Science*, 141:123–130.

502a. NANCE, W. E. (1964) Genetic tests with a sex-linked marker: Glucose-6-phosphate dehydrogenase. *Cold Spring Harbor Symposia on Quantitative Biology*, 29:415–425.

503. NANCE, W. E. and UCHIDA, I. (1964) Turner's syndrome, twinning, and an unusual variant of glucose-6-phosphate dehydrogenase. *American Journal of Human Genetics*, 16:380–392.

504. NAUDE, E. E. and NEAME, P. B. (1961) Sickle-cell trait in the Natal Indian. *South African Medical Journal*, 35:1026.

505. NEEB, H., BEIBOER, J. L., JONXIS, J. H. P., SIJPESTEIJN, J. A. K. and MULLER, C. J. (1961) Thalassemie met lepore hemoglobine bij twee Papoeakindern in Nederlands Nieuw Guinea. *Nederlandsch Tijdschrift voor Geneeskunde*, 105:8–14.

506. NEEL, J. V. (1951) The inheritance of the sickling phenomenon with particular reference to sickle cell disease. *Blood*, 6:389–412.

507. NEEL, J. V. (1954) Implications of some recent developments in hematological and serological genetics. *American Journal of Human Genetics*, 6:208–223.

507a. NEEL, J. V. (1966) Personal communication.

508. NEEL, J. V., HIERNAUX, J., LINHARD, J., ROBINSON, A. R., ZUELZER, W. W., and LIVINGSTONE, F. B. (1956) Data on the occurrence of hemoglobin C and other abnormal hemoglobins in some African populations. *American Journal of Human Genetics*, 8:138–150.

509. NEEL, J. V., ROBINSON, A. R., ZUELZER, W. W., LIVINGSTONE, F. B., and SUTTON, H. E. (1961) The frequency of elevations in the A_2 and fetal hemoglobin fractions in the natives of Liberia and adjacent regions, with data on haptoglobin and transferrin types. *American Journal of Human Genetics*, 13:262–278.

510. NEEL, J. V., SALZANO, F. M., JUNQUEIRA, P. C., KEITER, F., and MAYBURY-LEWIS, D. (1964) Studies on the Xavante Indians of the Brazilian Mato Grosso. *American Journal of Human Genetics*, 16:52–140.

511. NEGI, R. S. (1962) The incidence of sickle-cell trait in two Bastar tribes. *Man*, 62:142.

512. NEGI, R. S. (1963) The incidence of sickle-cell trait in Bastar, II. *Man*, 63:22.

513. NEGI, R. S. (1964) The incidence of sickle-cell trait in Bastar, III. *Man* 64:214.

514. NICOL, B. M. (1959) Fertility and food in Northern Nigeria. *West African Medical Journal,* 8:18–27.

515. NIJENHUIS, L. E. (1963) Blood group frequencies and haemoglobin types in Tibetans and Nepalese. *Vox Sanguinis,* 8:622–626.

516. NOGUEIRA, A. R. (1959) Hemoglobinas anormais nas provincias Portuguêsas de Africa. *Proceedings of the 6th International Congresses on Tropical Medicine and Malaria* (Lisbon, 1958). *Anais do Instituto de Medicina Tropical, Lisboa,* 16, Supplement 10:403–411.

516a. NUÑEZ MONTIEL, A., ARTEAGA PÉREZ, R., MONTILLA, L. G., and FERRER, A. (1962) Estudios hematológicos sobre la población de la Isla de Toas (Estado Zulia). *Acta Cientifica Venezolana,* 13:94–96.

517. NUÑEZ MONTIEL, J. T., ARTEAGA PÉREZ, R., and NUÑEZ MONTIEL, O. L. (1956) Estudio médico-social en indios de la Sierra de Perijá. *Acta Científica Venezolano,* 7:184.

518. NUYKEN, G. (1954) Thalassämie in Iran. *Medizinische Klinik,* 49:1955–1956.

519. O'BRIEN, C., GRAY, M. J., and JACOBS, A. S. (1964) A survey of cord bloods for abnormal hemoglobin, with further observations on hemoglobin $I_{Burlington}$. *American Journal of Obstetrics and Gynecology,* 88:816–822.

520. OEI, T. L. (1961) A genetic investigation arising from two cases of favism. *Acta Genetica et Statistica Medica,* 11:205–216.

521. OGDEN, M. A. (1943) Sickle cell anemia in the white race. *Archives of Internal Medicine,* 71:164–182.

522. OHTA, Y. (1963) An investigation of abnormal hemoglobins in Southern Japan. 1. A case of thalassemia minor discovered on Amami Islands. *Japanese Journal of Human Genetics,* 8:227–238.

523. OHTA, Y. (1964) An investigation of abnormal hemoglobins in Southern Japan. 2. Second case of thalassemia minor discovered in Fukuoka, Kyushu, Japan. *Japanese Journal of Human Genetics,* 9:10–17.

524. OHYA, I. (1963) Abnormal hemoglobins in North Kyushu Japan, with special reference to Hb-Kokura and Hb-Fukuoka. *Japanese Journal of Human Genetics,* 8:23–28.

525. OLIVER, R. and FAGE, J. D. (1962) *A Short History of Africa.* Penguin Books, Baltimore.

526. OLIVIA, J. and MYERSON, R. M. (1961) Hereditary persistence of fetal hemoglobin. *American Journal of Medical Sciences,* 241:215.

526a. OLUFEMI WILLIAMS, A. (1966) Haemoglobin genotypes, ABO blood groups, and Burkitt's tumour. *Journal of Medical Genetics,* 3:177–179.

527. OORT, M. (1964) Red cell glucose-6-phosphate dehydrogenase (G6PD) deficiency. Unpublished thesis, Central Laboratory of the Blood Transfusion Service of the Dutch Red Cross.

528. PALES, L. (1953) La sicklémie (sickle cell trait) en Afrique Occidentale Française (Haute Volta). *L'Anthropologie,* 57:61–67.

529. PALES, L., GALLAIS, P., BERT, J., and FOURQUET, R. (1954) La sicklémie (sickle cell trait) chez certaines populations nigéro-tchadiennes de l'Afrique Occidentale Française. *L'Anthropologie,* 58:472–480.

530. PALES, L. and LINHARD, J. (1952) La sicklémie (sickle cell trait) en Afrique Occidentale Française, vue de Dakar. *L'Anthropologie,* 56:53–86.

531. PARENT, J. (1950) Sickle cell anemia. *Annales de la Société Belge de Médecine Tropicale,* 30:47–52.

532. PARSONS, I. C. and RYAN, B. P. K. (1962) Observations on glucose-6-phosphate dehydrogenase deficiency in Papuans. *Medical Journal of Australia,* 2:585–587.

533. PARSONS, P. A. (1961) The initial progress of new genes with viability differences between sexes and with sex linkage. *Heredity,* 16:103–107.

534. PASTERNAK, C. A. and ROBERTS, D. F. (1956) Haemoglobin C in Berbers. *Man,* 56:52.

534a. PAULING, L., ITANO, H. A., SINGER, S. J., and WELLS, I. C. (1949) Sickle-cell anemia, a molecular disease. *Science,* 110:543–548.

535. PEDROSO FERREIRA, A. and TRINÇÃO, C. (1962) Abnormal haemoglobins in Portuguese Timor. *Man,* 62:49.

536. PERILLIE, P. E. and EPSTEIN, F. H. (1963) Sickling phenomenon produced by hypertonic solutions: a possible explanation for the hyposthenuria of sicklemia. *Journal of Clinical Investigations,* 42:570–580.

537. PETERS, W. (1965) Ecological factors limiting the extension of malaria in the Southwest Pacific—their bearing on malaria control or eradication programmes. *Acta Tropica,* 22:62–69.

538. PIERCE, L. E., RATH, C. E., and MCCOY, K. (1963) A new hemoglobin variant with sickling properties. *New England Journal of Medicine,* 268:862–866.

539. PIK, C., LOOS, J. A., JONXIS, J. H. P., and PRINS, H. K. (1965) Hereditary and acquired blood factors in the Negroid population of Surinam. II. The incidence of haemoglobin abnormalities and the deficiency of glucose-6-phosphate dehydrogenase. *Tropical and Geographical Medicine,* 17:61–68.

539a. DEPIÑANGO, C. L. A. and ARENDS, T. (1965) Abnormal hemoglobins in native blood donors of Bolivar State. *Acta Cientifica Venezolana,* 16:215–218.

540. PINTO NOGUEIRA, J., DE MATOS COITO, A., and ESPADA FERREIRA, A. (1950) Contribuição para o estudo das drepanocitemias nos naturais de Cabo Verde. *Anais do Instituto de Medicina Tropical, Lisboa,* 7:239–252.

540a. PLATO, C. C. and CRUZ, M. (1966) Blood group and haptoglobin frequencies of the Trukese of Micronesia. *Acta Genetica et Statistica Medica,* 16:74–83.

541. PLATO, C. C., CRUZ, M. T., and KURLAND, L. T. (1964) Frequency of G6PD deficiency, red-green colour blindness and Xg^a blood group among the Chamorros. *Nature,* 202:729.

542. PLATO, C. C., RUCKNAGEL, D. L., and GERSHOWITZ, H. (1964) Studies on the distribution of glucose-6-phosphate dehydrogenase deficiency, thalassemia, and other genetic traits in the coastal and mountain villages of Cyprus. *American Journal of Human Genetics,* 16:267–283.

542a. PLATO, C. C., RUCKNAGEL, D. L., and KURLAND, L. T. (1966) Blood group investigations on the Carolinians and Chamorros of Saipan. *American Journal of Physical Anthropology,* 24:147–154.

543. POINDEXTER, H. A. (1953) Epidemiological survey among the Gola tribe in Liberia. *American Journal of Tropical Medicine and Hygiene,* 2:30–38.

544. POLLITZER, W. S., (1958) The Negroes of Charleston (S. C.); a study of hemoglobin types, serology, and morphology. *American Journal of Physical Anthropology,* 16:241–263.

545. POLLITZER, W. S., CHERNOFF, A. I., HORTON, L. L., and FROELICH, M. (1959) Hemoglobin patterns in American Indians. *Science,* 129:216.

546. Pollitzer, W. S., Menegaz-Bock, R. M., and Herion, J. C. (1966) Factors in the microevolution of a triracial isolate. *American Journal of Human Genetics*, 18:26–38.

547. Pollitzer, W. S., Rucknagel, D. L., and Tashian, R. E. (1966) Unpublished observations.

548. Polosa, P. and Motta, L. (1963) On incidence of thalassemia and abnormal hemoglobins in the eastern part of Sicily—First results. *Proceedings of the 9th Congress of the European Society of Haematology* (Lisbon, 1963). S. Karger, New York. Pp. 530–534.

549. Polosa, P., Motta, L., Calcagno, G., and Lunetta, M. (1965) L'Hb C nella Sicilia orientale: rilievi popolazionistici. *Progresso Medico*, 21:41–47.

550. Polunin, I. (1953) The medical natural history of Malayan Aborigines. *Medical Journal of Malaya*, 8:55–114.

551. Polunin, I. and Sneath, P. H. A. (1953) Studies of blood groups in South-East Asia. *Journal of the Royal Anthropological Institute of Great Britain and Ireland*, 83:215–251.

552. Pons, J. A. and Oms, M. (1934) Incidencia del rasgo meniscocítico (Eritrocitos semilunares) en Puerto Rico. *Boletín de la Asociación Médica de Puerto Rico*, 26:367–371.

553. Porter, I. H., Boyer, S. H., Watson-Williams, E. J., Adam, A., Szeinberg, A., and Siniscalco, M. (1964) Variation of glucose-6-phosphate dehydrogenase in different populations. *Lancet*, 1:895–899.

554. Porter, I. H., Schulze, J., and McKusick, V. A. (1962) Genetical linkage between the loci for glucose-6-phosphate dehydrogenase deficiency and colour-blindness in American Negroes. *Annals of Human Genetics*, 26:107–122.

555. Portier, A., Cabannes, R., Massonat, J., and Thiebault, R. (1955) Enquête sur la drépanocytose chez l'indigène muselman algérien. *Proceedings of the 5th International Congress of Blood Transfusion*. Pp. 427–430.

556. Portier, A., Massonat, J., and Zevaco, P. (1952) Enquête sur la thalassémie en Afrique du Nord. *Algérie Médicale*, 1:23–29.

557. Pouya, Y. (1959) Thalassaemia in Iran. In J. H. P. Jonxis and J. F. Delafresnaye (Eds.), *Abnormal Haemoglobins*. C. C. Thomas, Springfield, Ill. Pp. 236–241.

557a. Pribilla, W., Klesse, P., Betke, K., Lehmann, H., and Beale, D. (1965) Hämoglobin-Köln-Krankheit: Familiäre hypochrome hämolytische Anämie mit Hämoglobinanomalie. *Klinische Wochenschrift*, 43:1049–1053.

558. Prins, A. H. J. (1952) *The Coastal Tribes of the Northeastern Bantu*. Ethnographic Survey of Africa, Part III, International African Institute, London.

559. Prins, H. K., Loos, J. A., and Meuwissen, J. H. E. Th. (1963) Glucose-6-phosphate dehydrogenase deficiency in West New Guinea. *Tropical and Geographical Medicine*, 15:361–370.

560. Quattrin, N., Dini, E., and Ventruto, V. (1964) Le emoglobinopatie in Campania. Studio triennale epidemiologico clinico e nosologico. *Annali Sclavo, Siena*, 6:3–58.

560a. Ragab, A. H., El-Alfi, O. S., and Abboud, M. A. (1966) Incidence of glucose-6-phosphate dehydrogenase deficiency in Egypt. *American Journal of Human Genetics*, 18:21–25.

561. RAMOT, B., ABRAHAMOV, A., FRAYER, Z, and GAFNI, D. (1964) The incidence and types of thalassaemia-trait carriers in Israel. *British Journal of Haematology*, 10:155–158.

562. RAMOT, B., BAUMINGER, S., BROK, F., GAFNI, D., and SHWARTZ, J. (1964) Characterization of glucose-6-phosphate dehydrogenase in Jewish mutants. *Journal of Laboratory and Clinical Medicine*, 64:895–904.

563. RAMOT, B. and BROK, F. (1964) A new G-6-PD mutant (Tel-Hashomer mutant). *Annals of Human Genetics*, 28:167–172.

564. RANNEY, H. M., JACOBS, A. S., BRADLEY, T. B., and CORDOVA, F. A. (1963) A 'new' variant of haemoglobin A_2 and its segregation in a family with haemoglobin S. *Nature*, 197:164–166.

564a. RAOULT, M. (n. d.) Unpublished observations.

565. RAPER, A. B. (1955) Malaria and the sickling trait. *British Medical Journal*, 1:1186–1189.

566. RAPER, A. B. (1956) Sickling in relation to morbidity from malaria and other diseases. *British Medical Journal*, 1:965–966.

567. RAPER, A. B. (1957) Unusual haemoglobin variant in a Gujerati Indian. *British Medical Journal*, 1:1285–1286.

568. RAPER, A. B. (1959) Further observations on sickling and malaria. *Transactions of the Royal Society of Tropical Medicine and Hygiene*, 53:110–117.

569. RAVISSE, P. (1952) Recherches sur la sicklémie chez les Pygmées de l'Afrique Equatoriale Française. *L'Anthropologie*, 56:491–493.

570. RAVISSE, P. (1955) Pathologie comparative des Babinga et leurs "patrons." *Médecine Tropicale*, 15:72–83.

571. RAY, R. N., CHATTERJEA, J. B., and CHANDHURI, R. N. (1964) Observations on the resistance in Hb E—thalassemia disease to induced infection with *Plasmodium vivax*. *Bulletin of the World Health Organization*, 30:51–55.

572. RESTREPO MESA, A. (1963) Hemoglobinas anormales y talasemia. *Antioquia Médica*, 13:580–593.

572a. REY, M., OUDART, J-L., CAMERLYNCK, P., DIOP MAR, I., and NOUHOUAYI, A. (1965) Paludisme, hémoglobinoses et déficit en glucose-6-phosphate-déshydrogénase (Note préliminaire). *Bulletin de la Société Médicale d'Afrique Noire de Langue Française (Dakar)*, 10:659–668.

573. RIBEIRO DO ROSÁRIO, M. and MAGALHÃES COLLAÇO, F. (1958) Nosografia da hemoglobian "S" em Portugal continental. Estudo familiar de dois casos de anemia de células. *Gazeta Médica Portuguêsa*, 11:541–554.

573a. RIEDER, R. F. and NAUGHTON, M. A. (1965) Hemoglobin G (Baltimore): a new abnormal hemoglobin and an additional individual with four hemoglobins. *Bulletin of the Johns Hopkins Hospital*, 116:17–32.

573b. RIESENBERG, S. H. (1965) Table of voyages affecting Micronesian Islands. *Oceania*, 36:155–170.

574. RIZZOTTI, G. (1955) Falcemia e malattia falcemica. Prime osservazioni circa la loro diffusione nella regione di Addis Abeba. *Archivio Italiano di Scienze Mediche Tropicali e di Parassitologia*, 36:555–563.

575. ROBERTS, D. F. and BOYO, A. E. (1960) On the stability of haemoglobin gene frequencies in West Africa. *Annals of Human Genetics*, 24:375–387.

576. ROBERTS, D. F. and BOYO, A. E. (1962) Abnormal haemoglobins in childhood among the Yoruba. *Human Biology*, 34:20–37.

577. ROBERTS, D. F. and LEHMANN, H. (1955) A search for abnormal haemoglobins in some Southern Sudanese peoples. *British Medical Journal*, 1:519–521.

578. Roberts, D. F., Lehmann, H., and Boyo, A. E. (1960) Abnormal hemoglobins in Bornu. *American Journal of Physical Anthropology*, 18:5–11.

579. Roberts, D. F., Luttrell, V., and Slater, C. P. (1965) Genetics and geography in Tinos. *Eugenics Review*, 56:185–193.

580. Robertson, D. H. H. (1961) Nitrofurazone-induced haemolytic anaemia in a refractory case of *Trypanosoma rhodesiense* sleeping sickness: the haemolytic trait and self-limiting haemolytic anaemia. *Annals of Tropical Medicine and Parasitology*, 55:49–63.

580a. vanRood, J. J., van de Beek, J., Gevers-Potgieser, H. H., Eernisse, J. G., Veeger, W., and Nieweg, H. O. (1962) Enzymdeficientie bij twee patienten met niet-sferocytaire hemolytische anemie. *Nederlandsch Tijdschrift voor Geneeskunde*, 106:1217–1220.

581. Rose, J. R. and Suliman, J. K. (1965) The sickle-cell trait in the Mende tribe of Sierra Leone. *West African Medical Journal*, 4:35–37.

582. Rosenblum, R., Kabakow, D., Lichtman, H. C., and Lyons, H. A. (1955) Sickle cell trait and disease in pulmonary tuberculosis. *Archives of Internal Medicine*, 95:540–542.

583. Rucknagel, D. L. (1957) Paper electrophoresis survey of hemoglobins of American Indians. *Journal of Laboratory and Clinical Medicine*, 49:896–899.

584. Rucknagel, D. L. (1964) The gene for sickle cell hemoglobin in the Wesorts: an extreme example of genetic drift and the founder effect. Unpublished Thesis, University of Michigan.

585. Rucknagel, D. L. (1966) Unpublished observations.

586. Rucknagel, D. L. and Neel, J. V. (1961) The hemoglobinopathies. In A. G. Steinberg (Ed.), *Progress in Medical Genetics*, Grune and Stratton, New York. Pp. 158–260.

586a. Ruffie, J., Vergnes, H., and Hobbe, T. (1966) Sur la réversibilité de le methémoglobinisation des hématies chez les populations indigenes du corridor interandin. Essai d'interpretation. *Comptes Rendus des Séances de l'Académie des Sciences (Paris) Serie D-Sciences Naturelles*, 262:1956–1958.

587. Ryan, B. P. K. and Parsons, I. C. (1961) Glucose-6-phosphate dehydrogenase activity in Papuans. *Nature*, 192:477.

588. Ryan, T. J., O'Connor, T. F., McCurdy, P. R., and Katz, S. (1960) Sickle cell trait and tuberculosis. *American Review of Respiratory Diseases*, 81:546–549.

589. Saha, N. and Banerjee, B. (1965) Incidence of abnormal haemoglobins in Punjab. *Calcutta Medical Journal*, 62:82–86.

590. Salazar Leite, A., Jorge, Janz, G., Gândara, A. F., Ré, L., Casaca, V., and Morais de Carvalho, A. (1955) Relatório da Missão do Instituto de Medicina Tropical a Angola (1954) em colaboração com a Missão de Prospecção de Endemias de Angola. *Anais do Instituto de Medicina Tropical, Lisboa*, 12:219–254.

591. Salazar Leite, A. and Ré, L. (1955) Contribution à l'étude ethnologique des populations africaines. *Archives de l'Institut Pasteur d'Algerie*, 33:344–349.

592. Saldanha, P. H. (1957) Gene flow from White into Negro populations in Brazil. *American Journal of Human Genetics*, 9:299–309.

592a. Salomon, H., Tatarski, I., Dance, N., Huehns, E. R., and Shooter, E. M. (1965) A new hemoglobin variant found in a Beduin tribe: hemoglobin "Rambam." *Israel Journal of Medical Sciences*, 1:836–840.

593. SALVIOLI, G. P. and BABINI, B. (1963) La fréquence de la déficience congénitale en G-6-P D chez les nouveau-nés de la ville de Bologne. *Archives Français de Pédiatrie,* 20:459–462.

594. SALZANO, F. M. (1965) Genetica de populações humanas Brasileiras. In *Homenaje a Juan Comas* (Mexico), 2:253–318.

595. SANGHVI, L. D. (1962) Hemoglobin survey of Maharashtra. Lecture, Department of Human Genetics, University of Michigan.

596. SANSARRICQ, H., MARILL, G., PORTIER, A., and CABANNES, R. (1959) Les hémoglobinopathies en Haute-Volta. *Sang,* 30:503–511.

597. SANSONE, G. and PIK, C. (1965) Familial haemolytic anaemia, with erythrocyte inclusion bodies, bilifuscinuria, and abnormal haemoglobin (haemoglobin Galliera Genova). *British Journal of Haematology,* 11:511–517.

598. SANSONE, G., SEGNI, G., and DECECCO, C. (1958) Il difetto biochimico eritrocitario predisponente all'emolisi favica. Prime ricerche sulla popolazione Ligure e su quella Sarda. *Bollettino de la Societa Italiana di Biologia Sperimentale,* 34:1558–1561.

599. SANTOS DAVID, J. H. (1960) *A Drepanocitemia e a Antropologia.* Companhia de Diamantes de Angola, Publicações Culturais No. 49. (Lisbon).

600. SANTOS DAVID, J., MOURA PIRES, F., and TRINÇÃO, C. (1962) Abnormal haemoglobins in the District of Lunda and the neighbouring District of Songo, Angola. *Man,* 62:48.

601. SANTOS DAVID, J. H. and TRINÇÃO, C. (1963) Drepanocitemia, deficiência da desidrogenase da glucose-6-fosfato (G-6-PD) eritrocitária e paludismo no posto do Cuango (Lunda-Angola). *Anais do Instituto de Medicina Tropical, Lisboa,* 20:5–16.

602. VAN DER SAR, A. (1949) De sikkelcelziekte. *Nederlandsch Tijdschrift voor Geneeskunde,* 93:1867–1874.

603. VAN DER SAR, A. (1959) The occurrence of carriers of abnormal haemoglobins S and C on Curaçao. Thesis, University of Groningen.

604. VAN DER SAR, A., SCHOUTEN, H., and STRUYKER, BOUDIER, A. M. (1964) Glucose-6-phosphate dehydrogenase deficiency in red cells. Incidence in the Curaçao population, its clinical and genetic aspects. *Enzymologia,* 27:289–310.

605. SARMENTO, A. (1944) Contribuição para o estudo da anemia de células falciformes nos negros de Angola. *Anais do Instituto de Medicina Tropical, Lisboa,* 1:345–350.

606. SARROUY, CH., CABANNES R., and ZEVACO, P. (1955) La thalassémie de l'enfant indigène nord-africain. *Toulouse Médical,* 56:195–219.

607. SAUGRAIN, J. (1957) Nouvelles recherches sur la drépanocytose à Madagascar. *Bulletin de la Société de Pathologie Exotique,* 50:480–486.

607a. SAUSSE, A. (1951) *Populations Primitives du Maroni (Guyane Française).* Institut Géographique National, Paris.

608. SAY, B., OZAND, P., BERKEL, I., and ÇEVK, N. (1965) Erythrocyte glucose-6-phosphate dehydrogenase deficiency in Turkey. *Acta Paediatrica Scandinavica,* 54:319–324.

609. SCHNEIDER, R. G. (1954) Incidence of hemoglobin C trait in 505 normal Negroes. A family with homozygous hemoglobin C and sickle-cell trait union. *Journal of Laboratory and Clinical Medicine,* 44:133–144.

610. SCHNEIDER, R. G. (1956) Incidence of electrophoretically distinct abnormalities of hemoglobin in 1550 Negro hospital patients. *American Journal of Clinical Pathology,* 26:1270–1276.

611. SCHNEIDER, R. G., ARAT, F., and HAGGARD, M. E. (1964) An inhomogeneous foetal haemoglobin variant (the Texas type). *Nature*, 202:1346–1347.

612. SCHNEIDER, R. G., HAGGARD, M. E., MCNUTT, C. W., JOHNSON, J. E., BOWMAN, B. H., and BARNETT, D. R. (1964) Hemoglobin $G_{Coushatta}$: a new variant in an American Indian family. *Science*, 143:697–698.

612a. SCHNEIDER, R. G., JONES, R. T., and SUZUKI, K. (1966) Hemoglobin $F_{Houston}$: a fetal variant. *Blood*, 27:670–676.

612b. SCHOKKER, R. C., WENT, L. N., and BOK, J. (1966) A new genetic variant of β thalassaemia. *Nature*, 209:44–46.

612c. SCHROEDER, W. A. and JONES, R. T. (1965) Some aspects of the chemistry and function of human and animal hemoglobins. *Fortschritte der Chemie Organischer Naturstoffe*, 23:113–194.

613. SCOTT, E. M. (1960) The relation of diaphorase of human erythrocytes to inheritance of methemoglobinemia. *Journal of Clinical Investigations*, 39:1176–1179.

614. SCOTT, E. M., GRIFFITH, I. V., HOSKINS, D. D., and SCHNEIDER, R. G. (1959) Lack of abnormal hemoglobins in Alaskan Eskimos, Indians and Aleuts. *Science*, 129:719–720.

615. SCOTT, E. M. and HOSKINS, D. D. (1958) Hereditary methemoglobinemia in Alaskan Eskimos and Indians. *Blood*, 13:795–802.

616. SENECAL, J., AUBRY, J., and FALADE, S. (1962) Infectious diseases in the child of pre-school age in Senegal. *West African Medical Journal*, 11:93–105.

617. SHAHID, M. J. (1963) Hemoglobinopathies in Lebanon. *Proceedings of the 9th Congress of the European Society of Haematology* (Lisbon, 1963). S. Karger, New York. Pp. 496–500.

618. SHAHID, M. and ABU HAYDAR, N. (1962) Sickle cell disease in Syria and Lebanon. *Acta Haematologica*, 27:268–273.

619. SHAHID, M., ABU HAYDAR, G., and ABU HAYDAR, N. (1963) Thalassaemia-haemoglobin E disease: a case report from Qatar (Persian Gulf). *Man*, 63:155.

620. SHARMA, R. S., PAREKH, J. G., and SHAH, K. M. (1963) Haemoglobinopathies in Western India. *Journal of the Association of Physicians of India*, 11:969–973.

621. SHEBA, C. (1962) Glucose-6-phosphate dehydrogenase (G-6-P-D) deficiency as a possible marker for studying ethnic origin and migration. *East African Medical Journal*, 39:261–263.

622. SHIBATA, S., IUCHI, I., MAZAGI, T., and TAKEDA, I. (1963) Hemoglobinopathy in Japan. *Bulletin of the Yamaguchi Medical School*, 10:1–9.

623. SHOWS, T. B., TASHIAN, R. E., BREWER, G. J., and DERN, R. J. (1964) Erythrocyte glucose-6-phosphate dehydrogenase in Caucasians: new inherited variant. *Science*, 145:1056–1057.

624. SHUKLA, R. N. and SOLANKI, B. R. (1958) Sickle-cell trait in Central India. *Lancet*, 1:297–298.

625. SIDDOO, J. K., SIDDOO, S. K., CHASE, W. H., MORGAN-DEAN, L., and PERRY, W. H. (1956) Thalassemia in Sikhs. *Blood*, 11:197–210.

626. SIGNORELLI, S., POLOSA, P., and MOTTA, L. (1964) Studies on haemoglobinopathies in Sicily. *Proceedings of the 9th International Congress of International Society of Hematology* (Mexico City, 1962), 3:51–64.

626a. SIJPESTEIJN, J. A. K. (1959) Thalassemia minor in een Nederlandse familie. *Nederlandsch Tijdschrift voor Geneeskunde*, 103:838–843.

627. DA SILVA, E. M. (1945) Estudos sobre indice de siclemia. *Memorias do Instituto Oswaldo Cruz,* 42:315–340.

628. DA SILVA, E. M. (1948) Absence of sickling phenomenon of the red blood corpuscle among Brazilian Indians. *Science,* 107:221–222.

629. SILVESTRONI, E. and BIANCO, I. (1950) Ricerche sulla frequenza della microcitemia in alcune citta dell'Italia continentale. *Rivista di Antropologia,* 38:172–178.

630. SILVESTRONI, E. and BIANCO, I. (1950) Ricerche sulla frequenza della microcitemia in Sicilia. *Rivista di Antropologia,* 38:179–182.

631. SILVESTRONI, E. and BIANCO, I. (1959) Nuovi dati sulla frequenza della microcitemia e delle malattie microcitemiche nella provincia di Lecce. *Nuovi Annali d'Igiene e Microbiologia,* 10:335–341.

632. SILVESTRONI, E. and BIANCO, I. (1960) Dati Statistici sulla frequenza della microcitemia e del morbo di Cooley nella Sardegna meridionale. *Nuovi Annali d'Igiene e Microbiologia,* 11:339–348.

633. SILVESTRONI, E. and BIANCO, I. (1962) Haemoglobin Barts in Italy. *Nature,* 195:394.

634. SILVESTRONI, E. and BIANCO, I. (1962) Diffusione e frequenza della microcitemia e della anemie microcitemiche nell'Italia continentale e in Sicilia. *Atti delle Giornate di Studio su "Il Problema sociale della Microcitemia e del Morbo di Cooley."* Istituto Italiano di Medicina Sociale, Roma. 1:51–63.

635. SILVESTRONI, E. and BIANCO, I. (1963) A new variant of human fetal hemoglobin: Hb F_{Roma}. *Blood,* 22:545–553.

636. SILVESTRONI, E., BIANCO, I., and BRANCATI, C. (1963) Haemoglobins N and P in Italian families. *Nature,* 200:658–659.

636a. SILVESTRONI, E., BIANCO, I., and MURATORE, F. (1965) Frequenza dei vari tipi di microcitemia e di emoglobine abnormi nella provincia di Lecce. *Progresso Medico,* 21:211–216.

637. SILVESTRONI, E., BIANCO, I., MUZZOLINI, M., and ROBERTI, L. (1958) Nuove indagini sulla presenza di emoglobine abnormi nelle popolazioni dell'Italia meridionale e insulare. *Progresso Medico,* 14:641.

638. SIMMONS, R. T., GRAYDON, J. J., and BIRDSELL, J. B. (1953) High R^z frequency in the blood of Australian Aborigines. *Nature,* 172:500.

639. SIMMONS, R. T. and GRAYDON, J. J. (1957) A blood group genetical survey in Eastern and Central Polynesians. *American Journal of Physical Anthropology,* 15:357–366.

639a. SINGER, K., CHERNOFF, A. I., and SINGER, L. (1951) Studies on abnormal hemoglobins. I. Their demonstration in sickle cell anemia and other hematologic disorders by means of alkali denaturation. *Blood,* 6:413–428.

639b. SINGER, R. (1960) Some biological aspects of the Bushman. *Zeitschrift für Morphologie und Anthropologie,* 51:1–6.

640. SINGER, R., BUDTZ-OLSEN, O. E., BRAIN, P., and SAUGRAIN, J. (1957) Physical features, sickling, and serology of the Malagasy of Madagascar. *American Journal of Physical Anthropology,* 15:91–124.

640a. SINISCALCO, M., BERNINI, L., FILIPPI, G., LATTE, B., MEERA KHAN, P., PIOMELLI, S., and RATTAZZI, M. (1966) Population genetics of haemoglobin variants, thalassaemia, and glucose-6-phosphate dehydrogenase deficiency with particular reference to the malaria hypothesis. *Bulletin of the World Health Organization,* 34:379–394.

641. SINISCALCO, M., BERNINI, L., LATTE, B., and MOTULSKY, A. G. (1961) Favism and thalassaemia in Sardinia and their relationship to malaria. *Nature*, 190:1179–1180.

641a. SINISCALCO, M., FILIPPI, G., and LATTE, B. (1964) Recombination between protan and deutan genes; data on their relative positions in respect of the G6PD locus. *Nature*, 204:1062–1064.

642. SJÖLIN, S., WALLENIUS, G., and WRANNE, L. (1964) Haemoglobin Barts and H in a Swedish boy. *Acta Haematologica*, 32:239–249.

642a. SMINK, D. A. and PRINS, H. K. (1965) Hereditary and acquired blood factors in the Negroid population of Surinam. V. Electrophoretic heterogeneity of glucose-6-phosphate dehydrogenase. *Tropical and Geographical Medicine*, 17:236–241.

643. SMITH, E. C. (1943) Child mortality in Lagos, Nigeria. *Transactions of the Royal Society of Tropical Medicine and Hygiene*, 36:287–303.

644. SMITH, E. W. and CONLEY, C. L. (1953) Filter paper electrophoresis of human hemoglobins with special reference to the incidence and clinical significance of hemoglobin C. *Bulletin of the Johns Hopkins Hospital*, 93:94–106.

644a. SMITH, G. D. and VELLA, F. (1960) Erythrocyte enzyme deficiency in unexplained kernicterus. *Lancet*, 1:1133.

645. SMITH, J. H. (1928) Sickle cell anemia. *Medical Clinics of North America*, 11:1171–1190.

646. SONNET, J. and MICHAUX, J. L. (1960) Glucose-6-phosphate dehydrogenase deficiency, haptoglobin groups, blood groups, and sickle cell trait in the Bantus of West Belgian Congo. *Nature*, 188:504–505.

647. SPITZ, A. J. W. (1960) Health and morbidity survey, Seychelles, 1956–1957. *Bulletin of the World Health Organization*, 22:439–467.

648. STAMATOYANNOPOULOS, G. and FESSAS, PH. (1964) Thalassaemia, glucose-6-phosphate dehydrogenase deficiency, sickling, and malarial endemicity in Greece: a study of five areas. *British Medical Journal*, 1:875–879.

648a. STAMATOYANNOPOULOS, G., PANAYOTOPOULOS, A., and MOTULSKY, A. G. (1966) The distribution of the glucose-6-phosphate dehydrogenase deficiency in Greece. *American Journal of Human Genetics*, 18:296–308.

648b. STAMATOYANNOPOULOS, G., PANAYOTOPOULOS, A., and PAPAYANNOPOULOU, TH. (1964) Mild glucose-6-phosphate dehydrogenase deficiency in Greek males. *Lancet*, 2:932–935.

649. STAVELY, J. M. and DOUGLAS, R. (1958) Blood groups in Maoris. *Journal of the Polynesian Society*, 67:239–247.

650. STAVELY, J. M. and DOUGLAS, R. (1959) Blood groups in Tongans (Polynesia). *Journal of the Polynesian Society*, 68:348–353.

651. STIJNS, J. and CHARLES, P. (1956) La tare thalassémique chez les Bantous d'Afrique centrale. *Annales de la Société Belge de Médecine Tropicale*, 36:763–780.

652. STRANGWAY, A. K. (1960) The hemoglobins, with a report on hemoglobins in four African tribes. *Canadian Medical Association Journal*, 83:1040–1046.

653. STRANSKY, E. and CAMPOS, P. I. (1957) On hemoglobin E in the Philippines. *Journal of the Philippine Medical Association*, 33:731–739.

654. SUAREZ, R. M., BUSO, R., MEYER, L. M., and OLAVARRIETA, S. T. (1959) Distribution of abnormal hemoglobins in Puerto Rico and survival studies of red blood cells using Cr^{51}. *Blood*, 14:255–261.

655. SUAREZ, R. M., OLAVERRIETA, S., BUSO, R., MEYER, L. M., and SUAREZ, JR., R. M. (1961) Glucose-6-phosphate dehydrogenase deficiency among certain Puerto Rican groups. *Boletín de la Asociación Médica de Puerto Rico,* 53:41–48.

656. SUKUMARAN, P. K. and PIK, C. (1965) Some observations on haemoglobin L_{Bombay}. *Biochimica et Biophysica Acta,* 104:290–292.

657. SUKUMARAN, P. K., SANGHVI, L. D., and VYAS, G. N. (1956) Sickle-cell trait in some tribes of Western India. *Current Science,* 25:290–291.

658. SUNDHARAGIATI, B. and VISESHAKUL, D. (1958) Paper electrophoretic studies on Hgb. E in the people of Northeast Thailand. *Medical Journal of the Medical Service Department, Bangkok,* 7:419–421.

659. SUNDHARAGIATI, B. and VISESHAKUL, D. (1959) Paper electrophoretic studies on Hgb. E in the people of Northern Thailand. *Medical Journal of the Medical Service Department, Bangkok,* 8:395–396.

660. SUNDHARAGIATI, B. and VISESHAKUL, D. (1959) Paper electrophoretic studies on Hgb. E in the people of Central Thailand. *Medical Journal of the Medical Service Department, Bangkok,* 8:405–407.

661. SUTTON, H. E., MATSON, G. A., ROBINSON, A. R., and KOUCKY, R. W. (1960) Distribution of haptoglobin, transferrin, and hemoglobin types among Indians of Southern Mexico and Guatemala. *American Journal of Human Genetics,* 12:338–347.

662. SUTTON, R. N. P. (1963) Erythrocyte glucose-6-phosphate dehydrogenase deficiency in Trinidad. *Lancet,* 1:855.

662a. SUTTON, R. N. P. (1966) Viral hepatitis in G-6-P. D. deficiency. *Lancet,* 1:550–551.

662b. SWARUP, S., BANERJI, P. G., GHOSH, S. K., and CHATTERJEA, J. B. (1965) Haemoglobin Barts in Bengalee blood. *Bulletin of the Calcutta School of Tropical Medicine,* 13:47–48.

663. SWARUP, S., GHOSH, S. K., KUNDU, H. B., and CHATTERJEA, J. B. (1959) Abnormal haemoglobins in Mysore. *Journal of the Indian Medical Association,* 33:209.

664. SWINDLER, D. R. (1955) The absence of the sickle cell gene in several Melanesian societies and its anthropologic significance. *Human Biology,* 27:284–293.

665. SWITZER, P. K. (1950) The incidence of the sickle cell trait in Negroes from the Sea Island Area of South Carolina. *Southern Medical Journal,* 43:48–49.

666. SWITZER, P. K. and FOUCHÉ, H. H. (1948) The sickle cell trait; incidence and influence in pregnant colored women. *American Journal of Medical Sciences,* 216:330–332.

667. SYDENSTRICKER, V. P. (1924) Sickle cell anemia. *Southern Medical Journal* 17:177–183.

668. SZEINBERG, A., OLIVER, M., SCHMIDT, R., ADAM, A., and SHEBA, C. (1963) Glucose-6-phosphate dehydrogenase deficiency and haemolytic disease of the new-born in Israel. *Archives of Diseases of Childhood,* 38:23–28.

669. TALEB, N., LOISELET, J., GHORRA, F., and SFEIR, H. (1964) Sur la déficience en glucose-6-phosphate déshydrogénase dans les populations autochtones du Liban. *Comptes Rendus des Séances de l'Académie des Sciences (Paris),* 258:5749–5751.

669a. TARGINO DE ARAUJO, J. and JAMRA, M. (1965) Incidência de hemoglobinas anormais em amostra da população da cidade de São Paulo, Brasil.

Revista do Hospital das Clinicas, Faculdade de Medicina Universidade de São Paulo, 20:310–319.

670. TEIXEIRA, W. G. (1944) Hematias falciformes nos indigênas de Angola. *Anais do Instituto de Medicina Tropical, Lisboa,* 1:365–374.

671. THEPHUSDIN, C., BLACKWELL, B-N., HUANG, J. T-H., and BLACKWELL, R. Q. (1964) Comparison of the distributions of haptoglobin and hemoglobin types in a Thai population. *U. S. Naval Medical Research Unit No. 2, Research Report MR005.09–1601.7.10.*

672. THOMPSON, G. R. (1962) Significance of haemoglobins S and C in Ghana. *British Medical Journal,* 1:682–685.

673. THOMPSON, G. R. (1963) Malaria and stress in relation to haemoglobins S and C. *British Medical Journal,* 2:976–978.

674. THOMPSON, R. B., LEGAN, S., and ODOM, J. (1964) A survey of hemoglobinopathies in Mississippi. *Journal of the Mississippi State Medical Association,* 5:461–465.

674a. THOMPSON, R. B., WARRINGTON, R., ODOM, J., and BELL, W. N. (1965) Interaction between genes for delta thalassemia and hereditary persistence of foetal hemoglobin. *Acta Genetica et Statistica Medica,* 15:190–200.

675. TIZIANELLO, A., PANNACCIULLI, I., SALVIDIO, E., and GAY, A. (1963) Erythrocytic glucose-6-phosphate dehydrogenase deficiency as a problem in the selection of blood donors. *Vox Sanguinis,* 8:47–50.

675a. TOBIAS, P. V. (1966) The peoples of Africa south of the Sahara. In P. T. Baker and J. S. Weiner (Eds.), *The Biology of Human Adaptability.* Oxford University Press, Oxford. Pp. 111–200.

676. TOMLINSON, W. J. (1941) Studies of sicklemia blood with a new method of rapid diagnosis. *American Journal of Clinical Pathology,* 11:835–841.

677. TOMLINSON, W. J. (1945) The incidence of sicklemia and sickle cell anemia in 3000 Canal Zone examinations upon natives of Central America. *American Journal of Medical Sciences,* 209:181–186.

678. TONDO, C. V. and SALZANO, F. M. (1960) Hemoglobin types of the Caingang Indians of Brazil. *Science,* 132:1893–1894.

679. TONDO, C. V. and SALZANO, F. M. (1962) Abnormal hemoglobins in a Brazilian Negro population. *American Journal of Human Genetics,* 14:401–409.

680. TONDO, C. V., SALZANO, F. M., and RUCKNAGEL, D. L. (1963) Hemoglobin Porto Alegre, a possible polymer of normal hemoglobin. *American Journal of Human Genetics,* 15:265–279.

681. TONGIORGI, E. (1947) Grano, miglio e fave in un focolare rituale dell 'eta' del bronzo a Grotta Misa (Bassa Valle della Fiora). *Nuovo Giornale Botanico Italiano,* 54:804–806.

682. TORREALBA, J. F. (1956) Algunas consideraciónes sobre la enfermedad de hematíes falciformes o enfermedad de Herrick en Venezuela (Addendum). *Gaceta Médica de Caracas,* 68:53–67.

683. TORREGROSA, M. V. V., RIVERA-TRUJILLO, A., ORTIZ, A., and RUIZ SOLER, O. (1957) Abnormal hemoglobins among Puerto Ricans. *Boletín de la Asociación Médica de Puerto Rico,* 49:145.

684. DETRAVERSE, P. M., COQUELET, M. L., and HENROTTE, J. G. (1963) Anomalie de l'hémoglobine dans la population de Madras. *Comptes Rendus de la Société de Biologie,* 157:38–41.

685. DE TRAVERSE, P. M., LE XUAN, CHAT, COQUELET, M. L. (1960) Les hémoglobinopathies au Viet-nam. *Proceedings of the 7th Congress of the*

European Society of Haematology (London, 1959). S. Karger, New York. Part II, Pp. 1053–1057.
685a. TRESCA, G. and LANZO, A. (1965) La microcitemia costituzionale in Eritrea. *Rassegna Italiana di Gastro-enterologia,* 11:169–173.
686. TRINÇÃO, C. (1948) Anemia de células falciformes. *Anais do Instituto de Medicina Tropical, Lisboa,* 5:357–400.
687. TRINÇÃO, C. (1957) Hemoglobinas anormais nos territórios Portuguêsas. *Boletim Clinico dos Hospitais Civis de Lisboa,* 21:813–827.
688. TRINÇÃO, C., DE ALMEIDA FRANCO, L. T., MARTINS DE MELO, J., and SURLACAR, L. (1963) Abnormal haemoglobins in Portuguese India (Goa and Diu Territories). *Proceedings of the 9th Congress of the European Society of Haematology* (Lisbon, 1963). S. Karger, New York. Pp. 474–476.
689. TRINÇÃO, C., DE ALMEIDA FRANCO, L. T., and NOGUEIRA, A. R. (1960) Abnormal haemoglobins in Portuguese Guinea. *Nature,* 185:326–327.
689a. TRINÇÃO, C. and CORDEIRO FERREIRA, N. (1962) Thalassaemia in Portugal. *Proceedings of the 8th Congress of the European Society of Haematology.* S. Karger, New York. Part 2, No. 307a.
689b. TRINÇÃO, C. and MARTINI DE MELO, J. (1965) Hemoglobin S rates in AS heterozygotes. *Israel Journal of Medical Sciences,* 1:772–776.
690. TRINÇÃO, C., PINTO, A. R., LEHMANN DE ALMEIDA, C., and GOUVEIA, E. (1950) A drepanocitémia entre a tribo papel da Guiné Portuguêsa. *Anais do Instituto de Medicina Tropical, Lisboa,* 7:125–130.
690a. TROWELL, H. C., RAPER, A. B., and WELLBOURN, A. F. (1957) The natural history of homozygous sickle-cell anaemia in Central Africa. *Quarterly Journal of Medicine,* 26:401–422.
691. TUCHINDA, S., BEALE, D., and LEHMANN, H. (1965) A new haemoglobin in a Thai family. A case of haemoglobin Siriraj-β thalassaemia. *British Medical Journal,* 1:1583–1585.
692. TUCHINDA, S., VAREENIL, C., BHANCHIT, P., and MINNICH, V. (1959) "Fast" hemoglobin component found in umbilical cord blood of Thai babies. *Pediatrics,* 24:43–56.
693. UDANI, P. M., PAREKH, J. G., and SHARMA, R. S. (1963) Haemoglobin "E"—thalassaemia. *Journal of the J. J. Group of Hospitals and Grant Medical College, Bombay,* 8:259–263.
694. VALSǏK, J. A., KOMENSKY, J. A., LEHMANN, H., and NICHOLS, J. (1960) Absence of abnormal haemoglobin in 274 children in South Slovakia (including 63 Gypsies). *Man,* 60:195.
695. VANDEPITTE, J. M. (1952) Sickle-cell anaemia in Africa. *British Medical Journal,* 1:920.
696. VANDEPITTE, J. M. and DELAISSE, J. (1957) Sicklémie et paludisme. Aperçu du problème et contribution personnelle. *Annales de la Société Belge de Médecine Tropicale,* 37:703–735.
697. VANDEPITTE, J. M. and DHERTE, P. (1959) Enquête sur les hémoglobines anormales à Stanleyville. *Annales de la Société Belge de Médecine Tropicale,* 39:711–715.
698. VANDEPITTE, J. and MOTULSKY, A. G. (1956) Abnormal haemoglobins in the Kasai Province of the Belgian Congo. *Nature,* 177:757.
699. VANDEPITTE, J. and STIJNS, J. (1963) Les hémoglobinoses au Congo (Léopoldville) et au Rwanda-Burundi. *Annales de la Société Belge de Médecine Tropicale,* 43:271–281.

700. VELLA, F. (1959) Haemoglobin A_2 estimations by starch block electrophoresis. *Medical Journal of Malaya*, 14:31–35.
701. VELLA, F. (1959) Favism in Asia. *Medical Journal of Australia*, 2:196–197.
702. VELLA, F. (1960) Abnormal haemoglobin variants in 10,441 Chinese subjects. *Acta Haematologica*, 23:393–397.
703. VELLA, F. (1960) Hereditary abnormalities in human haemoglobin synthesis. *Proceedings of the Centenary and Bicentenary Congress of Biology* (Singapore, 1958). University of Malaya Press. Pp. 193–204.
704. VELLA, F. (1961) Haemoglobin S in Khartoum. *East African Medical Journal*, 38:350–352.
705. VELLA, F., (1962) La microcitemia e il morbo di Cooley a Malta, Singapore, e Khartoum. *Atti delle Giornate di Studio su "Il Problema sociale della Microcitemia e del Morbo di Cooley."* Istituto Italiano di Medicina Sociale, Roma. 1:158–173.
706. VELLA, F. (1962) The frequency of thalassaemia minor in the Maltese Islands. *Acta Haematologica*, 27:278–288.
707. VELLA, F. (1962) Abnormal haemoglobins, thalassaemia, and erythrocyte glucose-6-phosphate dehydrogenase deficiency in Singapore and Malaya. *Oceania*, 32:219–225.
708. VELLA, F. (1963) Conditions associated with sickling and their laboratory diagnosis. *Sudan Medical Journal*, 2:77–87.
709. VELLA, F. (1964) Further data on the frequency of increased erythrocyte osmotic resistance in the Maltese Islands. *Tropical and Geographical Medicine*, 16:109–114.
710. VELLA, F. (1964) Sickling in the Western Sudan. *Sudan Medical Journal*, 3:16–20.
711. VELLA, F. (1965) The haemoglobinopathies in the Sudan. In J. H. P. Jonxis (Ed.), *Abnormal Haemoglobins in Africa*. F. A. Davis, Philadelphia. Pp. 339–355.
712. VELLA, F. (1965) Favism in Malta. *British Medical Journal*, 2:1002.
712a. VELLA, F. (1966) Haemoglobin S and sickling in Khartoum Province. *Transactions of the Royal Society of Tropical Medicine and Hygiene*, 60:48–52.
712b. VELLA, F. (1966) A search for electrophoretic variants of human haemoglobin. Paper presented at the Western Regional Group, M.R.C./N.C.I. Meeting, Suffield, March 20–23, 1966.
712c. VELLA, F., BEALE, D., and LEHMANN, H. (1966) Haemoglobin O Arab in Sudanese. *Nature*, 209:308–309.
713. VELLA, F. and HART, P. L. DEV. (1959) Sickle-cell anaemia in an Indian family in Malaya. *Medical Journal of Malaya*, 14:144–150.
714. VELLA, F. and IBRAHIM, S. A. (1961) The frequency of thalassaemia minor in a Greek community. *Journal of Tropical Medicine and Hygiene*, 64:202–206.
715. VELLA, F. and IBRAHIM, S. A. (1962) Erythrocyte glucose-6-phosphate dehydrogenase deficiency in Khartoum. *Sudan Medical Journal*, 1:136–137.
716. VELLA, F. and MOUSSA, W. G. (1962) Thalassaemia minor in schoolchildren of Egyptian Sudanese parentage. *Transactions of the Royal Society of Tropical Medicine and Hygiene*, 56:70–73.
717. VELLA, F. and SAINT CASSIA, M. (1961) Thalassaemia minor in a Maltese village. *Lancet*, 2:666–667.

718. VELLA, F. and TAVARIA, D. (1961) Haemoglobin variants in Sarawak and North Borneo. *Nature,* 190:729–730.

719. VELLA, F. and VERZIN, J. A. (1963) Fast foetal haemoglobin in Khartoum. *East African Medical Journal,* 40:9–10.

720. VERAS, S. and SKLAVUNU-ZURUKZOGLU, S. (1955) L'anémie falciforme chez les Nègres de la Thrace Occidentale. *Sang,* 26:326–327.

720a. VERGNES, H. (1965) La place de la glucose-6-phosphate déshydrogénase en anthropologie biologique. *Bulletins et Mémoires de la Société d'Anthropologie de Paris,* 11e série, 7:301–322.

721. VILAR, J. P., RAVISSE, P., SILVERIC, R., and SACCHARIN, H. (1963) Note sur les hémoglobinoses en Guiane française. *Bulletin de la Société de Pathologie Exotique,* 56:1083–1087.

722. VIVONA, S., BREWER, G. J., CONRAD, M., and ALVING, A. S. (1961) The concurrent weekly administration of chloroquine and primaquine for the prevention of Korean vivax malaria. *Bulletin of the World Health Organization,* 25:267–269.

722a. VOGEL, F. and ROHRBORN, G. (1965) Mutationsvorgänge bei der Entstehung von Hämoglobinvarianten. *Humangenetik,* 1:635–650.

722b. VORONOV, A. A. (1964) Anomalynye Gemoglobiny. *Voprosy Antropologii,* No. 17:131–143.

723. DEVRIES, A., JOSHUA, H., LEHMANN, H., HILL, R. L., and FELLOWS, R. E. (1963) The first observation of an abnormal haemoglobin in a Jewish family: haemoglobin Beilinson. *British Journal of Haematology,* 9:484–486.

724. VYAS, G. N., BHATIA, H. M., SUKUMARAN, P. K., BALKRISHNAN, V., and SANGHVI, L. D. (1962) Study of blood groups, abnormal hemoglobins, and other genetical characters in some tribes of Gujerat. *American Journal of Physical Anthropology,* 20:255–265.

725. WAGNER, G. (1949) *The Bantu of North Kavirondo. Volume 1.* Oxford University Press, London.

726. WALKER, D. G. and BOWMAN, J. E. (1959) Glutathione stability of the erythrocytes in Iranians. *Nature,* 184:1325.

727. WALKER, D. G. and BOWMAN, J. E. (1960) In vitro effect of *Vicia faba* extracts upon reduced glutathione of erythrocytes. *Proceedings of the Society of Experimental Biology and Medicine,* 103:476–477.

728. WALLACE, S. A. and KILLINGSWORTH, W. P. (1935) Sicklemia in the Mexican race. *American Journal of Diseases of Childhood,* 50:1208–1215.

729. WALSH, R. J. and COTTER, H. (1955) Sicklaemia in the Pacific. *Australian Journal of Science,* 17:175–176.

729a. WALTER, H. NEUMANN, S., and NEMESKERI, J. (1965) Populations-genetische Untersuchungen über die Verteilung von Hämoglobin S und Glucose-6-Phosphat-Dehydrogenasemangel im Bodrogköz (Nordost-ungarn). *Humangentik,* 1:651–567.

729b. WALTERS, J. H. (1954) Uncommon endemic diseases of the Persian Gulf Area. *Transactions of the Royal Society of Tropical Medicine and Hygiene,* 48:385–394.

730. WALTERS, J. H. and BRUCE-CHWATT, L. J. (1956) Sickle-cell anaemia and falciparum malaria. *Transactions of the Royal Society of Tropical Medicine and Hygiene,* 50:511–515.

731. WALTERS, J. H. and LEHMANN, H. (1956) Distribution of the S and C haemoglobin variants in two Nigerian communities. *Transactions of the Royal Society of Tropical Medicine and Hygiene,* 50:204–208.

732. WARREN, M. and WHARTON, R. H. (1963) The vectors of simian malaria: identity, biology, and geographical distribution. *Journal of Parasitology*, 49:892–904.

733. WATSON, J., STAHMAN, A. W., and BILELLO, F. P. (1948) The significance of the paucity of sickle cells in newborn Negro infants. *American Journal of Medical Sciences*, 215:419–423.

734. WATSON-WILLIAMS, E. J. (1965) Hereditary persistence of foetal haemoglobin and β-thalassaemia in Nigerians. In J. H. P. Jonxis (Ed.), *Abnormal Haemoglobins in Africa*. F. A. Davis, Philadelphia. Pp. 233–248.

735. WATSON-WILLIAMS, E. J., BEALE, D., IRVINE, D., and LEHMANN, H. (1965) A new haemoglobin, D Ibadan (β-87 threonine → lysine), producing no sickle-cell haemoglobin D disease with haemoglobin S. *Nature*, 205:1273–1276.

736. WEATHERALL, D. J. (1963) Abnormal haemoglobins in the neonatal period and their relationship to thalassaemia. *British Journal of Haematology*, 9:265–277.

737. WEATHERALL, D. J. (1964) Hemoglobin $J_{Baltimore}$ coexisting in a family with hemoglobin S. *Bulletin of the Johns Hopkins Hospital*, 114:1–12.

738. WEATHERALL, D. J., CLEGG, J. B., and NAUGHTON, M. A. (1965) Globin synthesis in thalassaemia: an in vitro study. *Nature*, 208:1061–1065.

738a. WEISMAN, A. I. (1966) Syphilis: was it endemic in pre-Columbian America or was it brought here from Europe? *Bulletin of the New York Academy of Medicine*, 42:284–300.

739. WEISS, W. and STECHER, W. (1952) Tuberculosis and the sickle-cell trait. *Archives of Internal Medicine*, 89:914–922.

740. WENT, L. N. (1957) Incidence of abnormal haemoglobins in Jamaica. *Nature*, 180:1131–1132.

741. WENT, L. N. and MACIVER, J. E. (1961) Thalassemia in the West Indies. *Blood*, 17:166–181.

741a. WHALLEY, P. J., PRITCHARD, J. A., and RICHARDS, J. R. (1963) Sickle cell trait and pregnancy. *Journal of the American Medical Association*, 186:1132–1135.

742. WHARTON, R. H., LAING, A. B. G., and CHEONG, W. H. (1963) Studies on the distribution and transmission of malaria and filariasis among Aborigines in Malaya. *Annals of Tropical Medicine and Parasitology*, 57:235–254.

743. WICKREMASINGHE, R. L., IKIN, E. W., MOURANT, A. E., and LEHMANN, H. (1963) The blood groups and haemoglobins of the Veddahs of Ceylon. *Journal of the Royal Anthropological Institute of Great Britain and Ireland*, 93:117–125.

744. WICKREMASINGHE, R. L. and PONNUSWAMY, N. E. L. (1963) Blood groups and haemoglobin types of Ceylonese. *Spolia Zeylanica (Bulletin of the National Museum of Ceylon)*, 30:149–154.

744a. WILSON, D. B., GARNHAM, P. C. C., and SWELLENGREBEL, N. H. (1950) A review of hyperendemic malaria. *Tropical Diseases Bulletin*, 47:677–698.

745. WOLFF, A. E. (1939) Sicklemia en sickle cell anemia (?) in Suriname. *Acta Leidensia*, 14:288–300.

746. WOLLSTEIN, M. and KREIDEL, K. V. (1928) Sickle cell anemia. *American Journal of Diseases of Children*, 36:998–1011.

746a. WONG HOCK BOON (1966) Viral hepatitis in G-6-P.D. deficiency. *Lancet* 1:882–883.

747. YAMAOKA, K. (1961) Studies on hemoglobinopathies observed in Japan. *Proceedings of the 8th International Congress of the International Society of Hematology* (Tokyo, 1960). Pan-Pacific Press, Tokyo. 2:1056–1063.

748. YUE, P. C. K. and STRICKLAND, M. (1965) Glucose-6-phosphate dehydrogenase deficiency and neonatal jaundice in Chinese male infants in Hong Kong. *Lancet,* 1:350–351.

749. YUSHKEVISH, L. B. and TSIRKINA, A. S. (1963) O znachenii geneticheskikh faktorov pri talassemii. *Problemy Gematologii i Perelivaniya Krovi,* 8:30–33.

750. ZANNOS-MARIOLEA, L. and KATTAMIS, C. (1961) Glucose-6-phosphate dehydrogenase deficiency in Greece. *Blood,* 18:34–47.

751. ZOUTENDYK, A. (1955) The blood groups of South African natives with particular reference to a recent investigation of the Hottentots. *Proceedings of the 5th International Congress of Blood Transfusion (Paris),* pp. 247–249.

752. ZOUTENDYK, A., KOPEC, A. C., and MOURANT, A. E. (1953) The blood groups of the Bushmen. *American Journal of Physical Anthropology,* 11:361–368.

753. ZUCKERKANDL, E. (1965) The evolution of hemoglobin. *Scientific American,* 212:110–118.

754. ZUCKERKANDL, E. and PAULING, L. (1965) Divergence and convergence in proteins. In V. Bryson and H. J. Vogel (Eds.), *Evolving Genes and Proteins.* Academic Press, New York. Pp. 99–166.

755. DEZULUETA, J. (1956) Malaria in Sarawak and Brunei. *Bulletin of the World Health Organization,* 15:651–671.

756. DEACQUATELLA, G. C. (1966) Glucose-6-phosphate dehydrogenase deficiency in different groups of Venezuela. *Acta Cientifica Venezolana,* 17:127.

757. BANK, A. and MARKS, P. A. (1966) Protein synthesis in a cell free human reticulocyte system: Ribosome function in thalassemia. *Journal of Clinical Investigations,* 45:330–336.

758. BEIGUELMAN, B., PINTO, W., DALL'AGLIO, F. F., DA SILVA, E., and VOZZA, J. (1966) Deficiência de desidrogenase de 6-fosfato de glicose (G-6-PD) e lepra. *Ciência e Cultura,* 18:95–96.

759. BONSIGNORE, A., FORNAINI, G., LEONCINI, G., and FANTONI, A. (1966) Electrophoretic heterogeneity of erythrocyte and leukocyte glucose-6-phosphate dehydrogenase in Italians from various ethnic groups. *Nature,* 211:876–878.

760. BOTHA, M. C., BEALE, D., ISAACS, W. A., and LEHMANN, H. (1966) Haemoglobin J Cape Town—α_2 92 Arginine → Glutamine β_2. *Nature,* 212:792–795.

761. BOWMAN, B. H., BARNETT, D. R., HODGKINSON, K. T., and SCHNEIDER, R. G. (1966) Chemical characterization of haemoglobin $G_{St.\text{-}L.}$. *Nature,* 211:1305–1306.

762. CAÑIZARES-PROAÑO, C. and VARELA-TORRES, R. (1965) Hemoglobin UNAM. Una nueva hemoglobina anormal. I. Estudio de identificación. *Boletín del Instituto de Estudios Medicos y Biologicos (Mexico City),* 23:75–87.

763. CHAN, T. K. (1966) Glucose-6-phosphate dehydrogenase in West Scotland. *Lancet,* 2:752.

764. DERN, R. J. (1966) A new hereditary quantitative variant of glucose-6-phosphate dehydrogenase characterized by a marked increase in

enzyme activity. *Journal of Laboratory and Clinical Medicine,* 68:560–565.

765. DOBBS, N. B., SIMMONS, J. W., WILSON, J. B., and HUISMAN, T. H. J. (1966) Hemoglobin Jenkins or Hemoglobin-N-Baltimore or $a_2\beta_2^{95glu}$ (BBA 23216). *Biochimica et Biophysica Acta,* 117:492–494.

766. GILES, E., CURTAIN, C. C., and BAUMGARTEN, A. (1966) Personal communication.

767. IFEKWUNIGWE, A. E. and LUZZATTO, L. (1966) Kernicterus in G-6-PD deficiency. *Lancet,* 1:667.

768. JONES, R. T., BRIMHALL, B., HUISMAN, T. H. J., KLEIHAUER, E., and BETKE, K. (1966) Hemoglobin Freiburg: abnormal hemoglobin due to deletion of a single amino acid residue. *Science,* 154:1024–1027.

769. KELLY, S. and ALMY, R. (1966) Glucose-6-phosphate dehydrogenase deficiency in Project Head Start children. *Public Health Reports,* 81:794–796.

770. KIRKMAN, H. N., DOXIADIS, S. A., VALAES, T., TASSOPOULOS, N., and BRINSON, A. G. (1965) Diverse characteristics of glucose-6-phosphate dehydrogenase from Greek children. *Journal of Laboratory and Clinical Medicine,* 65:212–221.

771. LABIE, D., SCHROEDER, W. A., and HUISMAN, T. H. J. (1966) The amino acid sequence of the δ-β chains of hemoglobin $\text{Lepore}_{\text{Augusta}}$ = $\text{Lepore}_{\text{Washington}}$. *Biochimica et Biophysica Acta,* 127:428–437.

772. LEWGOY, F. and SALZANO, F. M. (1966) Personal communication.

773. MATSON, G. A., SWANSON, J., and ROBINSON, A. (1966) Distribution of hereditary blood groups among Indians in South America. III. In Bolivia. *American Journal of Physical Anthropology,* 25:13–33.

774. MIYAJI, T., SUZUKI, H., OHBA, Y., and SHIBATA, S. (1966) Hemoglobin Agenogi ($\alpha_2\beta_2^{\text{Lys}}$), a slow moving hemoglobin of a Japanese family resembling HB-E. *Clinica Chimica Acta,* 14:624–629.

775. RESTREPO MARTIN, A. (1966) Frequency of abnormal hemoglobins in Colombia. *Acta Cientifica Venezolana,* 17:113–116.

776. RONALD, A. R., *et al.* (1966) Primaquine-sensitive haemolytic anaemia in West Pakistan. *Pakistan Journal of Medical Research,* 5:5–14.

777. VECCHIO, F., SCHETTINI, F., DIFRANCESCO, L., MELONI, T., and RUSSINO, G. (1966) Electrophoretic studies of erythrocyte glucose-6-phosphate dehydrogenase in normal and enzyme-deficient Sardinian subjects. *Acta Haematologica,* 35:46–51.

778. VENTRUTO, V., BAGLIONI, C., DEROSA, L., BIANCHI, P., COLOMBO, B., and QUATTRIN, N. (1965) Haemoglobin Caserta: an abnormal haemoglobin observed in a southern Italian family. *Scandinavian Journal of Haematology,* 2:118–125.

779. CABANNES, R. and SCHMIDT-BEURRIER, A. (1966) Recherches sur les hémoglobines des populations indiennes de l'Amerique du Sud. *L'Anthropologie,* 70:331–334.

780. DOEBLIN, T. and PINKERTON, P. H. (1966) Personal communication.

781. MOTULSKY, A. G., VANDEPITTE, J., and FRASER, G. R. (1966) Population genetic studies in the Congo. I. Glucose-6-phosphate dehydrogenase deficiency, hemoglobin S, and malaria. *American Journal of Human Genetics,* 18:514–537.

782. SHAKER, Y., ONSI, A., and AZIZ, R. (1966) The frequency of glucose-6-phosphate dehydrogenase deficiency in the newborns and adults in Kuwait. *American Journal of Human Genetics,* 18:609–613.

APPENDIX: THE FREQUENCIES OF THE RED CELL DEFECTS IN HUMAN POPULATIONS

The studies summarized in this appendix employed a great diversity of techniques, making it difficult to compare their results or to compile them on a standard table. This difficulty is particularly pronounced for the hemoglobin and thalassemia data. For the G6PD deficiency frequencies, the vast majority are based on Motulsky and Campbell-Kraut's (494a) dye test, although the methemoglobin reduction test of Brewer et al. (117a) is becoming prevalent. Male deficients are almost invariably detected with both these tests, so that the results for males are very comparable. For females, however, the number of heterozygotes detected does seem to differ. A few earlier studies used Beutler's (79) glutathione instability test, which is more difficult but does detect most male deficients. Where no studies with these tests have been done, the sex ratio of favism cases has been used to compute the frequency of the G6PD deficiency. These frequencies are surely not very accurate and in the future will be replaced by studies using the other tests. The frequencies recorded in the sickle-cell column were done by either the older sealed wet preparations with no artificial reducing agent, or by the newer methods that use some reducing agent such as sodium metabisulfite. In any case most variations on these two tests are extremely accurate; all results in this column should be comparable.

For the detection of β-thalassemia the most accurate method seems to be the measurement of the A_2 hemoglobin component, and all frequencies recorded in the A_2 column are reports of an elevation in this hemoglobin component. The most accurate method is starch block electrophoresis (276a), but the critical percentage point between normal and elevated is not the same for all studies. In addition, many have used some type of screening technique in which all samples are run on paper or starch gel electrophoresis, and those suspected of having an elevated A_2 hemoglobin component are checked on starch block electrophoresis. Furthermore, some of the frequencies recorded in this column are based simply on starch gel electrophoresis. Thus, the frequencies in this column are rather heterogeneous, but they should provide minimum estimates of the amount of β-thalassemia. For some populations many persons with a β-thalassemia gene do not seem to have an elevated A_2 fraction, so that this is indeed a minimum estimate. The F column is likewise a compilation of studies using diverse techniques. An elevated amount of fetal hemoglobin (hemoglobin F) is most easily and accurately determined by the alkali denaturation test of Singer et al. (639a), although various kinds of electrophoretic techniques will also detect fetal hemoglobin. However, an only slightly elevated amount is difficult to detect on paper. Since many of the frequencies in the F column are based solely on paper electrophoresis, they are estimates of genetic conditions with very appreciable amounts of fetal hemoglobin.

While the A_2 and F columns are estimates of β-thalassemia, the third column, Osm. Res., includes studies which estimate both α and β-thalassemias. The great majority of these frequencies are based on the osmotic resistance of the red cells in hypotonic salt solution. This property of the red cell is mostly a function of their size and shape, and persons with microcitemia have much more resistant cells. Hence the few frequencies based on red cell morphology estimate the same characteristic. While the other two columns are minimum estimates of thalassemia, the Osm. Res. column is closer to a maximum estimate, since there are many environmental conditions that can cause microcitemia.

The hemoglobin columns are self-explanatory. With the exceptions of the few estimates of the frequency of Barts hemoglobin, which is a variant of fetal hemoglobin, or of hemoglobin B_2, which is an A_2 variant, all of the hemoglobin frequencies are of variants of normal adult hemoglobin. When studies have found no abnormal variants, the number with hemoglobin A is recorded; otherwise only the numbers of individuals with abnormal hemoglobin genotypes are indicated.

Most of the population samples seem to be close to randomly determined. But there are many studies that include members of the same family. Only where this selection seemed to affect the results very significantly is it indicated. In addition, a great many of the studies are based on hospital patients or outpatient clinic visitors. When the patients were selected because they had a particular disease, this disease is indicated. Or when the patients most likely to have an abnormal hemoglobin (such as those with anemia) were selected, the sample is shown as patients. This is a definite bias for many of the studies, but an examination of the frequencies for hospital patients and other individuals in the same population, where these are available, does not seem to indicate as much discrepancy or difference as might be expected.

No attempt to calculate gene frequencies has been made, since each study seemed to have its own special problems. The percentage of individuals with the trait or abnormal hemoglobin has been computed. Although this includes both presumed homozygotes and heterozygotes for any abnormal hemoglobin, one-half of this percentage is a rough estimate of the gene frequency. The percentage for any particular abnormal hemoglobin is centered in parentheses in the column containing individuals with both the abnormal and normal hemoglobin. In some studies only the "number with" an abnormal hemoglobin is recorded with no indication of whether some have only the abnormal hemoglobin and others a mixture of normal and abnormal hemoglobin. In this case the number with an abnormal hemoglobin is shown in square brackets. In other cases the number of individuals tested is not given, so that only percentages in parentheses are shown in the appropriate columns. When both A_2 and F hemoglobin fractions were determined, the percentage below these columns is of the number with either of these two fractions elevated. If the numbers in the two columns are added and the percentage of the total subtracted from this, the difference is the number of individuals with both the A_2 and F hemoglobin fractions elevated.

In compiling these tables a great many petty decisions had to be made in order to standardize the results of these many diverse investigations, and I hope these decisions did not distort the original data too badly. But before unexpected conclusions are drawn from these frequencies, the original sources should be consulted. I have attempted to consult the original sources for the data, but in a few cases this was not possible. In most cases the designations for the populations used in the original work are included in the tables, but some have been anglicized. When a more common name is used for the same group, as for example the tribes of Africa, this appears as the first citation with the original designation in parentheses. I have also attempted to include all published data for the frequencies of the abnormal hemoglobins, thalassemia, and the G6PD deficiency. I apologize to anyone who finds their data are missing. And since this is a continuing project, I would appreciate knowing of any such lacunae. In an attempt to keep the data as current as possible, several additions have been made during the publication of the book. The last group were too late to be alphabetized and appear in the back of the bibliography, and the inclusion of some in the major bibliography have resulted in slight departures from alphabetical order. But since the numbers of the bibliography entries are most important, this should not detract from the bibliography's utility.

REF.	POPULATION	PLACE	NUMBER TESTED	G6PD DEF.	SICKLE CELL	THALASSEMIA			HEMOGLOBIN TYPES							
						A_2	F	OSM. RES.								A
POLYNESIA																
299	Easter Islanders		183	0												
639	Easter Islanders		33		0											
	Tubuai Islanders		11		0											
	Mangareva Islanders		22		0											
	Rapaiti Islanders		17		0											
	Raivavae Islanders		6		0											
	Nukuhiva Islanders		23		0											
	Hivaoa Islander		1		0											
100	Tahitians		250		0											
215	North Cook Islanders		127													127
	South Cook Islanders		87													87
214a	South Cook Islanders	Atiu Island	100			0										100

REF.	POPULATION	PLACE	NUMBER TESTED	G6PD DEF.	SICKLE CELL	THALASSEMIA			HEMOGLOBIN TYPES							
						A_2	F	OSM. RES.	S	AS		AC				A
POLYNESIA (CONT.)																
214a	South Cook Islanders	Rarotonga	323			0										323
650	Maori (Tuhoe)	New Zealand	163													163
410	Maori	North Island New Zealand	92													92
707	Maori	New Zealand	85													85
649	Tongans	Tonga Islands	200													200
359	Puerto Ricans	Hawaii	138						1	3 (2.9)		1 (0.7)				
	Negroes	Hawaii	28							1 (3.6)						
	Japanese	Hawaii	889													889
	Portuguese	Hawaii	222													222
	Filipinos	Hawaii	190													190
	Hawaiians	Hawaii	157													157
	Chinese	Hawaii	152													152
	Koreans	Hawaii	51													51
	Caucasians	Hawaii	23													23
	Spaniards	Hawaii	19													19
	Mexicans	Hawaii	13													13

REF.	POPULATION	PLACE	NUMBER TESTED	G6PD DEF.	SICKLE CELL	THALASSEMIA			HEMOGLOBIN TYPES							
						A_2	F	OSM. RES.		AS		AE		AJ		A
POLYNESIA (CONT.)																
359	Samoans	Hawaii	11													11
	Italians	Hawaii	5													5
	Russians	Hawaii	3													3
	Guamanians	Hawaii	2													2
	Oriental-Caucasians	Hawaii	227													227
	Hawaiian-Caucasian-Orientals	Hawaii	868							4 (0.5)		2 (0.2)		1		
MICRONESIA																
214	Ellice Islanders		108													108
213	Gilbert Islanders		236													236
182	Marshall Islanders	Rongelap	308	0												308
376	Palau Islanders	Angaur	58M	5 (8.6)												
	Palau Islanders	Koror	24M	2 (8.3)												

REF.	POPULATION	PLACE	NUMBER TESTED	G6PD DEF.	SICKLE CELL	THALASSEMIA			HEMOGLOBIN TYPES							
						A_2	F	OSM. RES.								A
MICRONESIA (CONT.)																
376	Yap Islanders	Ifalik	34M	2 (5.9)												
	Ulithi Islanders		117M	0												
541	Chamorros	Guam	246M	1 (0.4)												
542a	Chamorros	Saipan	142	0		2 (1.4)										142
	Caroline Islanders	Saipan	144	0		0										144
540a	Trukese	Truk	78													78
	Trukese	Losap	70													70
	Trukese	Mortlocks Island	88													88
	Trukese	Pulap and Puluwat	48													48
	Trukese	Lamotrek and Satawal	73													73
MELANESIA																
211	New Hebrideans	Efate Island	200			0										200
212	Solomon Islanders	New Georgia, Simbo, Ganongga, and Kolombangara Islands	101			0										101

REF.	POPULATION	PLACE	NUMBER TESTED	G6PD DEF.	SICKLE CELL	THALASSEMIA A_2	THALASSEMIA F	THALASSEMIA OSM. RES.	HEMOGLOBIN TYPES							
										A Lepore						A
MELANESIA (CONT.)																
212	Solomon Islanders	Choiseul Island	24			0										24
	Solomon Islanders	Vella Lavella Island	30			0										30
	Solomon Islanders	Shortland, Treasury and Faure Islands	33			0										33
729	Solomon Islanders		39		0											
664	West Nakanai	New Britain	156		0											
	Bakovi	New Britain	45		0											
	Kambi	New Britain	38		0											
	Bulu	New Britain	17		0											
	Melanesians	New Britain	21		0											
195	Tolai	Gazelle Peninsula New Britain	154			6 (3.9)										
287	Tolai	Gazelle Peninsula New Britain	122M	1 (0.8)												
195	Sulka	Gazelle Peninsula New Britain	72			4 (5.6)				1						
287	Sulka	Gazelle Peninsula	102M	15 (14.7)												

REF.	POPULATION	PLACE	NUMBER TESTED	G6PD DEF.	SICKLE CELL	THALASSEMIA			HEMOGLOBIN TYPES							
						A_2	F	OSM. RES.								A
MELANESIA (CONT.)																
195	Baining	Gazelle Peninsula New Britain	52			3 (5.8)										
287	Baining	Gazelle Peninsula New Britain	108M	13 (12.0)												
195	Taulil	Gazelle Peninsula New Britain	39			3 (7.7)										
287	Taulil	Gazelle Peninsula New Britain	25M	1 (4.0)												
	Kilenge	New Britain	133M	10 (7.5)												
	Mansing	New Britain	27M	5 (18.5)												
	Arawe	New Britain	13M	3 (23.1)												
AUSTRALIA																
325	Aborigines	Queensland	72		0											
326	Aborigines	Mona-mona Queensland	55													55
	Aborigines	Daintree Queensland	55													55
	Aborigines	Yarrabah Queensland	56													56

REF.	POPULATION	PLACE	NUMBER TESTED	G6PD DEF.	SICKLE CELL	THALASSEMIA			HEMOGLOBIN TYPES							
						A_2	F	OSM. RES.								A
AUSTRALIA (CONT.)																
638	Aborigines	Western Australia	125		0											
126	Aborigines	Central Australia	100													100
	Aborigines	Northern Australia	123													123
	Caucasians		100													100
128	Aborigines	Edward River Cape York	88	0												
	Aborigines	Mitchell River Cape York	146	0												
	Aborigines	Lockhart River Cape York	27	0												
	Aborigines	Aurukun Cape York	76	0												
	Aborigines	Weipa Cape York	41	0												
	Aborigines	Wrotham Park Cape York	23	0												
	Aborigines	Alice Springs Central Australia	140	0												
	Aborigines	Port Hedland Western Australia	99	0												
	Aborigines	Marble Bar Western Australia	24	0												

REF.	POPULATION	PLACE	NUMBER TESTED	G6PD DEF.	SICKLE CELL	THALASSEMIA			HEMOGLOBIN TYPES							
						A_2	F	OSM. RES.		AE						
AUSTRALIA (CONT.)																
128	Aborigines	Nullagine Western Australia	58	0												
338	Greeks		308			21 (6.8)										
	Italians		445			9 (2.0)										
	Cypriots		23			2 (8.7)										
NEW GUINEA																
729	New Guineans	Port Moresby	161		0											
375	New Guineans	Port Moresby	39	1 (2.6)												
195	New Guineans	Port Moresby	?							1						
532	Papuans	Rigo District	95M	9 (9.5)												
	Papuans	Kerema District	97M	10 (10.3)												
	Papuans	Orokolo Kerema District	42M	0												
	Papuans	Milne Bay District	33M	3 (9.1)												
195	Bukawa	Markham River Valley	64			5 (7.8)										

REF.	POPULATION	PLACE	NUMBER TESTED	G6PD DEF.	SICKLE CELL	THALASSEMIA			HEMOGLOBIN TYPES							
						A_2	F	OSM. RES.								A
NEW GUINEA (CONT.)																
287	Bukawa	Markham River Valley	31M	9 (29.0)												
195	Wampur	Markham River Valley	64			1 (1.6)										64
287	Wampur	Markham River Valley	29M	6 (20.7)												
195	Mumeng	Markham River Valley	118			1 (0.8)										118
287	Mumeng	Markham River Valley	90M	3 (3.3)												
766	Melanesians	Labubutu, Markham River Valley	33M	6 (18.2)												
	Melanesians	Labubutu, Markham River Valley	72			12 (16.6)										
	Papuans	Tumbuna, Markham River Valley	105M	2 (1.9)												
	Papuans	Tumbuna, Markham River Valley	180			5 (2.8)										
	Papuans	Mamamban, Markham River Valley	47M	4 (8.5)												
	Papuans	Mamamban, Markham River Valley	100			9 (9.0)										

REF.	POPULATION	PLACE	NUMBER TESTED	G6PD DEF.	SICKLE CELL	THALASSEMIA A$_2$	THALASSEMIA F	THALASSEMIA OSM. RES.	HEMOGLOBIN TYPES								
NEW GUINEA (CONT.)																	
766	Melanesians	Wankum, Markham River Valley	96M	11 (11.4)													
	Melanesians	Wankum, Markham River Valley	150			0											
	Melanesians	Kaiapit, Markham River Valley	17M	2 (11.8)													
	Melanesians	Kaiapit, Markham River Valley	30			0											
	Melanesians	Sukurum-Dumlinan Markham Valley	17M	2 (11.8)													
	Melanesians	Sukurum-Dumlinan Markham Valley	35			8 (22.9)											
	Melanesians	Gnarowein, Markham River Valley	67M	1 (1.5)													
	Melanesians	Gnarowein, Markham Valley	105			0											
	Papuans	Binumarien Markham Valley	41M	1 (2.0)													
	Papuans	Binumarien Markham Valley	60			0											
	Melanesians	Tsile-Tsile Markham River Valley	53M	1 (1.9)													

REF.	POPULATION	PLACE	NUMBER TESTED	G6PD DEF.	SICKLE CELL	THALASSEMIA			HEMOGLOBIN TYPES							
						A_2	F	OSM. RES.								
NEW GUINEA (CONT.)																
766	Melanesians	Tsile-Tsile, Markham River Valley	78			10 (12.8)										
375	Papuans	Wewak	69	2 (2.9)												
195	Sause	Numboruan, Sepik River Valley	41			3 (7.3)										
287	Sause	Numboruan, Sepik River Valley	24M	1 (4.2)												
195	Sause	Marambanja, Sepik River Valley	40			3 (7.5)										
287	Sause	Marambanja, Sepik River Valley	31M	0												
195	Sause	Kiaruvu, Sepik River Valley	52			6 (11.5)										
287	Sause	Kiaruvu, Sepik River Valley	40M	1 (2.5)												
195	Sause	Kwaian, Sepik River Valley	46			2 (4.3)										
287	Sause	Kwaian, Sepik River Valley	44M	0												
195	Sause	Kuvari, Sepik River Valley	12			3 (25.0)										

REF.	POPULATION	PLACE	NUMBER TESTED	G6PD DEF.	SICKLE CELL	THALASSEMIA			HEMOGLOBIN TYPES							
						A_2	F	OSM. RES.								
NEW GUINEA (CONT.)																
287	Sause	Kuvari, Sepik River Valley	12M	0												
195	Sause	Ambukwon, Sepik River Valley	13			0										
287	Sause	Ambukwon, Sepik River Valley	14M	0												
195	Sause	Humburu, Sepik River Valley	22			0										
287	Sause	Humburu, Sepik River Valley	22M	0												
195	Sause	Winjuan, Sepik River Valley	24			2 (8.3)										
287	Sause	Winjuan, Sepik River Valley	24M	0												
195	Sause	Bukinera, Sepik River Valley	32			2 (6.3)										
287	Sause	Bukinera, Sepik River Valley	32M	1 (3.1)												
195	Sause	Buruan, Sepik River Valley	5			0										
287	Sause	Buruan, Sepik River Valley	5M	0												
195	Sause	Alisu, Sepik River Valley	42			4 (9.5)										

REF.	POPULATION	PLACE	NUMBER TESTED	G6PD DEF.	SICKLE CELL	THALASSEMIA			HEMOGLOBIN TYPES							
						A_2	F	OSM. RES.		A Lepore						A
NEW GUINEA (CONT.)																
287	Sause	Alisu, Sepik River Valley	41M	0												
195	Sause	Kumun, Sepik River Valley	34			2 (5.9)										
287	Sause	Kumun, Sepik River Valley	35M	0												
195	Sause	Sepik River Valley	354							1						
	Abelam	Kuminibus I, Sepik River Valley	62			1 (1.6)										
287	Abelam	Kuminibus I, Sepik River Valley	31M	1 (3.2)												
195	Abelam	Neligum, Sepik River Valley	51			1 (2.0)										
287	Abelam	Neligum, Sepik	18M	3 (16.7)												
195	Abelam	Sepik River Valley	113													113
729	Chimbu	Eastern Highlands	280		0											
195	Gadsup	Eastern Highlands	22			0										22

REF.	POPULATION	PLACE	NUMBER TESTED	G6PD DEF.	SICKLE CELL	THALASSEMIA			HEMOGLOBIN TYPES							
						A_2	F	OSM. RES.								A
NEW GUINEA (CONT.)																
287	Gadsup	Eastern Highlands	39M	0												
195	Kukukuku	Eastern Highlands	24			0										24
287	Kukukuku	Eastern Highlands	116M	0												
	Awa	Eastern Highlands	16M	0												
195	Tairora	Eastern Highlands	131			0										131
287	Tairora	Eastern Highlands	88M	1 (1.1)												
	Auyana	Eastern Highlands	40M	2 (5.0)												
195	Usurufa	Eastern Highlands	53			0										53
194	Usurufa	Eastern Highlands	1													1
	Yate	Eastern Highlands	3													3
287	Yate	Eastern Highlands	5M	0												
194	Fore	Eastern Highlands	75													75

REF.	POPULATION	PLACE	NUMBER TESTED	G6PD DEF.	SICKLE CELL	THALASSEMIA			HEMOGLOBIN TYPES							
						A_2	F	OSM. RES.								A
NEW GUINEA (CONT.)																
287	Fore	Eastern Highlands	39M	0												
195	Kamano	Eastern Highlands	4			0										4
194	Keiagana	Eastern Highlands	12													12
	Yagaria	Eastern Highlands	1													1
	Gimi	Eastern Highlands	11													11
195	Gimi	Eastern Highlands	4			0										4
195	Enga	Western Highlands	95			2 (2.1)										95
365	Papuans	West Irian	250													250
239	Papuans	Klamono West Irian	115		0											
287	Papuans	Asmat West Irian	18M	3 (16.7)												
	Papuans	Merauke West Irian	25M	2 (8.0)												
377	Dani	Mulia West Irian	69	0												

REF.	POPULATION	PLACE	NUMBER TESTED	G6PD DEF.	SICKLE CELL	THALASSEMIA			HEMOGLOBIN TYPES							
						A_2	F	OSM. RES.								
NEW GUINEA (CONT.)																
559	Papuans	Wor,Arso District West Irian	43M	14 (32.6)												
	Papuans	Kwini, Arso District West Irian	41M	2 (4.9)												
	Papuans	Arso, Arso District West Irian	119M	11 (9.2)												
	Papuans	Genjem Nimboran District West Irian	50M	1 (2.0)												
	Papuans	Benjom Nimboran District West Irian	57M	4 (7.0)												
	Papuans	Pobajin,Kwimeno Nimboran District West Irian	68M	5 (7.4)												
	Papuans	Imeno, Sarmai Nimboran District West Irian	71M	10 (14.1)												
	Papuans	Sarmi, Sarmi District West Irian	77M	5 (6.5)												
	Papuans	Bageisewar Sarmi District West Irian	79M	1 (1.3)												

REF.	POPULATION	PLACE	NUMBER TESTED	G6PD DEF.	SICKLE CELL	THALASSEMIA			HEMOGLOBIN TYPES							
						A_2	F	OSM. RES.								A
NEW GUINEA (CONT.)																
559	Papuans	Airmati Sarmi District West Irian	80M	3 (3.8)												
	New Guineans	Biak	114M	5 (4.4)												
	Dani Papuans	Bokondini West Irian	234M	5 (2.1)												
	Kapauka Papuans	Enarotali West Irian	222M	0												
PHILIPPINES																
153a	Filipino (Infants)	Manila	157	4 (2.5)												
492	Filipino Sailors	Seattle Washington	73													73
359	Filipinos	Hawaii	190													190
496	Filipinos	Alaska	112													112
729	Filipinos		52		0											
496	Filipinos	Manila	403			5	4 (1.2)	20 (5.0)								

REF.	POPULATION	PLACE	NUMBER TESTED	G6PD DEF.	SICKLE CELL	THALASSEMIA			HEMOGLOBIN TYPES							
						A_2	F	OSM. RES.		AE		AG				
PHILIPPINES (CONT.)																
496	Filipinos	Northern Luzon (Ilocos Norte, Ilocos Sur, La Union, Pangasinan, Mountain, Cagayan, Isabela, Neuva Ecija, Neuva Vizcaya, Zambales, Pampanga, Bataan, Tarlac, Bulacan)	169M	19 (11.2)												
	Filipinos	Manila	100M	5 (5.0)												
	Filipinos	Southern Luzon (Cavite, Batanga, Laguna, Rizal, Abbay, Camarines Norte, Camarines Sur, Sorsogon)	67M	1 (1.5)												
91a	Filipinos	Luzon	1709							10 (0.6)		1				
496	Filipinos	Central Philippines (Mindoro, Marinduque, Romblin, Capiz, Antique, Iloilo, Negros, Masbate, Leyte, Bohol, Cebu)	55M	2 (3.7)												
91a	Filipinos	Western Visayas	854							12 (1.4)						

REF.	POPULATION	PLACE	NUMBER TESTED	G6PD DEF.	SICKLE CELL	THALASSEMIA			HEMOGLOBIN TYPES							
						A_2	F	OSM. RES.		AE						A
PHILIPPINES (CONT.)																
496	Filipinos	Mindanao and Sulu (Misamis, Sulu, Zamboanga, Lanao, Bukidnon, Surigao, Davao)	16M	0												
INDONESIA																
365	Maluku (Ambon) Islanders		135													135
428	Maluku (Ambon) Islanders		295							1						
	Maluku Islanders		430							1 (0.2)						
527	Malaku (Ambon) Islanders		100M	3												
580a	Malaku (Ambon) Islanders		100M	2												
	Malaku Islanders		200M	5 (2.5)												
535	Timorese	Portuguese Timor	2213							5 (0.2)						
432	Indonesians	Djarkarta	368M	5 (1.4)												

REF.	POPULATION	PLACE	NUMBER TESTED	G6PD DEF.	SICKLE CELL	THALASSEMIA			HEMOGLOBIN TYPES							
						A_2	F	OSM. RES.		AE		AO		AJ		A
INDONESIA (CONT.)																
428	Buginese	Sulawesi (Celebes)	448							7 (1.6)		5 (1.1)				
	Makassarese	Sulawesi (Celebes)	134							3 (2.2)		3 (2.2)				
	Toradja	Sulawesi (Celebes)	77									1 (1.3)				
	Mandar	Sulawesi (Celebes)	54													54
	Gorontalo	Sulawesi (Celebes)	104									1 (1.0)				
	Menado	Sulawesi (Celebes)	186											1		
	Timorese	Indonesian Timor	52							6 (11.5)						
	Sumbawa Islanders		44							9 (20.5)						
	Sumba Islanders		26							5 (19.2)						
	Bali Islanders		219							8 (3.7)						
	Madurese	Madura	319							42 (13.2)						
	Javanese	East Java	500							23 (4.6)						

REF.	POPULATION	PLACE	NUMBER TESTED	G6PD DEF.	SICKLE CELL	THALASSEMIA			HEMOGLOBIN TYPES							
						A_2	F	OSM. RES.		AS		AE				A
INDONESIA (CONT.)																
428	Sundanese	West Java	2126									53 (2.5)				
	Sumatrans	Palembang	293									6 (2.0)				
	Minangkabau	Central Sumatra	235							1 (0.4)		5 (2.1)				
	Batak	Central Sumatra	98									3 (3.1)				
	Atjehnese	Northern Sumatra	38									3 (7.9)				
	Indonesians	Dajak Kalimantan (Borneo)	108													108
	Indonesians	Bandjar Kalimantan (Borneo)	23									1 (4.3)				
	Chinese	Djakarta	75													75
	Indonesian-Chinese	Djakarta	116							1 (0.9)		4 (3.4)				
	Indonesian-Dutch	Djakarta	20									1 (5.0)				

REF.	POPULATION	PLACE	NUMBER TESTED	G6PD DEF.	SICKLE CELL	THALASSEMIA			HEMOGLOBIN TYPES							
						A_2	F	OSM. RES.		AE						A
BORNEO																
179	Land Dyaks	Sarawak	101							1						
718	Land Dyaks	Sarawak	341													341
	Land Dyaks	Sarawak	442							1 (0.2)						
431	Land Dyaks	Sarawak	24M	0												
179	Sea Dyaks	Sarawak	85													85
718	Sea Dyaks	Sarawak	68													68
	Sea Dyaks	Sarawak	153													153
431	Sea Dyaks	Sarawak	80M	1 (1.3)												
	Iban	Sarawak	56M	3 (5.4)												
718	Malays	Sarawak	166							5 (3.0)						
431	Malays	Sarawak	95M	11 (11.6)												
718	Chinese	Sarawak	742							2 (0.3)						
431	Others	Sarawak	38M	0												
	Malays	Brunei	317M	20 (6.3)												

REF.	POPULATION	PLACE	NUMBER TESTED	G6PD DEF.	SICKLE CELL	THALASSEMIA			HEMOGLOBIN TYPES							
						A_2	F	OSM. RES.		AE						
BORNEO (CONT.)																
718	Muruts	Sabah	53							3 (5.7)						
431	Muruts	Sabah	33M	8 (24.2)												
	Kadazan	Sabah	165M	20 (12.1)												
	Bajan	Sabah	58M	2 (3.4)												
	Bisaya	Sabah	6M	1												
	Malays	Sabah	73M	3 (4.1)												
	Others	Sabah	63M	0												
MALAYA																
551	Negrito	Lanoh Perak River	34		0											
	Negrito	Jahai Perak River	119		0											
	Negrito	Kensui	15		0											
	Negrito	Kinta-Bong	10		0											
	Aboriginal Malay	Orang Darat	46		0											

REF.	POPULATION	PLACE	NUMBER TESTED	G6PD DEF.	SICKLE CELL	THALASSEMIA			HEMOGLOBIN TYPES							
						A_2	F	OSM. RES.	E	AE						
MALAYA (CONT.)																
430	Senoi	Semai	111						4	26 (27.0)						
	Senoi	Semai	181M	40 (22.1)												
	Senoi	Temiar	62						11	18 (46.8)						
	Senoi	Temiar	137M	25 (18.2)												
	Senoi	Temuan	37							3 (8.1)						
	Senoi	Temuan	114M	18 (15.8)												
	Senoi	Jahut	13M	3 (23.1)												
	Senoi	Jakun	4M	0												
	Senoi	Not Known	102M	12 (11.8)												
430	Senoi	Not Known	29						1	8						
416	Senoi	Not Known	3						—	1						
	Senoi	Not Known	32						1	9 (31.3)						

REF.	POPULATION	PLACE	NUMBER TESTED	G6PD DEF.	SICKLE CELL	THALASSEMIA			HEMOGLOBIN TYPES							
						A_2	F	OSM. RES.	E	AE						A
MALAYA (CONT.)																
707	Semelai	Fort Iskandar and Sinibai	41						1	12 (31.7)						
430	Aboriginal Malay	Semelai	29							6 (20.7)						
	Aboriginal Malay	Semelai	56M	9 (16.1)												
	Aboriginal Malay	Jakun	9													9
	Aboriginal Malay	Lanok	1													1
	Aboriginal Malay	Not Known	607M	103 (17.0)												
416	Malays	Kedah Province	33							1 (3.0)						
	Malays	Penang and Wellesley Provinces	26							2 (7.7)						
	Malays	Perak Province	25							2 (8.0)						
	Malays	Selangor Province	101							6 (5.9)						
	Malays	Negri-Sambilan Province	26													26

REF.	POPULATION	PLACE	NUMBER TESTED	G6PD DEF.	SICKLE CELL	THALASSEMIA A_2	THALASSEMIA F	THALASSEMIA OSM. RES.	HEMOGLOBIN TYPES E	AE		AD	AK	AJ		Barts
MALAYA (CONT.)																
701	Malays	Singapore	126M	0												
434	Malays	Malaya	353M	7												
	Malays		479M	7 (1.5)												
707	Malays	Malaya	4984						7	240 (5.0)		7	4	1		
	Malays	Penang Province	296							2 (0.7)			1			
	Malays	Kuala Lumpur	304							6 (2.0)						
	Malays	Malacca	52							2 (3.9)						
	Malays	Johore Bahru	651							44 (6.8)						
	Malays	Singapore	3681							158 (4.3)		6	3	1		
707	Malay (cord blood)	Malaya	162													2
433	Malay (cord blood)	Malaya	157													5
	Malay (cord blood)	Malaya	319													7 (2.2)
700	Malays	Malaya	15			0										

REF.	POPULATION	PLACE	NUMBER TESTED	G6PD DEF.	SICKLE CELL	THALASSEMIA			HEMOGLOBIN TYPES							
						A_2	F	OSM. RES.		AE	AD	AJ	AG	AQ		A
MALAYA (CONT.)																
416	Malays	Johore Province	21													21
	Malays	Malacca Province	7							1 (14.3)						
	Malays	Kelantan Province	78							8 (10.3)						
	Malays	Tiengganu Province	16							2 (12.5)						
	Malays	Pahang Province	13							4 (30.8)						
702	Chinese	Singapore	7101							17	1	2	1	2		
	Chinese	Johore Bahru	913							4		1				
	Chinese	Malacca	152							4						
	Chinese	Kuala	738							1						
	Chinese	Lumpur	103													103
	Chinese	Penang	566													566
	Chinese	Sarawak	458							1	—	—	—	1		
	Chinese	Malaysia	10031							27 (0.3)	1	3	1	3		

REF.	POPULATION	PLACE	NUMBER TESTED	G6PD DEF.	SICKLE CELL	THALASSEMIA A_2	THALASSEMIA F	THALASSEMIA OSM. RES.	HEMOGLOBIN TYPES		HEMOGLOBIN TYPES		HEMOGLOBIN TYPES				
										AE		AD	AJ	AK	AL	Barts
MALAYA (CONT.)																
707	Chinese (cord blood)	Malaya	1962													63
433	Chinese (cord blood)	Malaya	592													30
	Chinese (cord blood)	Malaya	2554													93 (3.6)
700	Chinese	Malaya	32			3 (9.4)										
434	Chinese	Malaya	212M	5												
701	Chinese	Malaya	225M	5												
	Chinese	Malaya	437M	10 (2.3)												
707	Indians	Penang	421							2				1		
	Indians	Kuala Lumpur	448							5		1			1	
	Indians	Johore Bahru	320									3				
	Indians	Singapore	2117							8		11	1	4	1	
	Indians	Malaya	3341							15 (0.4)		15 (0.4)	1	5	2	
700	Indians	Malaya	17			0										

REF.	POPULATION	PLACE	NUMBER TESTED	G6PD DEF.	SICKLE CELL	THALASSEMIA			HEMOGLOBIN TYPES							
						A_2	F	OSM. RES.		AE			AJ			Barts
MALAYA (CONT.)																
707	Indians (cord blood)	Malaya	222													2
433	Indians (cord blood)	Malaya	278													3
	Indians (cord blood)	Malaya	500													5 (1.0)
701	Indians	Malaya	92M	3												
434	Indians	Malaya	206M	2												
	Indians	Malaya	298M	5 (1.7)												
707	Europeans	Malaya	4153							4			1			
700	Europeans	Malaya	16			0										
701	Europeans	Malaya	76M	0												
707	Europeans (cord blood)	Malaya	142													1 (0.7)
701	Sephardic Jews	Singapore	15M	6 (40.0)												
707	Eurasians	Malaya	710							11 (1.5)						
434	Eurasians	Malaya	22M	0												

REF.	POPULATION	PLACE	NUMBER TESTED	G6PD DEF.	SICKLE CELL	THALASSEMIA			HEMOGLOBIN TYPES							
						A_2	F	OSM. RES.	E	AE						A
BURMA																
417	Burmese Students	London	80						2	12 (17.5)						
82	Burmese		2	0												
47	Burmese		?							(28.0)						
THAILAND																
501	Chinese	Bangkok	213													213
251	South Chinese	Thailand	66			3 (24.2)	13									
252	South Chinese	Thailand	66													66
254	South Chinese	Thailand	62M	2 (3.2)												
	South Chinese	Thailand	68F	3 (4.4)												
251	Thai	Urban Bangkok	149			4 (6.0)	5									
252	Thai	Urban Bangkok	149						1	14 (10.1)						
251	Thai	Rural Bangkok	135			4 (10.4)	10									
252	Thai	Rural Bangkok	121						1	21 (18.2)						

REF.	POPULATION	PLACE	NUMBER TESTED	G6PD DEF.	SICKLE CELL	THALASSEMIA A_2	THALASSEMIA F	THALASSEMIA OSM. RES.	HEMOGLOBIN TYPES E	AE						
THAILAND (CONT.)																
254	Thai	Central Thailand	628M	61 (9.7)												
	Thai	Central Thailand	26F	4 (15.4)												
501	Thai	Central Thailand	554							74 (13.4)						
	Thai	South Thailand	126							16 (12.7)						
659	Thai	Hard-Yai, South Thailand	333						[30]	(9.0)						
252	Thai	Nakorn Sawan Province Central Thailand	93			2 (2.2)			1	18 (20.4)						
	Thai	Pisanulok District	106			4 (3.8)			1	18 (17.9)						
253	Thai	Hill Areas Pisanulok District	219						9	66 (34.2)						
	Thai	Plains Areas Pisanulok District	417						6	68 (17.7)						
	Thai	Hill Areas Lamphun and Chiengmai Districts Northern Thailand	374						1	45 (12.3)						

REF.	POPULATION	PLACE	NUMBER TESTED	G6PD DEF.	SICKLE CELL	THALASSEMIA A_2	THALASSEMIA F	THALASSEMIA OSM. RES.	HEMOGLOBIN TYPES E	AE						
THAILAND (CONT.)																
253	Thai	Plains Areas Lamphun and Chiengmai Districts	487							39 (8.0)						
501	Thai	North Thailand	99							8 (8.1)						
254	Thai	North Thailand	821M	129 (15.7)												
	Thai	North Thailand	106F	24 (22.6)												
251	Thai (Pregnant)	Chiengmai Province	131F			5	27 (24.4)									
252	Thai (Pregnant)	Chiengmai Province	131F							9 (6.9)						
659	Thai	Chiengmai Province	352						1	23 (6.8)						
252	Thai	Chiengmai City	119M			11 (9.2)			1	13 (11.8)						
	Thai	Chiengdao and Fang, Chiengmai Province	110			5 (4.5)				13 (11.8)						
	Thai	Doi Saked District Chiengmai Province	159			7 (4.4)				11 (6.9)						

REF.	POPULATION	PLACE	NUMBER TESTED	G6PD DEF.	SICKLE CELL	THALASSEMIA			HEMOGLOBIN TYPES						
						A_2	F	OSM. RES.	E	AE					
THAILAND (CONT.)															
252	Thai	Sanpatong and Hod, Chiengmai Province	219			12 (5.5)			1	21 (10.0)					
	Thai	Lamphun Province	225			17 (7.6)				17 (7.6)					
659	Thai	Lampoon Province	102				2			8 (7.8)					
252	Thai	Chiengrai Province	32			2 (6.3)				3 (9.4)					
659	Thai	Chiengrai Province	125							4 (3.2)					
251	Thai	Chiengmai Province	607			34 (9.7)	25								
	Thai	Lamphun and Chiengmai Provinces	225			17 (20.9)	30								
659	Thai	Lampang Province	53							6 (11.3)					
	Thai	Prae Province	30							7 (23.3)					
	Thai	Narn Province	39							4 (10.3)					
254	Thai Yong	Lamphun Province	134M	15 (11.2)											

REF.	POPULATION	PLACE	NUMBER TESTED	G6PD DEF.	SICKLE CELL	THALASSEMIA			HEMOGLOBIN TYPES							
						A_2	F	OSM. RES.		AE						A
THAILAND (CONT.)																
254	Thai Yong	Lamphun Province	84F	17 (20.2)												
252	Thai Yong	Lamphun Province	166			15 (9.0)										166
254	Thai Lue	North Thailand	57M	7 (12.3)												
	Thai Lue	North Thailand	15F	2 (13.3)												
	Thai Ya	Chiengrai Province	45M	9 (20.0)												
	Thai Ya	Chiengrai Province	15F	5 (33.3)												
252	Thai Lue Thai Ya and Thai Kuen	North Thailand	122			9 (7.4)										122
251	Thai Yong Thai Ya and Thai Lue	North Thailand	288			24	20 (15.3)									
254	Mon	Lamphun Province	31M	4 (12.9)												
	Mon	Lamphun Province	58F	16 (27.6)												
252	Mon	Lamphun Province	89			3 (3.4)				12 (13.5)						

REF.	POPULATION	PLACE	NUMBER TESTED	G6PD DEF.	SICKLE CELL	THALASSEMIA			HEMOGLOBIN TYPES							
						A_2	F	OSM. RES.	E	AE						A
THAILAND (CONT.)																
254	Lawa	Chiengmai Province	106M	4 (3.8)												
	Lawa	Chiengmai Province	24F	2 (8.3)												
252	Lawa	Chiengmai Province	75			5 (6.7)				2 (2.7)						
	Mrabri	North Thailand	18			1 (5.6)				6 (33.3)						
251	Mon-Khmer and Mon-Lawa	North Thailand	171			7 (10.5)	11									
254	Lahu	North Thailand	52M	1 (1.9)												
	Lahu	North Thailand	9F	0												
	Lissu	North Thailand	37M	1 (2.7)												
	Lissu	North Thailand	4F	0												
251	Lahu and Lissu	North Thailand	111			10 (13.5)	5									
252	Lahu and Lissu	North Thailand	61													61
254	Karen	North Thailand	24M	3 (12.5)												
	Karen	North Thailand	13F	1 (7.7)												

REF.	POPULATION	PLACE	NUMBER TESTED	G6PD DEF.	SICKLE CELL	THALASSEMIA A_2	THALASSEMIA F	THALASSEMIA OSM. RES.	HEMOGLOBIN TYPES E	AE						A
THAILAND (CONT.)																
254	Miao (Hmung)	North Thailand	102M	0												
	Miao (Hmung)	North Thailand	21F	0												
251	Miao (Hmung)	North Thailand	62			6	5 (17.7)									
252	Miao (Hmung)	North Thailand	62													62
659	Thai	Utaradit Province	38							7 (18.4)						
660	Thai	Tark Province	100						[20]	(20.0)						
	Thai	Sukothai Province	123						[20]	(16.3)						
	Thai	Pichit Province	145						[31]	(21.4)						
	Thai	Phetchaboon Province	91						[19]	(20.9)						
501	Thai	Northeast Thailand	49							16 (32.7)						
254	Thai	Northeast Thailand	784M	109 (13.9)												
658	Thai	Srisaket Province	44						6	10 (36.4)						
	Thai	Other Provinces Northeast Thailand	18						3	5 (44.4)						

REF.	POPULATION	PLACE	NUMBER TESTED	G6PD DEF.	SICKLE CELL	THALASSEMIA			HEMOGLOBIN TYPES							
						A_2	F	OSM. RES.	E	AE						
THAILAND (CONT.)																
251	Thai	Udon and Konkaen Provinces	88			5 (6.8)	1									
252	Thai	Udon and Konkaen Provinces	88						4	31 (39.8)						
660	Vietnamese	Ubol Province	49						[5]	(10.2)						
251	Thai	Ubol Province	130			3 (6.2)	5									
658	Thai	Ubol Province	324						16	104						
252	Thai	Ubol Province	130						10	45						
	Thai	Ubol Province	454						26	149 (38.5)						
660	Khmer	Surin Province	103						[37]	(35.9)						
251	Khmer	Surin Province	138			1 (0.7)										
252	Khmer	Surin Province	133						8	71 (59.4)						
254	Khmer and Suay	Surin Province	174M	29 (16.7)												
	Khmer and Suay	Surin Province	80F	22 (27.5)												

REF.	POPULATION	PLACE	NUMBER TESTED	G6PD DEF.	SICKLE CELL	THALASSEMIA			HEMOGLOBIN TYPES							
						A_2	F	OSM. RES.	E	AE		AJ	JE	JD		Barts
THAILAND (CONT.)																
658	Thai	Surin Province	11						1	5						
252	Thai	Surin Province	<u>151</u>						<u>12</u>	<u>69</u>						
	Thai	Surin Province	162						13	74 (53.7)						
251	Thai	Surin Province	125			2 (3.2)	2									
671	Thai Soldiers	Korat Province	662						39	242 (42.4)		1				
90a	Thai Soldiers	Korat Province	1923							?		6	2	1		
251	Thai Soldiers		188			15 (10.1)	4			18 (9.6)						
	Thai	Nakhon Ratchasima Korat Province	180			3 (6.1)	8									
252	Thai	Nakhon Ratchasima Korat Province	180						7	63 (38.9)						
501	Thai	Southeast Thailand	48							9 (18.8)						
391	Thai	Rayong Province	412						[93]	(22.6)						
389	Thai	Rayong Province	243M	37 (15.2)												
692	Thai (cord blood)	Thailand	414													21 (5.1)

REF.	POPULATION	PLACE	NUMBER TESTED	G6PD DEF.	SICKLE CELL	THALASSEMIA			HEMOGLOBIN TYPES							
						A_2	F	OSM. RES.	E	AE						A
LAOS																
57	Vietnamese	Laos	100							7 (7.0)						
	Chinese	Laos	72													72
	Meo-Yao	Xieng-Kouang Hills	159													159
	Phon-Theng (Khas)	Thamou, Luang Prabang	130						1	21 (16.9)						
	Phon-Theng (Khas)	Kha Tahoy Saravane	41						4	15 (46.3)						
	Thai Lao	Haut Mekong	10							1 (10.0)						
	Thai Lao	Luang Prabang	93						[23]	(24.7)						
	Thai Lao	Houa Phan	11							1						
	Thai Lao	Xieng Kouang	7													7
	Thai Lao	Sayaboury	33						[16]	(48.5)						
	Thai Lao	Vientiane	376						[104]	(27.7)						
	Thai Lao	Borikhane	29						[9]	(31.0)						
	Thai Lao	Khammovane	38						[17]	(44.7)						

REF.	POPULATION	PLACE	NUMBER TESTED	G6PD DEF.	SICKLE CELL	THALASSEMIA			HEMOGLOBIN TYPES							
						A_2	F	OSM. RES.	E	AE						
LAOS (CONT.)																
57	Thai Lao	Savannakhet	139						[66]	(47.5)						
	Thai Lao	Saravane	23						[11]	(47.8)						
	Thai Lao	Wapi Khanthong	7						[5]							
	Thai Lao	Sedone	42						[14]	(33.3)						
	Thai Lao	Champassac	25						[12]	(48.0)						
	Thai Lao	Attopeu	21						[5]	(23.8)						
	Thai Lao	Sthandone	15						[5]	(33.3)						
CAMBODIA																
311	Cambodian Students	Paris	100							12 (12.0)						
120	Cambodians	Pnom-Penh	69						2	18 (29.0)						
118a	Moi Khas	Pnom-Penh	10							5						
	Moi Phnong	Pnom-Penh	10						1	5						
119	Cambodians	Kandal Province	220						14	64 (35.5)						

REF.	POPULATION	PLACE	NUMBER TESTED	G6PD DEF.	SICKLE CELL	THALASSEMIA			HEMOGLOBIN TYPES							
						A_2	F	OSM. RES.	E	AE						
CAMBODIA (CONT.)																
119	Cambodians	Takeo Province	94						4	26 (31.9)						
	Cambodians	Prey-Veng Province	43						2	14 (37.2)						
	Cambodians	Kompong-Cham Province	50						1	15 (32.0)						
	Cambodians	Kompong-Speu Province	50						3	15 (36.0)						
	Cambodians	Srai Rieng Province	54						1	11 (22.2)						
	Cambodians	Kampot Province	32						3	6 (28.1)						
	Cambodians	Kompong-Chuang Province	11							5 (45.5)						
	Cambodians	Kompong-Thom Province	15							1 (6.7)						
	Cambodians	Battambang Province	18							4 (22.2)						
	Cambodians	Siem-Reap Province	6							2						
	Cambodians	Pursat Province	9						1	3						
	Cambodians	Kratie Province	3							2						
	Cambodians	Stung-Treng Province	27						1	11 (44.4)						

REF.	POPULATION	PLACE	NUMBER TESTED	G6PD DEF.	SICKLE CELL	THALASSEMIA			HEMOGLOBIN TYPES							
						A_2	F	OSM. RES.	E	AE		AQ				
VIETNAM																
15	Vietnamese	South Vietnam	113							3 (2.7)		20 (17.7)				
94	South Vietnamese	Saigon	482							17 (3.5)						
685	Vietnamese	South Vietnam	255			4 (1.6)			[21]	(8.2)						
	Vietnamese	Central Vietnam	43			0			[1]	(2.3)						
36a	Vietnamese	Hoa Vang District DaNang Province	127							4 (3.1)						
685	Vietnamese	North Vietnam	161			3 (1.9)			[5]	(3.1)						
CHINA																
82	Chinese		41M	0												
	Chinese		36F	0												
154	Chinese	Kwantung Province	200M	11 (5.5)												
495	Chinese	Fukien Province	300M	9 (3.0)												
748	Chinese (cord blood)	Hong Kong	1177M	44 (3.7)												

REF.	POPULATION	PLACE	NUMBER TESTED	G6PD DEF.	SICKLE CELL	THALASSEMIA A$_2$	THALASSEMIA F	THALASSEMIA OSM. RES.	HEMOGLOBIN TYPES	AE		AD				A
CHINA (CONT.)																
93	Chinese	Kwangtung Province	190													190
	Chinese	Fukien Province	225													225
495	Chinese	Fukien Province	300			9 (3.0)		28 (9.3)								
93	Chinese	Szechuan Province	51													51
	Chinese	Yunnan Province	472							3 (0.6)						
	Chinese	Hunan Province	140													140
	Chinese	Kiangsi Province	75													75
	Chinese	Chekiang	279													279
	Chinese	Anhwei Province	88													88
	Chinese	Hupei Province	84							2 (2.4)						
	Chinese	Kiangsu Province	344													344
	Chinese	Honan Province	67									1				
	Chinese	Shantung Province	113													113
	Chinese	Hopei Province	111													111
	Chinese	Liaoning Province	36													36
471	Chinese	Canton	1000's					(2.0)								

REF.	POPULATION	PLACE	NUMBER TESTED	G6PD DEF.	SICKLE CELL	THALASSEMIA			HEMOGLOBIN TYPES							
						A_2	F	OSM. RES.				AJ				A
TAIWAN																
93	Fukienese		1658													1658
	Hakkanese		1244									2				
405	Hakka Hsin-Pu		442M	30 (6.8)												
	Hakka Hsin-Pu		218F	3 (1.4)												
	Hakka Hu-Kou		242M	16 (6.6)												
	Hakka Hu-Kou		78F	4 (5.1)												
	Hakka Mei-Nung		851M	38 (4.5)												
	Hakka Mei-Nung		359F	8 (2.2)												
	Mainland Chinese		282M	5 (1.8)												
	Mainland Chinese		163F	2 (1.2)												
	Taiwanese Chinese		343M	1 (0.3)												
	Taiwanese Chinese		258F	1 (0.4)												
94a	Atayal		354			0										354

REF.	POPULATION	PLACE	NUMBER TESTED	G6PD DEF.	SICKLE CELL	THALASSEMIA			HEMOGLOBIN TYPES							
						A_2	F	OSM. RES.		AG						A
TAIWAN (CONT.)																
94a	Saisiat		184			0										184
	Bunan		684			0										684
	Tsou		309			0										309
	Ami		1571			0				9 (0.6)						
	Puyuma		329			0										329
	Rukai		129			0										129
	Paiwan		941			0										941
KOREA																
729	Koreans		50		0											
359	Koreans		51													51
JAPAN																
465	Japanese	Hiroshima and Nagasaki	2231				2									
522	Japanese	Kagoshima Prefecture	2200			1										2200
523	Japanese	North Kyushu	10000			1										
263	Japanese	Mishima Island	739				0									739
622	Japanese	Yamaguchi Prefecture	30000						13 Abnormal Hemoglobins (0.04)							

REF.	POPULATION	PLACE	NUMBER TESTED	G6PD DEF.	SICKLE CELL	THALASSEMIA A_2	THALASSEMIA F	THALASSEMIA OSM. RES.	HEMOGLOBIN TYPES E	AE						A
JAPAN (CONT.)																
304	Japanese	Japan	89825						30	Abnormal Hemoglobins (0.03)						
464a	Japanese	Shichikawa Wakayama Prefecture	535M	1 (0.2)												
	Japanese	Shichikawa Wakayama Prefecture	568F	0												
483a	Japanese	Tokyo	2107M	0												
	Japanese	Tokyo	721F	0												
	Japanese	Tokyo	161	0												
	Japanese	Tokyo	614	0												
CEYLON																
744	Ceylonese	Colombo	2060													2060
202	Ceylonese	Colombo	800		0											
11	Veddas		167							5 (3.0)						
743	Veddas	Pollebedde Central Ceylon	38						1	4 (13.2)						
	Veddas	Dambana Central Ceylon	27													27

REF.	POPULATION	PLACE	NUMBER TESTED	G6PD DEF.	SICKLE CELL	THALASSEMIA			HEMOGLOBIN TYPES							
						A_2	F	OSM. RES.	E	AE		AK				A
CEYLON (CONT.)																
743	Veddas	Ginidamana-Dalukana Central Ceylon	87						2	26 (32.2)						
	Veddas	Adampane-Bukmikade Northern Ceylon	32							5 (15.6)						
ANDAMAN ISLANDS																
407	Andamanese (mixed)		16		0											
	Onge	Little Andaman Island	52		0											
INDIA																
684	Indians	Madras City	101			0	0					3 (3.0)				
393	Higher Castes	Pondichery Madras	28			5 (17.9)										28
	Lower Castes	Pondichery Madras	114			16 (14.0)						3 (2.6)				
	Untouchables	Pondichery Madras	11			0										11
	Nairs	Pondichery Madras	3			1										3

REF.	POPULATION	PLACE	NUMBER TESTED	G6PD DEF.	SICKLE CELL	THALASSEMIA			HEMOGLOBIN TYPES							
						A_2	F	OSM. RES.		AS				AK		A
INDIA (CONT.)																
393	Moslems	Pondichery Madras	1													1
	Khorwas	Pondichery Madras	1													1
	Unknown	Pondichery Madras	12			2								1		
123	Pallar	Tinnevelly, Madras	112		1 (0.9)											
407	Paniyan	Nilgiri District Madras	61		21											
122	Paniyan	Wynad, Nilgiri District, Madras	74		22											
196	Paniyan	Wynad, Nilgiri District, Madras	955		265											
	Paniyan		1090		308 (28.2)											
125	Kurumba	Nilgiri District Madras	112		20											
407	Kurumba	Nilgiri District Madras	16		3											
381	Kurumba	Nilgiri District Madras	43		10					10						
418	Kurumba	Nilgiri District Madras	26		7					7						
	Kurumba	Nilgiri District Madras	197		40 (20.3)											

REF.	POPULATION	PLACE	NUMBER TESTED	G6PD DEF.	SICKLE CELL	THALASSEMIA			HEMOGLOBIN TYPES							
						A_2	F	OSM. RES.		AS						A
INDIA (CONT.)																
158	Kotas	Nilgiri District Madras	12		0											12
407	Kotas	Nilgiri District Madras	86		0											
418	Kotas	Nilgiri District Madras	22		0											22
	Kotas	Nilgiri District Madras	120													
407	Irulas	Nilgiri District Madras	124		39											
381	Irulas	Nilgiri District Madras	15		6					6						
418	Irulas	Nilgiri District Madras	18		4					4						
	Irulas	Nilgiri District Madras	157		49 (31.2)											
407	Badagas	Nilgiri District Madras	191		16											
418	Badagas	Nilgiri District Madras	30		2					2						
	Badagas	Nilgiri District Madras	221		18 (8.1)											

REF.	POPULATION	PLACE	NUMBER TESTED	G6PD DEF.	SICKLE CELL	THALASSEMIA A_2	THALASSEMIA F	THALASSEMIA OSM. RES.	HEMOGLOBIN TYPES	AS						A
INDIA (CONT.)																
158	Todas	Nilgiri District Madras	12		0											
407	Todas	Nilgiri District Madras	84		3											
381	Todas	Nilgiri District Madras	60		2					2						
418	Todas	Nilgiri District Madras	50		1					1						
	Todas	Nilgiri District Madras	206		6 (2.9)											
158	Indians	Kerala	35													35
88	Malayalam	Kerala	190													190
407	Malayalam	Kerala	111		0											
	Malayalam	Kerala	301													
	Tamils	Kerala	128		0											
	Telegus	Kerala	109		0											
	Canarese	Kerala	95		0											
122	Malapantaram	Quilon District Kerala	116		0											
	Kuruvan	Quilon District Kerala	36		0											

REF.	POPULATION	PLACE	NUMBER TESTED	G6PD DEF.	SICKLE CELL	THALASSEMIA			HEMOGLOBIN TYPES							
						A_2	F	OSM. RES.		AD	AS		AK	AQ		A
INDIA (CONT.)																
122	Ulladan	Quilon District Kerala	142		0											
	Malavedan	Quilon District Kerala	69		0											
	Kadar	Trichur District Kerala	167		0											
561	Cochin Jews from Kerala	Israel	66			9 (15.2)	2									
621	Cochin Jews from Kerala	Israel	58M	6 (10.3)												
422	Indians	Goa	684		0											
688	Indians	Goa	1843							5 (0.3)			2	4		
	Indians	Goa	833				20	20 (2.4)								
663	Indians	Shimoga District Mysore	550		1 (0.2)											
	Indians	Shimoga District Mysore	68							1 (1.5)	1					
158	Chenchu	Andra Pradesh	9													9
473	Hindus	Polavaram Andhra Pradesh	75M	1 (1.3)												

REF.	POPULATION	PLACE	NUMBER TESTED	G6PD DEF.	SICKLE CELL	THALASSEMIA			HEMOGLOBIN TYPES							
						A_2	F	OSM. RES.								
INDIA (CONT.)																
473	Koya Doras	Thallavaram Andhra Pradesh	131M	16 (12.2)												
	Other Tribes	Thallavaram Andhra Pradesh	93M	3 (3.2)												
511	Dorla	Konta Tahsil Bastar District Madhya Pradesh	20[illegible]		26 (11.8)											
	Dhurwa	Jagdalpur Tahsil Bastar District	218		7 (3.2)											
	Northern Dhurwa	Jagdalpur Tahsil Bastar District	60		10 (16.7)											
512	Bade Bhatra	Jagdalpur Tahsil Bastar District	153		25 (16.3)											
	Manjhela Bhatra	Jagdalpur Tahsil Bastar District	64		7 (10.9)											
	San Bahtra	Jagdalpur Tahsil Bastar District	88		17 (19.3)											
	Mahra Caste	Jagdalpur Tahsil Bastar District	123		47 (38.2)											
	Eastern Muria	Kondagaon Tahsil Bastar District Madya Pradesh	143		15 (10.5)											

REF.	POPULATION	PLACE	NUMBER TESTED	G6PD DEF.	SICKLE CELL	THALASSEMIA			HEMOGLOBIN TYPES								
						A_2	F	OSM. RES.									
INDIA (CONT.)																	
512	Western Muria (Jhoria)	Kondagaon Tahsil Bastar District Madya Pradesh	169		27 (16.0)												
513	Bison-horned Maria	Bijapur Tahsil Bastar District Madya Pradesh	185		29 (15.7)												
	Raj Gond	Bastar District	68		8 (11.8)												
	Dorla	Bastar District	27		3 (11.1)												
	Mahra Caste	Bhopalpatnam Bastar District	30		12 (40.0)												
	Halba	Bastar District	34		9 (26.5)												
	Telanga (Telugu)	Bastar District	19		0												
	Others	Bastar District	34		3 (8.8)												
392a'	Mehtar	Ujjain District Madhya Pradesh	72		1 (1.4)												
	Nayta Muslim	Ujjain and Dewas Districts, Madhya Pradesh	65		1 (1.5)												
	Brahmin	Ujjain District	28		0												
	Chamar	Ujjain and Dewas Districts	27		0												

REF.	POPULATION	PLACE	NUMBER TESTED	G6PD DEF.	SICKLE CELL	THALASSEMIA			HEMOGLOBIN TYPES							
						A_2	F	OSM. RES.								
INDIA (CONT.)																
392a'	Rajput	Ujjain District Madhya Pradesh	42		0											
	Jain and Vaishya	Ujjain District	15		0											
	Dhakar	Dewas District Madhya Pradesh	25		0											
	Muslim	Ujjain and Dewas Districts	12		0											
	Others	Ujjain and Dewas Districts	17		0											
	Balai	Ujjain and Dewas Districts	10		0											
196	Balai	Madhya Pradesh	104		5 (4.8)											
	Bhilala	Madhya Pradesh	139		39 (28.1)											
	Bhil	Madhya Pradesh	174		21 (12.1)											
197	Mahar Caste	Nagpur Maharashtra	482		87											
624	Mahar Caste	Nagpur Maharashtra	450		100											
	Mahar Caste	Nagpur Maharashtra	932		187 (20.0)											

REF.	POPULATION	PLACE	NUMBER TESTED	G6PD DEF.	SICKLE CELL	THALASSEMIA			HEMOGLOBIN TYPES							
						A_2	F	OSM. RES.		AS						A
INDIA (CONT.)																
624	Kunbi Caste	Nagpur Maharashtra	116		11 (9.4)											
	Teli Caste	Nagpur Maharashtra	80		9 (11.3)											
	Koshti Caste	Nagpur Maharashtra	46		0											
	Gond	Nagpur Maharashtra	53		0											
	Muslim	Nagpur Maharashtra	68		0											
	Brahmin Caste	Nagpur Maharashtra	26		0											
	Others	Nagpur Maharashtra	171		0											
420	Caste Students	Aurangabad Maharashtra	700		36 (5.1)											
595	Maratha Caste	Maharashtra	201													201
	Gujar Caste	Maharashtra	203													203
	Pajna Caste	Maharashtra	200													200
	Chamar Caste	Maharashtra	208													208
	Mahar Caste	Maharashtra	200							4 (2.0)						
	Mixed Castes	Maharashtra	222													222

REF.	POPULATION	PLACE	NUMBER TESTED	G6PD DEF.	SICKLE CELL	THALASSEMIA			HEMOGLOBIN TYPES							
						A_2	F	OSM. RES.		AS		AD		AJ		A
INDIA (CONT.)																
595	Thakur Tribe	Sahyadri Section Maharashtra	264													264
	Kokna Tribe	Sahyadri Section Maharashtra	190							8 (4.2)						
	Katkari Tribe	Sahyadri Section Maharashtra	262							21 (8.0)						
	Warli Tribe	Sahyadri Section Maharashtra	225							36 (16.0)						
567	Indians from Bombay	Uganda	326									2 (0.6)		1		
58	Indians	Bombay	81M	6 (7.4)												
	Indians	Bombay	29F	9 (31.0)												
	Hindus	Maharashtra	35M	0												
	Hindus	Maharashtra	8F	2												
	Hindus	Maharashtra	43	2 (4.7)												
	Konkan Hindus	Saraswats Maharashtra	10M	2												
	Konkan Hindus	Saraswats Maharashtra	5F	1												
	Konkan Hindus	Saraswats Maharashtra	15	3 (20.0)												

REF.	POPULATION	PLACE	NUMBER TESTED	G6PD DEF.	SICKLE CELL	THALASSEMIA			HEMOGLOBIN TYPES							
						A_2	F	OSM. RES.	S	AS						
INDIA (CONT.)																
58	Indian Christians	Bombay	12M	0												
	Indian Christians	Bombay	1F	0												
	Others	Bombay	21M	4 (19.0)												
	Others	Bombay	6F	1												
59	Parsees	Bombay	100M	19 (19.0)												
	Parsees	Bombay	116F	15 (12.9)												
561	Bnai Israel Jews from Bombay	Israel	172			24 (16.9)	9									
621	Bnai Israel Jews from Bombay	Israel	102M	2 (2.0)												
620	Sorathis	near Palgar Gujerat	326						17	82 (30.4)						
724	Bhils	Panchmahal District, Gujerat	206							32 (15.5)						
	Gamit	Surat District Gujerat	207		65 (31.4)				2	26	(many not tested)					
	Dubla	Surat District Gujerat	211							20 (9.5)						

REF.	POPULATION	PLACE	NUMBER TESTED	G6PD DEF.	SICKLE CELL	THALASSEMIA			HEMOGLOBIN TYPES							
						A_2	F	OSM. RES.	S	AS		AD	AJ	AL		
INDIA (CONT.)																
724	Koli	Surat District Gujerat	182							8 (4.4)						
	Naika	Surat District Gujerat	174		28 (16.1)					26						
	Dhodia	Surat District Gujerat	213							38 (17.8)						
	Dhanka	Broach District Gujerat	215						3	41 (20.5)						
595	Brahmins	Gujerat	203		0											
	Lohana	Gujerat	603									5	2	3		
657	Anavil Brahman Caste	Surat District Gujerat	53		0											
	Leva Patidar Caste	Kheda District Gujerat	150		0											
688	Indians	Diu, Gujerat	379							1 (0.3)		2 (0.5)				
56	Oriahs from Orissa	Assam	100		15 (15.0)											
	Griza Oriahs from Orissa	Assam	100		29 (29.0)											
196	Bado Gadaba	Koraput District Orissa	99		0											

REF.	POPULATION	PLACE	NUMBER TESTED	G6PD DEF.	SICKLE CELL	THALASSEMIA			HEMOGLOBIN TYPES							
						A_2	F	OSM. RES.		AS						A
INDIA (CONT.)																
196	Pareng Gadaba	Koraput District Orissa	225		28 (12.4)											
	Ollaro Gadaba	Koraput District Orissa	225		6 (2.7)											
	Bareng Paroja	Koraput District Orissa	104		0											
	Konda Paroja	Koraput District Orissa	225		30 (13.3)											
159	Santals	Midnapore West Bengal	119	Families						2 Families (1.7)						
160	Anglo-Indians	Kharagpore West Bengal	89				0									89
392	Duley	Hooghly District West Bengal	69		0											
	Tentulia Bagdi	Hooghly District West Bengal	89		0											
86	Rarhi Brahimin Caste	Hooghly District West Bengal	100		0											
	Muslims	Hooghly District West Bengal	100		0											
157	Indians	Bengal	10000		0											
122	Indians	Calcutta	400		0											

REF.	POPULATION	PLACE	NUMBER TESTED	G6PD DEF.	SICKLE CELL	THALASSEMIA A_2	THALASSEMIA F	THALASSEMIA OSM. RES.	HEMOGLOBIN TYPES		E	AE				A Barts
INDIA (CONT.)																
157	Indians	Bengal	700					26 (3.7)			2	25 (3.9)				
662b	Indian (cord blood)	Bengal	100													4 (4.0)
196	Rajbanshi	Midnapur, Jalpaiguri and Cooch Behar	300		0											
	Padmaraj (Pods)	24-Parganas Bengal	100		0											
	Mahishyas	24-Parganas Bengal	60		0											
158	Totos	Totopara, Assam	116									23 (19.8)				
157	Indians	Bihar	54													54
407	Oraons	Bihar	100		0											
380	Oraons	Bihar	56		0											56
	Oraons	Bihar	156													
407	Kharias	Bihar	23		0											
85	Danukh Caste	Mainpuri District Uttar Pradesh	335		32 (9.6)											
701	Indians	Singapore	92M	3 (3.3)												

REF.	POPULATION	PLACE	NUMBER TESTED	G6PD DEF.	SICKLE CELL	THALASSEMIA A_2	THALASSEMIA F	THALASSEMIA OSM. RES.	HEMOGLOBIN TYPES	AD		AE	AL	AJ	AK	A	Barts
INDIA (CONT.)																	
481	Indians	Agra, Uttar Pradesh	250													250	
466	Indians (anemic)	Agra, Uttar Pradesh	410					7 (1.7)				1 (0.2)					
224	Indians	Uttar Pradesh	235													235	
466	Indians	Western Uttar Pradesh	102													102	
707	Indians in Singapore		3341							15 (0.4)		15 (0.4)	2	1	5		
	Indians (cord blood)	Singapore	222														2 (0.9)
157	Nepalese	Calcutta	109									1 (0.9)					
515	Nepalese	Pokhara, Nepal	14													14	
89	Gorkhas from Nepal	Poona Maharashtra	200													200	
703	Gurkhas from Nepal	Singapore	560									3 (0.5)					
515	Tibetans	Nepal	47													47	
343	Khumbu (Sherpas)	Tibet	128			1 (0.8)	1									128	
589	Hindus	Punjab	100							1 (1.0)							

REF.	POPULATION	PLACE	NUMBER TESTED	G6PD DEF.	SICKLE CELL	THALASSEMIA			HEMOGLOBIN TYPES						
						A_2	F	OSM. RES.	D	AD	AJ	AE	AS	JD	A
INDIA (CONT.)															
589	Sikhs	Punjab	250							3 (2.4)					
90	Sikhs	Northwest India	279						1	4 (1.8)					
625	Sikhs	Vancouver,Canada	80					5 (6.3)							
48a	Indians	Seattle Washington	87M	5 (5.7)											
PAKISTAN															
415	East Pakistanis		23									2 (8.7)			
	West Pakistanis	Karachi	76										1 (1.3)		
99	Brahui	Northwest Pakistan	4							1					
	Sindi	Northwest Pakistan	6								1				
	Baluchi	Northwest Pakistan	9							2					
	Pathans	Northwest Pakistan	18								2			1	
	Others	Northwest Pakistan	18												18
775	Pakistanis	Lahore	450M	(2-3)											

REF.	POPULATION	PLACE	NUMBER TESTED	G6PD DEF.	SICKLE CELL	THALASSEMIA			HEMOGLOBIN TYPES							
						A_2	F	OSM. RES.								
IRAN																
727	Mamassani	Southwest Iran	69M	14 (20.3)												
	Mamassani	Southwest Iran	44F	3 (6.8)												
726	Iranians	Shiraz	275	26 (9.5)												
	Iranians	Fars District Except Shiraz	89	10 (11.2)												
	Iranians	Iran	358M	35 (9.8)												
	Iranians	Iran	198F	12 (6.1)												
103	Armenians from Soviet Armenia	New Julfa Isfahan	152M	1 (0.7)												
	Armenians from Soviet Armenia	New Julfa Isfahan	11F	0												
518	Iranian Patients	Gorgan and Khorasan Provinces	121					43 (35.5)								
	Turkmen Patients	Gorgan and Khorasan Provinces	71					29 (40.8)								

REF.	POPULATION	PLACE	NUMBER TESTED	G6PD DEF.	SICKLE CELL	THALASSEMIA			HEMOGLOBIN TYPES							
						A_2	F	OSM. RES.								
IRAN (CONT.)																
518	Baluchi Patients	Gorgan and Khorasan Provinces	8					3								
561	Persian Jews	Israel	182			5 (2.7)	1									
621	Iranian Jews	Israel	557M	84 (15.1)												
	Persian Jews from West Iran	Israel	45M	20 (44.4)												
	Persian Jews from Central Iran	Israel	370M	40 (10.8)												
AFGHANISTAN																
621	Jews from Afghanistan	Israel	29M	3 (10.3)												
U. S. S. R.																
621	Jews from Bukhara	Israel	46M	0												
IRAQ																
621	Iraqi Jews	Israel	902M	224 (24.8)												

REF.	POPULATION	PLACE	NUMBER TESTED	G6PD DEF.	SICKLE CELL	THALASSEMIA			HEMOGLOBIN TYPES							
						A_2	F	OSM. RES.								
IRAQ (CONT.)																
621	Iraqi Jews from Baghdad	Israel	286M	70 (24.5)												
	Iraqi Jews from Mosul, Erbil and Kirkuk	Israel	34M	18 (53.0)												
	Kurdish Jews from Mosul, Erbil, Kirkuk and West Iran	Israel	59M	21 (35.6)												
	Kurdish Jews from Zahko, Dahok, Sindor, Amadia, and North Iraq	Israel	126M	89 (70.6)												
IRAQ AND TURKEY																
621	Kurdish Jews from Kurdistan	Israel	196M	114 (58.2)												
561	Kurdish Jews from Kurdistan	Israel	110			20 (20.0)	15									
TURKEY AND U. S. S. R.																
621	Jews from Caucasus	Israel	25M	7 (28.0)												

REF.	POPULATION	PLACE	NUMBER TESTED	G6PD DEF.	SICKLE CELL	THALASSEMIA			HEMOGLOBIN TYPES							
						A_2	F	OSM. RES.	S	AS			AD	E		
TURKEY																
324	Kurdish Jews from Urfa	Israel	167M	60 (35.9)												
	Kurdish Jews from Urfa	Israel	102					10 (9.8)								
621	Sephardic Jews from Turkey	Israel	256M	5 (2.0)												
608	Kurdish Turks	Diyarbakir	208M	4 (1.9)												
	Turks	Rize(Coruh)	109M	0												
	Turks	Rize(Coruh)	43F	0												
722	Turkish Soldiers		104M	1 (1.0)												
14	Turks		400										1			
9	Turks	Southwest Turkey	440			1		1		1						
	Turks	Southeast Turkey	330			1				1						
	Turks	Elsewhere	578						3					2		
13	Turks	Southern Turkey	240			1							1			
6	Turks	Mersin	181		25 (13.8)											
	Turks	Catalkeli	195		25 (12.8)											

REF.	POPULATION	PLACE	NUMBER TESTED	G6PD DEF.	SICKLE CELL	THALASSEMIA			HEMOGLOBIN TYPES							
						A_2	F	OSM. RES.	AS	AE						
TURKEY (CONT.)																
7	Eti-Turks	Mersin	131						?	1						
	Eti-Turks	Kelahmed	150						?	3						
	Eti-Turks	Tarsus and Mersin	155						?	2						
	Eti-Turks		436							6 (1.4)						
13	Eti-Turks		60				4 (6.7)									
8	Eti-Turks	Fernek Iskenderun	114		30 (26.3)											
	Eti-Turks	Nesli Iskenderun	150		18 (12.0)											
	Eti-Turks	Harbiye,Antakya	74		4 (5.4)											
	Eti-Turks	Karatas,Adana	102		20 (19.6)											
	Eti-Turks	Kelahmet,Mersin	150		41 (27.3)											
608	Eti-Turks	Adana and Tarsus	105M	12 (11.4)												
	Eti-Turks	Adana and Tarsus	53F	1 (1.9)												
	Turks	Izmir	212M	2 (0.9)												

REF.	POPULATION	PLACE	NUMBER TESTED	G6PD DEF.	SICKLE CELL	THALASSEMIA			HEMOGLOBIN TYPES							
						A_2	F	OSM. RES.								
	TURKEY (CONT.)															
608	Turks (Newborns)	Ankara	1000M	5 (0.5)												
	Cyprus Turks		200M	7 (3.5)												
	Greeks	Istanbul	37M	0												
	Greeks	Istanbul	70F	0												
	Jews	Istanbul	29M	0												
	Jews	Istanbul	64F	0												
	Armenians	Istanbul	44M	0												
	Armenians	Istanbul	57F	0												
705	Armenians	Khartoum, Sudan	59					16 (27.1)								
	LEBANON AND SYRIA															
621	Jews from Lebanon and Syria	Israel	80M	5 (6.3)												
	LEBANON															
8	Allewits	Tripoli	101		4 (4.0)											

REF.	POPULATION	PLACE	NUMBER TESTED	G6PD DEF.	SICKLE CELL	THALASSEMIA			HEMOGLOBIN TYPES							
						A_2	F	OSM. RES.		AS		AC				
LEBANON (CONT.)																
144a	Lebanese	Beirut	849			16 (2.3)	20			1 (0.1)						
669	Lebanese	Beirut	155M	4 (2.6)												
144a	Lebanese	North Lebanon	340			10 (5.3)	17			3 (0.8)						
669	Lebanese	North Lebanon	29M	0												
144a	Lebanese	Lebanon Mountains	863			23 (3.0)	16			2 (0.2)						
669	Lebanese	Lebanon Mountains	210M	6 (2.9)												
144a	Lebanese	South Lebanon	518			14 (3.9)	16			1 (0.2)		1 (0.2)				
669	Lebanese	South Lebanon	88M	6 (6.8)												
144a	Lebanese	Bekaa	368			8 (3.3)	10			2 (0.5)						
669	Lebanese	Bekaa	67M	1 (1.5)												

REF.	POPULATION	PLACE	NUMBER TESTED	G6PD DEF.	SICKLE CELL	THALASSEMIA A_2	THALASSEMIA F	THALASSEMIA OSM. RES.	HEMOGLOBIN TYPES	AS		AC				A
	LEBANON (CONT.)															
	Same Data as Previous Lebanese Groups by Religion															
144a	Sunnite Moslems		547			16 (4.4)	20			3 (0.5)		1 (0.2)				
669	Sunnite Moslems		97M	6 (6.2)												
144a	Shiite Moslems		507			11 (2.8)	10			4 (0.8)						
669	Shiite Moslems		101M	5 (5.0)												
144a	Druzes		202			11 (5.9)	7									202
669	Druzes		105M	0												
144a	Maronite Christians		996			19 (2.6)	20			1 (0.1)						
669	Maronite Christians		117M	5 (4.3)												
144a	Greek Orthodox Christians		452			10 (4.0)	17			1 (0.2)						
669	Greek Orthodox Christians		87M	1 (1.1)												

REF.	POPULATION	PLACE	NUMBER TESTED	G6PD DEF.	SICKLE CELL	THALASSEMIA			HEMOGLOBIN TYPES							
						A_2	F	OSM. RES.								A
LEBANON (CONT.)																
	Same Data By Religion															
144a	Armenians		234			4	5 (2.6)									234
699	Armenians		36M	0												
	Others		6M	0												
SYRIA																
618	Arabs	Khazramah	20		10 (50.0)											
705	Syrians	Khartoum, Sudan	85					10 (11.8)								
249	Syrians	Nigeria	188		0											
ISRAEL																
222	Oriental and Sephardic Jews		357													357
221	Yemenite Jews		104		0											
621	Aden and Yemen Jews		415M	22 (5.3)												
	Black Jews from Cochin		58M	6 (10.3)												

REF.	POPULATION	PLACE	NUMBER TESTED	G6PD DEF.	SICKLE CELL	THALASSEMIA A_2	THALASSEMIA F	THALASSEMIA OSM. RES.	HEMOGLOBIN TYPES							
ISRAEL (CONT.)																
561	Black Jews from Cochin		66			9 (15.2)	2									
621	Bnai Israel Jews from Bombay		102M	2 (2.0)												
	Persian Jews from Central Iran		370M	40 (10.8)												
	Persian Jews from Western Iran		45M	20 (44.4)												
561	Persian Jews		182			5 (2.7)	1									
621	Kurdish Jews from Northern Iraq		126M	89 (70.6)												
	Kurdish Jews from Mosul, Erbil, Kirkuk, Salamaiya and West Iraq		59M	21 (35.6)												
561	Kurdish Jews from Iraq		110			20 (20.0)	15									
621	Iraqi Jews from Baghdad		286M	70 (24.5)												

REF.	POPULATION	PLACE	NUMBER TESTED	G6PD DEF.	SICKLE CELL	THALASSEMIA			HEMOGLOBIN TYPES							
						A_2	F	OSM. RES.								
ISRAEL (CONT.)																
621	Iraqi Jews from Mosul, Kirkuk and Erbil		34M	18 (53.0)												
	Non-Ashkenazim Jews from Iraq		902M	224 (24.8)												
	Non-Ashkenazim Jews from Iran		557M	84 (15.1)												
	Non-Ashkenazim Jews from Kurdistan		196M	114 (58.2)												
	Non-Ashkenazim Jews from Caucasus		25M	7 (28.0)												
	Non-Ashkenazim Jews from Afghanistan		29M	3 (10.3)												
	Non-Ashkenazim Jews from Bukhara		46M	0												
	Non-Ashkenazim Jews from Egypt		112M	4 (3.6)												
	Non-Ashkenazim Jews from Morocco		219M	1 (0.5)												

REF.	POPULATION	PLACE	NUMBER TESTED	G6PD DEF.	SICKLE CELL	THALASSEMIA			HEMOGLOBIN TYPES							
						A_2	F	OSM. RES.								
	ISRAEL (CONT.)															
561	Non-Ashkenazim Jews from Morocco		147			2 (2.7)	2									
621	Non-Ashkenazim Jews from the Atlas Mountains Morocco		23M	1 (4.3)												
	Non-Ashkenazim Jews from Algeria and Tunisia		112M	1 (0.9)												
	Non-Ashkenazim Jews from Libya		219M	2 (0.9)												
	Non-Ashkenazim Jews from Djerba		52M	0												
	Sephardic Jews from Turkey		256M	5 (2.0)												
	Sephardic Jews from Greece and Bulgaria		152M	1 (0.7)												
	Sephardic Jews from Elsewhere		93M	2 (2.2)												
	Falasha Jews from Ethiopia		208M	0												

REF.	POPULATION	PLACE	NUMBER TESTED	G6PD DEF.	SICKLE CELL	THALASSEMIA			HEMOGLOBIN TYPES							
						A_2	F	OSM. RES.								A
ISRAEL (CONT.)																
621	Ashkenazim Jews		819M	3 (0.4)												
	Karaites		18M	0												
	Circassians		57M	0												
	Druses		92M	4 (4.3)												
	Arabs		264M	12 (4.5)												
220	Palestine Arabs		118		1 (0.8)											
621	Samaritans		69M	0												
99a	Samaritans		132	0												
	Samaritans		104			14 (13.5)										104
JORDAN																
617	Jordanian Patients		68		0											
	Gaza Patients		37		0		2									
21	Bedouin Arabs		308		1 (0.3)											

REF.	POPULATION	PLACE	NUMBER TESTED	G6PD DEF.	SICKLE CELL	THALASSEMIA			HEMOGLOBIN TYPES							
						A_2	F	OSM. RES.	S	AS						Barts
JORDAN (CONT.)																
21	Palestine Arabs		111		0											
SAUDI ARABIA																
429	Arab Newborns		33													3 (9.1)
409	Shi'i Arabs	Qatif Oasis	394						2	97 (25.1)						
	Sunni Arabs	Qatif Oasis	22							1 (4.5)						
275	Arabs	Qatif Oasis	111M	38 (34.2)												
	Arabs	Safwah Qatif Oasis	51M	33 (64.7)												
	Arabs	Al Ajam Qatif Oasis	104M	68 (65.4)												
409	Shi'i Arabs	Al'Hasa Oasis	65							16 (24.6)						
	Sunni Arabs	Al'Hasa Oasis	217							26 (12.0)						
275	Arabs	Al'Hasa Oasis	64M	3 (4.7)												
	Arabs	Qarah Al'Hasa Oasis	104M	25 (24.0)												

REF.	POPULATION	PLACE	NUMBER TESTED	G6PD DEF.	SICKLE CELL	THALASSEMIA			HEMOGLOBIN TYPES							
						A_2	F	OSM. RES.		AS						A
SAUDI ARABIA (CONT.)																
275	Arabs	Mansurah Al'Hasa Oasis	92M	49 (53.3)												
	Arabs	Eastern Province	34M	1 (2.9)												
409	Sunni Arabs (Settled on Oases)	Eastern Province	83							6 (7.2)						
	Sunni Arabs (Bedouin Nomads)	Eastern Province	79													79
275	Arabs	Western Province	97M	4 (4.1)												
409	Sunni Arabs (Settled)	Hejaz Western Province	102													102
	Sunni Arabs (Settled)	'Asir Western Province	30													30
	Sunni Arabs (Settled)	Najran Western Province	44							2 (4.5)						
	Sunni Arabs (Settled)	Nejd Central Province	179							2 (1.1)						
	Sunni Arabs (Bedouin Nomads)	West and Central Provinces	99													99
	Arabs	Elsewhere	62							6 (9.7)						

REF.	POPULATION	PLACE	NUMBER TESTED	G6PD DEF.	SICKLE CELL	THALASSEMIA			HEMOGLOBIN TYPES							
						A_2	F	OSM. RES.								
KUWAIT																
782	Kuwaiti (Newborn)		93M	18 (19.4)												
	Kuwaiti		118M	22 (18.6)												
	Jordanians (Newborn)		72M	17 (23.6)												
	Jordanians		70M	16 (22.9)												
	Iraqi (Newborn and Adult)		27M	9 (33.3)												
	Lebanese (Newborn and Adult)		11M	1 (9.1)												
	Syrian (Newborn and Adult)		11M	4 (36.4)												
	Saudi (Newborn and Adult)		6M	4												
	Other Nationalities (Newborn and Adult)		53M	7 (13.2)												

REF.	POPULATION	PLACE	NUMBER TESTED	G6PD DEF.	SICKLE CELL	THALASSEMIA			HEMOGLOBIN TYPES							
						A_2	F	OSM. RES.								
ADEN																
407	Arabs		111		2 (1.8)											
	Zabidis	Achdam Western Province	114		26 (22.8)											
YEMEN																
621	Yemen and Aden Jews	Israel	415M	22 (5.3)												
221	Yemen Jews	Israel	104		0											
CYPRUS																
750	Cypriots	Greece	310M	10 (3.2)												
608	Turkish Cypriots	Turkey	200M	7 (3.5)												
49	Greek Cypriots		78					22 (28.2)								
	Turkish Cypriots		21					5 (23.8)								
	Armenian Cypriot		1					1								
	Greek Cypriots	Limassol	417					71 (17.0)								

REF.	POPULATION	PLACE	NUMBER TESTED	G6PD DEF.	SICKLE CELL	THALASSEMIA			HEMOGLOBIN TYPES							
						A_2	F	OSM. RES.	S	AS						
CYPRUS (CONT.)																
49	Turkish Cypriots	Limassol	115					24 (20.9)								
542	Cypriots	Yialousa	339M	36 (10.6)												
	Cypriots	Yialousa	69			1 (1.4)				1 (1.4)						
	Cypriots	Yialousa	164					44 (26.8)								
	Cypriots With Abnormal Blood Films (26.8%)	Yialousa	23			6 (7.0)										
	Cypriots	Syrianochori	229M	16 (7.0)												
	Cypriots	Syrianochori	184					48 (26.1)								
	Cypriots With Abnormal Blood Films (26.1%)	Syrianochori	25			8 (6.3)			1	1						
49	Greek Cypriots	Alithinou Troodos Mountains	65					31 (47.7)								
542	Cypriots	Troodos Mountains	476M	0												
	Cypriots	Troodos Mountains	46			4 (8.7)										

REF.	POPULATION	PLACE	NUMBER TESTED	G6PD DEF.	SICKLE CELL	THALASSEMIA			HEMOGLOBIN TYPES							
						A_2	F	OSM. RES.								A2 Sphakia
CYPRUS (CONT.)																
542	Cypriots	Troodos Mountains	130					32 (24.6)								
	Cypriots With Abnormal Blood Films (24.6%)	Troodos Mountains	19			4 (5.2)										
GREECE																
53	Greeks	Sphakia District Crete	125M	3 (2.4)												
	Greeks	Sphakia District Crete	171			10 (7.0)	4									1
648a	Greeks	Chanea Province Crete	107M	8 (7.5)												
	Greeks	Rethymnon Province Crete	61M	1 (1.6)												
29	Greeks	Pombia Crete	51M	5 (9.8)												

REF.	POPULATION	PLACE	NUMBER TESTED	G6PD DEF.	SICKLE CELL	THALASSEMIA			HEMOGLOBIN TYPES							
						A_2	F	OSM. RES.								A
GREECE (CONT.)																
51	Greeks	Pombia Crete	131			12 (9.2)										131
750	Greeks	Herakleion Crete	206M	6												
29	Greeks	Herakleion Crete	107M	8												
	Greeks	Herakleion Crete	313M	14 (4.5)												
51	Greeks	Herakleion Crete	107			5 (4.7)										107
648a	Greeks	Heraclion Province Crete	163M	3 (1.8)												
	Greeks	Lassithi Province Crete	59M	3 (5.0)												
456	Greeks	Aegean Islands Crete and Dodecaneses	172					13 (7.6)								
648a	Greeks	Dodecannese	97M	6 (6.2)												
29	Greeks	Rhodes Rhodes	93M	20 (21.5)												

REF.	POPULATION	PLACE	NUMBER TESTED	G6PD DEF.	SICKLE CELL	THALASSEMIA			HEMOGLOBIN TYPES							
						A_2	F	OSM. RES.								A
GREECE (CONT.)																
51	Greeks	Rhodes Rhodes	93			12 (12.9)										93
29	Greeks	Massari Rhodes	47M	16 (34.0)												
51	Greeks	Massari Rhodes	47			13 (27.7)										47
29	Greeks	Laerma Rhodes	58M	27 (46.6)												
51	Greeks	Laerma Rhodes	58			15 (25.9)										58
648a	Greeks	Cyclades	92M	2 (2.1)												
648	Greeks	Serifos	167				5	23 (13.8)								167
579	Greeks	Tinos Tinos	68M	1 (1.5)												
	Greeks	Foothill Villages Tinos	58M	2 (3.4)												
	Greeks	Hill Villages Tinos	88M	1 (1.1)												
648a	Greeks	Samos	42M	0												
	Greeks	Chios	50M	0												

REF.	POPULATION	PLACE	NUMBER TESTED	G6PD DEF.	SICKLE CELL	THALASSEMIA			HEMOGLOBIN TYPES							
						A_2	F	OSM. RES.								
GREECE (CONT.)																
648a	Greeks	Lesbos	97M	3												
216	Greeks	Lesbos	939M	41												
	Greeks	Lesbos	1036M	44 (4.2)												
261	Greeks	Lemnos	200M	27 (13.5)												
648a	Greeks	Coast of Black Sea	72M	0												
	Greeks	Asia Minor	225M	4 (1.7)												
	Greeks	Immigrants to Greece	54M	0												
	Greeks	Eastern Thrace	127M	3 (2.3)												
261	Greeks and Turks	Thrace	200M	4 (2.0)												
200	Slavs	Vrahia Macedonia	92		0											
	Slavs	Kimina Macedonia	162		0											
	East Rumanians	Trikalla Macedonia	168		0											

REF.	POPULATION	PLACE	NUMBER TESTED	G6PD DEF.	SICKLE CELL	THALASSEMIA			HEMOGLOBIN TYPES							
						A_2	F	OSM. RES.								
GREECE (CONT.)																
200	Smyrnans	Vathylakos Macedonia	162		0											
	Refugees	Neon Petritsi Macedonia	238		0											
	Christian Gypsies	Fitoki-Flamburos Macedonia	181		0											
	Refugees	Stavrupolis Macedonia	108		2 (1.9)											
	Refugees	Lekani Macedonia	160		0											
	Refugees	Kechrocampos Macedonia	102		0											
	Refugees	Paranestion Macedonia	86		0											
	Refugees	Komotini Macedonia	143		0											
	East Thracians	Arisvi Macedonia	82		0											
	West Thrace Turks	Aratos Macedonia	163		0											
	East Thracians	Elafochori Macedonia	97		0											

REF.	POPULATION	PLACE	NUMBER TESTED	G6PD DEF.	SICKLE CELL	THALASSEMIA			HEMOGLOBIN TYPES							
						A_2	F	OSM. RES.								
GREECE (CONT.)																
200	Moslem Gypsies	Elafochori Macedonia	111		0											
456	Greeks	Macedonia and Thrace	337					11 (3.3)								
720	Greeks (Negroid)	West Thrace	49		6 (12.2)											
648a	Greeks	Xanthi Thrace	41M	1 (2.4)												
	Greeks	Rodhopi Thrace	40M	1 (2.5)												
	Greeks	Evros Thrace	122M	3 (2.4)												
	Greeks	Kavalla Macedonia	129M	8 (6.2)												
	Greeks	Drama Macedonia	101M	6 (5.9)												
	Greeks	Serrae Macedonia	225M	15 (6.7)												
	Greeks	Thessaloniki Macedonia	262M	25 (9.5)												
	Greeks	Kilkis Macedonia	101M	2 (1.9)												

REF.	POPULATION	PLACE	NUMBER TESTED	G6PD DEF.	SICKLE CELL	THALASSEMIA			HEMOGLOBIN TYPES							
						A_2	F	OSM. RES.								
GREECE (CONT.)																
648a	Greeks	Pierria Macedonia	63M	4 (6.3)												
	Greeks	Emathia Macedonia	103M	14 (13.5)												
	Greeks	Pella Macedonia	121M	7 (5.7)												
	Greeks	Florina Macedonia	51M	0												
	Greeks	Kozani Macedonia	151M	3 (2.0)												
	Greeks	Kastoria Macedonia	39M	0												
200	Greeks	Epanomi Macedonia	183		5 (2.7)											
	Greeks	St. Prodromos Macedonia	177		0											
	Greeks	Zangliveri Macedonia	172		0											
	Greeks	Hortiatis Macedonia	159		0											
	Greeks	Xylopolis Macedonia	90		0											
	Greeks	Halastra Macedonia	108		4 (3.7)											

REF.	POPULATION	PLACE	NUMBER TESTED	G6PD DEF.	SICKLE CELL	THALASSEMIA			HEMOGLOBIN TYPES							
						A_2	F	OSM. RES.								
GREECE (CONT.)																
200	Greeks	Klidi Macedonia	67		4 (6.0)											
	Greeks	Tsinaforon Macedonia	151		14 (9.3)											
	Greeks	Korifi Macedonia	142		18 (12.7)											
	Greeks	Loutros Macedonia	102		6 (5.9)											
	Greeks	Leptokaria Macedonia	106		3 (2.8)											
	Greeks	Fytia Macedonia	150		0											
	Greeks	Aidonochorion Macedonia	136		4 (2.9)											
	Greeks	Paleokomi Macedonia	100		6 (6.0)											
	Greeks	Prosotsani Macedonia	220		0											
	Greeks	Gratini Macedonia	86		0											
	Greeks	Kosmion Macedonia	76		0											
	Greeks	Soufli Macedonia	205		0											

REF.	POPULATION	PLACE	NUMBER TESTED	G6PD DEF.	SICKLE CELL	THALASSEMIA			HEMOGLOBIN TYPES							
						A_2	F	OSM. RES.		AS						
GREECE (CONT.)																
648a	Greeks	Chalkidhiki Macedonia	72M	6 (8.3)												
29	Greeks	Ormylia Chalkidhiki Macedonia	21M	3 (14.3)												
16	Greeks	Ormylia Chalkidhiki Macedonia	238		55											
200	Greeks	Ormylia Chalkidhiki Macedonia	103		18											
51	Greeks	Ormylia Chalkidhiki Macedonia	21		3	1 (4.8)				3						
	Greeks	Ormylia Chalkidhiki Macedonia	362		76 (21.0)											
29	Greeks	Nikiti Chalkidhiki Macedonia	52M	22 (42 3)												
51	Greeks	Nikiti Chalkidhiki Macedonia	52		13	2 (3.8)				13						

REF.	POPULATION	PLACE	NUMBER TESTED	G6PD DEF.	SICKLE CELL	THALASSEMIA			HEMOGLOBIN TYPES							
						A_2	F	OSM. RES.		AS						
GREECE (CONT.)																
16	Greeks	Nikiti Chalkidhiki Macedonia	122		11											
200	Greeks	Nikiti Chalkidhiki Macedonia	143		27											
	Greeks	Nikiti Chalkidhiki Macedonia	317		51 (16.1)											
29	Greeks	St. Nicholas Chalkidhiki Macedonia	29M	8 (27.6)												
51	Greeks	St. Nicholas Chalkidhiki Macedonia	29		8	1 (3.4)				8						
16	Greeks	St. Nicholas Chalkidhiki Macedonia	211		54											
200	Greeks	St. Nicholas Chalkidhiki Macedonia	101		24											
	Greeks	St. Nicholas Chalkidhiki Macedonia	341		86 (25.2)											
16	Greeks	Athytos Chalkidhiki Macedonia	167		20 (12.0)											

REF.	POPULATION	PLACE	NUMBER TESTED	G6PD DEF.	SICKLE CELL	THALASSEMIA			HEMOGLOBIN TYPES							
						A_2	F	OSM. RES.								
GREECE (CONT.)																
16	Greeks	Cassandra Chalkidhiki Macedonia	137		21 (15.3)											
	Greeks	Cryopighi Chalkidhiki Macedonia	57		12 (21.1)											
	Greeks	Ag. Mamas Chalkidhiki Macedonia	115		31 (27.0)											
16	Greeks	Kapsochora Chalkidhiki Macedonia	92		4											
200	Greeks	Kapsochora Chalkidhiki Macedonia	96		1											
	Greeks	Kapsochora Chalkidhiki Macedonia	188		5 (2.7)											
16	Greeks	Furka Chalkidhiki Macedonia	119		19											
200	Greeks	Furka Chalkidhiki Macedonia	92		2											
	Greeks	Furka Chalkidhiki Macedonia	211		21 (10.1)											

REF.	POPULATION	PLACE	NUMBER TESTED	G6PD DEF.	SICKLE CELL	THALASSEMIA			HEMOGLOBIN TYPES						
						A_2	F	OSM. RES.							
GREECE (CONT.)															
16	Greeks	Kassandrinon Chalkidhiki Macedonia	84		2										
200	Greeks	Kassandrinon Chalkidhiki Macedonia	46		0										
	Greeks	Kassandrinon Chalkidhiki Macedonia	120		2 (1.7)										
16	Greeks	Paliouri Chalkidhiki Macedonia	123		16										
200	Greeks	Paliouri Chalkidhiki Macedonia	160		16										
	Greeks	Paliouri Chalkidhiki Macedonia	283		32 (11.3)										
16	Greeks	Chanoti Chalkidhiki Macedonia	70		0										
200	Greeks	Chanoti Chalkidhiki Macedonia	62		0										
	Greeks	Chanoti Chalkidhiki Macedonia	132												

REF.	POPULATION	PLACE	NUMBER TESTED	G6PD DEF.	SICKLE CELL	THALASSEMIA			HEMOGLOBIN TYPES							
						A_2	F	OSM. RES.								
GREECE (CONT.)																
16	Greeks	Polychronon Chalkidhiki Macedonia	133		7											
200	Greeks	Polychronon Chalkidhiki Macedonia	160		13											
	Greeks	Polychronon Chalkidhiki Macedonia	293		20 (6.8)											
16	Greeks	Kallandra Chalkidhiki Macedonia	133		7											
200	Greeks	Kallandra Chalkidhiki Macedonia	90		2											
	Greeks	Kallandra Chalkidhiki Macedonia	223		9 (4.0)											
16	Greeks	St. Paraskovi Chalkidhiki Macedonia	100		6											
200	Greeks	St. Paraskovi Chalkidhiki Macedonia	50		0											
	Greeks	St. Paraskovi Chalkidhiki Macedonia	150		6 (4.0)											

REF.	POPULATION	PLACE	NUMBER TESTED	G6PD DEF.	SICKLE CELL	THALASSEMIA A_2	THALASSEMIA F	THALASSEMIA OSM. RES.	HEMOGLOBIN TYPES							
	GREECE (CONT.)															
16	Greeks	Nea Skioni Chalkidhiki Macedonia	109		7											
200	Greeks	Nea Skioni Chalkidhiki Macedonia	40		0											
	Greeks	Nea Skioni Chalkidhiki Macedonia	149		7 (4.7)											
16	Greeks	Sikia Chalkidhiki Macedonia	265		78											
200	Greeks	Sikia Chalkidhiki Macedonia	846		265											
	Greeks	Sikia Chalkidhiki Macedonia	1111		343 (30.9)											
16	Greeks	Parthenon Chalkidhiki Macedonia	108		35											
200	Greeks	Parthenon Chalkidhiki Macedonia	153		49											
	Greeks	Parthenon Chalkidhiki Macedonia	261		84 (32.2)											

REF.	POPULATION	PLACE	NUMBER TESTED	G6PD DEF.	SICKLE CELL	THALASSEMIA			HEMOGLOBIN TYPES							
						A_2	F	OSM. RES.								A
GREECE (CONT.)																
200	Greeks	Valta Chalkidhiki Macedonia	196		25 (12.8)											
	Greeks	Kallithea Chalkidhiki Macedonia	90		8 (8.9)											
	Greeks	Pazarakia Chalkidhiki Macedonia	150		21 (14.0)											
648a	Greeks	Salonica	74M	4 (5.4)												
456	Greeks	Thessaly	244					28 (11.5)								
648	Greeks	Mountain Villages Elasson, Thessaly	78					8 (10.3)								78
	Greeks	Mountain Villages Elasson, Thessaly	55M	2 (3.6)												
	Greeks	Foothill Villages Elasson, Thessaly	139M	11 (7.9)												
	Greeks	Foothill Villages Elasson, Thessaly	165					13 (7.9)								165
648a	Greeks	Larissa District Thessaly	189M	21 (11.1)												
	Greeks	Trikkala District, Thessaly	112M	9 (8.0)												

REF.	POPULATION	PLACE	NUMBER TESTED	G6PD DEF.	SICKLE CELL	THALASSEMIA A_2	THALASSEMIA F	THALASSEMIA OSM. RES.	HEMOGLOBIN TYPES	AS						A
	GREECE (CONT.)															
648a	Greeks	Magnessia District, Thessaly	128M	5 (3.9)												
648	Greeks	Mountain Villages, Karditsa Thessaly	122M	4 (3.3)				14 (11.5)								122
	Greeks	Foothill Villages Karditsa, Thessaly	88M	4 (4.5)												
	Greeks	Foothill Villages Karditsa, Thessaly	98					6 (6.1)		1 (1.0)						
	Greeks	Plains Villages Karditsa, Thessaly	182M	36 (19.8)												
	Greeks	Plains Villages Karditsa, Thessaly	208					41 (19.7)		5 (2.4)						
51	Greeks	Karditsa District, Thessaly	102			10 (9.8)				2 (2.0)						
29	Greeks	Karditsa District, Thessaly	102M	8												
648a	Greeks	Karditsa District, Thessaly	124M	15												
	Greeks	Karditsa District, Thessaly	226M	23 (10.2)												
456	Greeks	Central Greece and Euboea	423					32 (7.6)								

REF.	POPULATION	PLACE	NUMBER TESTED	G6PD DEF.	SICKLE CELL	THALASSEMIA			HEMOGLOBIN TYPES							
						A_2	F	OSM. RES.	S	AS						
GREECE (CONT.)																
29	Greeks	Atalanti Phthiotis	105M	5 (4.8)												
51	Greeks	Atalanti Phthiotis	105			8 (7.6)				5 (4.8)						
648a	Greeks	Phthiotis District	137M	11 (8.0)												
172	Greeks	Lake Copais Boeotia	119							32 (26.9)						
173	Greeks	Petromagula Boeotia	200M	29 (14.5)												
	Greeks	Petromagula Boeotia	175						2	34 (20.6)						
648	Greeks	Petromagula Boeotia	183					23 (12.6)								
648a	Greeks	Boeotia District	103M	6 (5.8)												
	Greeks	Euboea District	140M	4 (2.8)												
	Greeks	Attica District	160M	3 (1.8)												
750	Greek Newborns	Athens	300M	3 (1.0)												
648a	Greeks	Athens	120M	3 (2.5)												

REF.	POPULATION	PLACE	NUMBER TESTED	G6PD DEF.	SICKLE CELL	THALASSEMIA			HEMOGLOBIN TYPES							
						A_2	F	OSM. RES.								
GREECE (CONT.)																
750	Greeks	Athens	280M	1												
379a	Greeks	Athens	<u>986M</u>	<u>33</u>												
	Greeks	Athens	1266M	34 (2.7)												
648a	Greeks	Phocis District	67M	4 (5.9)												
	Greeks	Eurytania District	34M	0												
	Greeks	Aetolo and Acarnania Districts	186M	18 (9.6)												
456	Greeks	Peloponnesus	300					19 (6.3)								
648a	Greeks	Achaia Peloponnese	186M	16 (8.6)												
	Greeks	Corinthia Peloponnese	90M	5 (5.5)												
	Greeks	Argolis Peloponnese	71M	2 (2.8)												
	Greeks	Arcadia Peloponnese	128M	2 (1.5)												
	Greeks	Laconia Peloponnese	112M	1 (0.9)												

REF.	POPULATION	PLACE	NUMBER TESTED	G6PD DEF.	SICKLE CELL	THALASSEMIA			HEMOGLOBIN TYPES							
						A_2	F	OSM. RES.		AS						
GREECE (CONT.)																
648a	Greeks	Messenia Peloponnese	180M	16 (8.8)												
	Greeks	Ileia Peloponnese	144M	12 (8.3)												
173	Greeks	Pygros and Amalia Ileia Peloponnese	290M	18 (6.2)						2 (0.7)						
456	Greeks	Ionian Islands	50			7 (14.0)										
648a	Greeks	Zante Island	30M	0												
	Greeks	Cephalonia Island	37M	0												
	Greeks	Leukada Island	25M	1 (4.0)												
456	Greeks	Epirus	74					9 (12.2)								
171	Greeks	Aneza, Gavria and Aghios Spyridon Villages Arta District Epirus	91M	16 (17.6)				12 (13.2)		13 (14.3)						
648a	Greeks	Arta Epirus	86M	6 (7.0)												

REF.	POPULATION	PLACE	NUMBER TESTED	G6PD DEF.	SICKLE CELL	THALASSEMIA			HEMOGLOBIN TYPES								
						A_2	F	OSM. RES.	S	AS		A Lepore				A	Alpha Thal.
GREECE (CONT.)																	
262	Greeks	Ghavria and Kalovatos Villages Arta Epirus	443M	61 (13.8)													
	Greeks	Ghavria and Kalovatos Villages Arta Epirus	904			98 (11.7)	3		8	92 (11.1)		8 (0.9)					50 (5.5)
171	Greeks	Lowland Villages Arta Epirus	171M	28 (16.4)				26 (15.2)		11 (6.4)							
	Greeks	Foothill Villages Arta Epirus	94M	4 (4.3)				10 (10.6)								94	
	Greeks	Mountain Villages Arta Epirus	176M	5 (2.8)				17 (9.7)								176	
648a	Greeks	Preveza District Epirus	54M	4 (7.4)													
	Greeks	Thesprotia District Epirus	41M	0													
	Greeks	Ioannina District Epirus	124M	1 (0.8)													
	Greeks	Corfu Island	79M	4 (5.0)													

REF.	POPULATION	PLACE	NUMBER TESTED	G6PD DEF.	SICKLE CELL	THALASSEMIA			HEMOGLOBIN TYPES							
						A_2	F	OSM. RES.								A
GREECE (CONT.)																
648	Greeks	Sokraki Corfu	146					23 (15.8)								146
	Greeks	Sokraki Corfu	116M	1 (0.9)												
	Greeks	Lowland Villages Corfu	976					128 (13.1)								976
	Greeks	Lowland Villages Corfu	772M	48 (6.2)												
YUGOSLAVIA																
261a	Yugoslavs	Gevgelija Macedonia	24M	0												24
	Yugoslavs	Gevgelija Macedonia	15F	0												15
	Yugoslavs	Stip Macedonia	26M	0												26
	Yugoslavs	Stip Macedonia	15F	2 (13.3)												15
	Yugoslavs	Stip Macedonia	16					2 (12.5)								
	Yugoslavs	Skopje Macedonia	22M	2 (9.1)												22
	Yugoslavs	Skopje Macedonia	7					0								

REF.	POPULATION	PLACE	NUMBER TESTED	G6PD DEF.	SICKLE CELL	THALASSEMIA			HEMOGLOBIN TYPES							
						A_2	F	OSM. RES.								A
YUGOSLAVIA (CONT.)																
261a	Gypsies	Skopje Macedonia	34M	0												34
	Gypsies	Skopje Macedonia	8F	2												8
	Gypsies	Skopje Macedonia	42	2 (4.8)												
	Gypsies	Skopje Macedonia	25					2 (8.0)								
	Yugoslavs	Dubrovnik Dalmatia	34M	0												34
	Yugoslavs	Dubrovnik Dalmatia	27F	0												27
	Yugoslavs	Dubrovnik Dalmatia	23					2 (8.7)								
	Yugoslavs	Ston Dalmatia	55M	0												55
	Yugoslavs	Ston Dalmatia	11F	0												11
	Yugoslavs	Ston Dalmatia	60					1 (1.6)								
	Yugoslavs	Metkovic Dalmatia	19M	2 (10.5)												19
	Yugoslavs	Metkovic Dalmatia	19F	0												19

REF.	POPULATION	PLACE	NUMBER TESTED	G6PD DEF.	SICKLE CELL	THALASSEMIA			HEMOGLOBIN TYPES							
						A_2	F	OSM. RES.		A Lepore						A
YUGOSLAVIA (CONT.)																
261a	Yugoslavs	Metkovic Dalmatia	29					2 (6.9)								
	Yugoslavs	Split Dalmatia	62M	0												62
	Yugoslavs	Split Dalmatia	19F	0												19
	Yugoslavs	Split Dalmatia	67					4 (6.0)								
	Yugoslavs	Zadar Dalmatia	27M	0												27
	Yugoslavs	Zadar Dalmatia	1F	0												1
	Yugoslavs	Zadar Dalmatia	19					3 (15.8)								
	Yugoslavs	Biograd Dalmatia	61M	0												61
	Yugoslavs	Biograd Dalmatia	37F	0												37
	Yugoslavs	Biograd Dalmatia	93					2 (2.2)								
	Yugoslavs	Rijeka Dalmatia	126M	1 (0.8)			1 (0.8)			1 (0.8)						
	Yugoslavs	Rijeka Dalmatia	119					5 (4.2)								

REF.	POPULATION	PLACE	NUMBER TESTED	G6PD DEF.	SICKLE CELL	THALASSEMIA			HEMOGLOBIN TYPES							
						A_2	F	OSM. RES.								A
YUGOSLAVIA (CONT.)																
261a	Yugoslavs	Mavrovo (Nr. Rijeka) Dalmatia	3M	0												3
	Yugoslavs	Mavrovo (Nr. Rijeka) Dalmatia	11F	0												11
	Yugoslavs	Mavrovo (Nr. Rijeka) Dalmatia	12					1 (8.3)								
BULGARIA																
39	Bulgarians With Favism	Sofia	9F/65M	(13.8)												
HUNGARY																
729a	Hungarians	Bodrog Northeast Hungary	363		0											
	Hungarians	Bodrog Northeast Hungary	233	9 (3.9)												
MALTA																
712	Maltese Students		208M	9 (4.3)												

REF.	POPULATION	PLACE	NUMBER TESTED	G6PD DEF.	SICKLE CELL	THALASSEMIA A_2	THALASSEMIA F	THALASSEMIA OSM. RES.	HEMOGLOBIN TYPES							
MALTA (CONT.)																
706	Maltese	Birkirkara	608					27 (4.4)								
	Maltese	Gzira	104					2 (1.9)								
	Maltese	Hamrun	236					12 (5.1)								
	Maltese	Msida	209					5 (2.4)								
	Maltese	Qormi	351					12 (3.4)								
	Maltese	Sliema	433					14 (3.2)								
	Maltese	"Three Cities"	54					2 (3.7)								
	Maltese	Valletta	117					4 (3.4)								
	Maltese	Zabbar	56					1 (1.8)								
	Maltese	Floriana	174					6 (3.4)								
	Maltese	Gargur	145					3 (2.1)								
	Maltese	Marsa	233					18 (7.7)								

REF.	POPULATION	PLACE	NUMBER TESTED	G6PD DEF.	SICKLE CELL	THALASSEMIA			HEMOGLOBIN TYPES							
						A_2	F	OSM. RES.								
MALTA (CONT.)																
706	Maltese	Mellieha	741					164 (22.1)								
	Maltese	Mosta	218					13 (6.0)								
	Maltese	Naxxar	185					4 (2.2)								
	Maltese	Pawla	248					26 (10.5)								
	Maltese	Rabat	526					22 (4.2)								
	Maltese	St. Paul's Bay	254					13 (5.1)								
	Maltese	Tarxien	208					14 (6.7)								
	Maltese	Zebbug	233					22 (9.4)								
	Maltese	Elsewhere	1027					58 (5.6)								
709	Maltese	Dingli	250					3 (1.2)								
	Maltese	Mgarr	348					35 (10.1)								
	Maltese	Vittoriosa	191					5 (2.6)								

REF.	POPULATION	PLACE	NUMBER TESTED	G6PD DEF.	SICKLE CELL	THALASSEMIA			HEMOGLOBIN TYPES							
						A_2	F	OSM. RES.								
MALTA (CONT.)																
709	Maltese	Senglea	207					8 (3.9)								
	Maltese	Cospicua	426					47 (11.0)								
	Maltese	Kalkara	189					10 (5.3)								
	Maltese	Zabbar	230					2 (0.9)								
	Maltese	Birsebbugia	210					10 (4.8)								
	Maltese	Marsascala	130					8 (6.2)								
	Maltese	Fgura	147					7 (4.8)								
	Maltese	Kirkop	121					6 (5.0)								
	Maltese	Qrendi	155					17 (11.0)								
	Maltese	Luqa	192					4 (2.1)								
	Maltese	Zejtun	142					1 (0.7)								
	Maltese	Gudja	150					12 (8.0)								

REF.	POPULATION	PLACE	NUMBER TESTED	G6PD DEF.	SICKLE CELL	THALASSEMIA			HEMOGLOBIN TYPES							
						A_2	F	OSM. RES.								
MALTA (CONT.)																
709	Maltese	Ghaxaq	160					1 (0.6)								
	Maltese	Safi	104					3 (2.9)								
	Maltese	Mqabba	143					9 (6.3)								
	Maltese	Siggiewi	178					8 (4.5)								
	Maltese	Zurrieq	171					14 (8.2)								
	Maltese	Marsaxlokk	181					28 (15.5)								
	Maltese	Sannat Gozo Island	198					2 (1.0)								
	Maltese	San Lawrenz Gozo Island	73					2 (2.7)								
706	Maltese	Nadur Gozo Island	297					7 (2.4)								
	Maltese	Xewkija Gozo Island	372					26 (7.0)								
	Maltese	Zebbug Gozo Island	184					45 (24.5)								
	Maltese	Elsewhere Gozo Island	23					6 (26.1)								

REF.	POPULATION	PLACE	NUMBER TESTED	G6PD DEF.	SICKLE CELL	THALASSEMIA			HEMOGLOBIN TYPES							
						A_2	F	OSM. RES.		AS	AK	AC				
ITALY																
637	Sicilians	Sicily	397							1	1					
626	Sicilians	Catania Sicily	100					7 (7.0)		1 (1.0)						
	Sicilians	Gela Caltanissetta Province	140					10 (7.1)		6 (4.3)						
548	Sicilians	Gela, Catania and Connalucata	934					45 (4.8)		16 (1.7)		2 (0.2)				
630	Sicilians	Catania Province	960					35 (3.7)								
	Sicilians	Paterno Catania Province	343					14 (4.1)								
	Sicilians	Adrano Catania Province	154					9 (5.8)								
	Sicilians	Scordia Catania Province	127					7 (5.5)								
	Sicilians	Caltanissetta Province	643					18 (2.8)								
	Sicilians	Gela Caltanissetta Province	227					20 (8.8)								
	Sicilians	S. Cataldo Caltanissetta Province	94					1 (1.1)								

REF.	POPULATION	PLACE	NUMBER TESTED	G6PD DEF.	SICKLE CELL	THALASSEMIA A_2	THALASSEMIA F	THALASSEMIA OSM. RES.	HEMOGLOBIN TYPES							
ITALY (CONT.)																
630	Sicilians	Borgo Petilia Caltanissetta Province	111					3 (2.7)								
	Sicilians	Colonia Palermo Province	972					43 (4.4)								
	Sicilians	Bagheria Palermo Province	172					5 (2.9)								
	Sicilians	Aspra Palermo Province	284					13 (4.6)								
	Sicilians	Agrigento Agrigento Province	100					8 (8.0)								
	Sicilians	S. Leone Agrigento Province	110					8 (7.3)								
	Sicilians	Naro Agrigento Province	269					12 (4.5)								
	Sicilians	Porto Empedocle Agrigento Province	123					7 (5.7)								
	Sicilians	Ribera Agrigento Province	111					12 (10.8)								

REF.	POPULATION	PLACE	NUMBER TESTED	G6PD DEF.	SICKLE CELL	THALASSEMIA			HEMOGLOBIN TYPES							
						A_2	F	OSM. RES.								
ITALY (CONT.)																
630	Sicilians	Menfi Agrigento Province	110					8 (7.3)								
	Sicilians	Sciacca Agrigento Province	174					8 (4.6)								
	Sicilians	Elsewhere Agrigento Province	35					2 (5.7)								
	Sicilians	Siracusa Province	517					22 (4.3)								
	Sicilians	Noto Siracusa Province	215					8 (3.7)								
	Sicilians	Lentini Siracusa Province	145					12 (8.3)								
	Sicilians	Francofonte Siracusa Province	115					8 (7.0)								
634	Sicilians	Ragusa Ragusa Province	132					17 (12.9)								
	Sicilians	Ispica Ragusa Province	62					6 (9.7)								
	Sicilians	Pozzallo Ragusa Province	203					24 (11.8)								

REF.	POPULATION	PLACE	NUMBER TESTED	G6PD DEF.	SICKLE CELL	THALASSEMIA A_2	THALASSEMIA F	THALASSEMIA OSM. RES.	HEMOGLOBIN TYPES	AS		A Lepore	AJ	AD	AN	
ITALY (CONT.)																
634	Sicilians	Regalbuto Enna Province	64					5 (7.8)								
630	Sicilians	Messina Province	628					18 (2.9)								
634	Sicilians	Messina Messina Province	765					23 (3.0)								
	Sicilians	Giardini Messina Province	61					6 (9.8)								
	Sicilians	Milazzo Messina Province	90					5 (5.6)								
637	Calabrians		856							3 (0.4)			1	1		
113	Calabrians		825				1	58 (7.0)				1			4	
634	Calabrians	Reggio Calabria	371					13 (3.5)								
112	Calabrians	Cosenza Cosenza Province						(4.0)								
	Calabrians	Piane Crati Cosenza Province						(4.4)								
	Calabrians	Castrovillari Cosenza Province						(10.0)								
	Calabrians	Amantea Cosenza Province						(4.7)								

REF.	POPULATION	PLACE	NUMBER TESTED	G6PD DEF.	SICKLE CELL	THALASSEMIA			HEMOGLOBIN TYPES							
						A_2	F	OSM. RES.								
ITALY (CONT.)																
112	Calabrians	Roseto Capo Spulico Cosenza Province						(12.8)								
	Calabrians	Rocca Imperiale Cosenza Province						(6.6)								
	Calabrians	Amendolara Cosenza Province						(9.6)								
	Calabrians	Trebisacce Cosenza Province						(6.8)								
	Calabrians	Cassano Ionio Cosenza Province						(10.8)								
	Calabrians	Paola Cosenza Province						(3.6)								
	Calabrians	Cariati Cosenza Province						(6.8)								
	Calabrians	Terranova di Sibari Cosenza Province						(12.2)								
	Albanians	Spezzano Albanese Cosenza Province						(9.2)								
	Calabrians	Corigliano Calabro Cosenza Province						(8.1)								
	Calabrians	Rossano Cosenza Province						(5.6)								

REF.	POPULATION	PLACE	NUMBER TESTED	G6PD DEF.	SICKLE CELL	THALASSEMIA A_2	THALASSEMIA F	THALASSEMIA OSM. RES.	HEMOGLOBIN TYPES							
ITALY (CONT.)																
112	Calabrians	S. Lucido Cosenza Province						(4.1)								
	Calabrians	Acri Cosenza Province						(3.4)								
	Albanians	S. Demetrio Corone Cosenza Province						(7.5)								
	Albanians	Rota Greca Cosenza Province						(8.0)								
	Calabrians	S. Giovanni in Fiore Cosenza Province						(6.6)								
	Albanians	S. Martino di Finita Cosenza Province						(9.1)								
	Calabrians	Panettieri Cosenza Province						(3.8)								
	Calabrians	Scalea Cosenza Province						(10.0)								
	Albanians	Lungro Cosenza Province						(1.2)								
	Albanians	Frascineto Cosenza Province						(3.6)								
	Calabrians	Bisignano Cosenza Province						(6.7)								

REF.	POPULATION	PLACE	NUMBER TESTED	G6PD DEF.	SICKLE CELL	THALASSEMIA			HEMOGLOBIN TYPES							
						A_2	F	OSM. RES.								
ITALY (CONT.)																
112	Calabrians	Montalto Uffugo Cosenza Province						(3.5)								
	Calabrians	Cerchiara di Calabria Cosenza Province						(16.0)								
	Calabrians	Francavilla Cosenza Province						(12.7)								
	Calabrians	Villapiana Cosenza Province						(13.5)								
	Albanians	Plataci Cosenza Province						(5.5)								
	Calabrians	Calopezzati Cosenza Province						(16.0)								
	Calabrians	Montegiordano Cosenza Province						(5.3)								
	Albanians	Civita Cosenza Province						(7.8)								
	Calabrians	Roggiano Gravina Cosenza Province						(2.2)								
	Calabrians	Torano Castello Cosenza Province						(13.2)								
	Calabrians	Praia a Mare Cosenza Province						(4.1)								

REF.	POPULATION	PLACE	NUMBER TESTED	G6PD DEF.	SICKLE CELL	THALASSEMIA			HEMOGLOBIN TYPES							
						A_2	F	OSM. RES.								
ITALY (CONT.)																
112	Calabrians	Sartano Cosenza Province						(18.1)								
	Calabrians	Mongrassano Cosenza Province						(6.3)								
	Albanians	Cerzeto Cosenza Province						(14.1)								
	Albanians	Cavallerizzo Cosenza Province						(7.4)								
	Albanians	S. Caterina Albanese Cosenza Province						(3.5)								
	Calabrians	Malvito Cosenza Province						(2.7)								
	Calabrians	Mottafollone Cosenza Province						(5.2)								
	Calabrians	Fagnano Castello Cosenza Province						(1.4)								
	Calabrians	Guardia Piemontese Cosenza Province						(1.6)								
	Calabrians	Lattarico Cosenza Province						(2.4)								
	Calabrians	S. Marco Argentano Cosenza Province						(2.2)								

REF.	POPULATION	PLACE	NUMBER TESTED	G6PD DEF.	SICKLE CELL	THALASSEMIA			HEMOGLOBIN TYPES							
						A_2	F	OSM. RES.								
ITALY (CONT.)																
112	Calabrians	S. Pietro in Guarano Cosenza Province						(4.8)								
	Calabrians	Castiglione Cosentino Cosenza Province						(17.7)								
	Albanians	Vaccarizzo Albanese Cosenza Province						(7.1)								
	Albanians	S. Cosmo Albanese Cosenza Province						(2.5)								
	Albanians	S. Basile Cosenza Province						(4.1)								
	Albanians	S. Lorenzo del Vallo Cosenza Province						(10.7)								
	Calabrians	Saracena Cosenza Province						(2.3)								
	Calabrians	Tarsia Cosenza Province						(4.0)								
	Albanians	S. Benedetto Ulbano Cosenza Province						(6.5)								
	Calabrians	Lauropoli Cosenza Province						(5.2)								

REF.	POPULATION	PLACE	NUMBER TESTED	G6PD DEF.	SICKLE CELL	THALASSEMIA			HEMOGLOBIN TYPES							
						A_2	F	OSM. RES.								
ITALY (CONT.)																
112	Calabrians	Doria Cosenza Province						(3.7)								
	Calabrians	Oriolo Calabro Cosenza Province						(8.4)								
	Albanians	S. Sofia D'Epiro Cosenza Province						(5.7)								
	Albanians	Firmo Cosenza Province						(3.3)								
	Calabrians	S. Domenica Talao Cosenza Province						(1.6)								
	Calabrians	Nocara Cosenza Province						(10.0)								
	Calabrians	Canna Cosenza Province						(3.8)								
	Calabrians	Casole Bruzio Cosenza Province						(1.4)								
	Calabrians	Trenta Cosenza Province						(6.2)								
	Calabrians	Crosia Cosenza Province						(6.3)								
	Calabrians	Dipignano Cosenza Province						(0.7)								

REF.	POPULATION	PLACE	NUMBER TESTED	G6PD DEF.	SICKLE CELL	THALASSEMIA			HEMOGLOBIN TYPES							
						A_2	F	OSM. RES.								
ITALY (CONT.)																
112	Calabrians	Mirto Cosenza Province						(7.3)								
	Calabrians	Altomonte Cosenza Province						(5.4)								
	Calabrians	Cleto Cosenza Province						(4.5)								
	Calabrians	S. Agata D'Esaro Cosenza Province						(2.9)								
	Calabrians	Bianchi Cosenza Province						(2.2)								
	Calabrians	Colosimi Cosenza Province						(1.3)								
	Calabrians	Mandatoriccio Cosenza Province						(4.6)								
	Calabrians	Castroregio Cosenza Province						(10.3)								
	Calabrians	Pietrapaola Cosenza Province						(3.5)								
	Calabrians	Campana Cosenza Province						(13.3)								
	Calabrians	Albidona Cosenza Province						(6.6)								

REF.	POPULATION	PLACE	NUMBER TESTED	G6PD DEF.	SICKLE CELL	THALASSEMIA A$_2$	THALASSEMIA F	THALASSEMIA OSM. RES.	HEMOGLOBIN TYPES							
ITALY (CONT.)																
112	Calabrians	Bocchigliero Cosenza Province						(5.7)								
	Calabrians	Caloveto Cosenza Province						(9.4)								
	Calabrians	Scala Coeli Cosenza Province						(9.9)								
	Calabrians	Longobucco Cosenza Province						(4.5)								
	Calabrians	Terravecchia Cosenza Province						(10.1)								
	Calabrians	S. Lorenzo Bellizzi Cosenza Province						(12.5)								
	Calabrians	Paludi Cosenza Province						(2.6)								
	Calabrians	Cropalati Cosenza Province						(5.8)								
	Calabrians	Fiumefreddo Bruzio Cosenza Province						(1.6)								
	Calabrians	Longobardi Cosenza Province						(4.6)								
	Calabrians	Malito Cosenza Province						(5.4)								

REF.	POPULATION	PLACE	NUMBER TESTED	G6PD DEF.	SICKLE CELL	THALASSEMIA A_2	THALASSEMIA F	THALASSEMIA OSM. RES.	HEMOGLOBIN TYPES							
ITALY (CONT.)																
112	Calabrians	Grimaldi Cosenza Province						(1.1)								
	Calabrians	Morano Calabro Cosenza Province						(3.1)								
	Albanians	S. Giorgio Albanese Cosenza Province						(3.1)								
	Calabrians	Diamante Cosenza Province						(2.8)								
	Total Examined	Cosenza Province	26230					1624 (6.2)								
	Calabrians	Soveria Mannelli Catanzaro Province						(7.1)								
	Calabrians	Crotone Catanzaro Province						(6.6)								
	Calabrians	Isola Capo Rizzuto Catanzaro Province						(15.2)								
	Calabrians	Cutro Catanzaro Province						(6.9)								
	Calabrians	Roccabernarda Catanzaro Province						(19.7)								
	Calabrians	Ciro Superiore Catanzaro Province						(10.0)								

REF.	POPULATION	PLACE	NUMBER TESTED	G6PD DEF.	SICKLE CELL	THALASSEMIA			HEMOGLOBIN TYPES							
						A_2	F	OSM. RES.								
ITALY (CONT.)																
112	Calabrians	Ciro Marina Catanzaro Province						(8.4)								
	Calabrians	Mesoraca Catanzaro Province						(10.0)								
	Calabrians	Petilia Policastro Catanzaro Province						(5.3)								
	Calabrians	Belvedere Spinelli Catanzaro Province						(11.1)								
	Calabrians	Rocca Di Neto Catanzaro Province						(13.0)								
	Calabrians	Caccuri Catanzaro Province						(4.1)								
	Calabrians	Cerenzia Catanzaro Province						(9.0)								
	Calabrians	S. Severina Catanzaro Province						(15.9)								
	Calabrians	S. Mauro Marchesato Catanzaro Province						(17.5)								
	Calabrians	Savelli Catanzaro Province						(2.1)								
	Calabrians	Botricello Catanzaro Province						(14.5)								

REF.	POPULATION	PLACE	NUMBER TESTED	G6PD DEF.	SICKLE CELL	THALASSEMIA			HEMOGLOBIN TYPES							
						A_2	F	OSM. RES.								B_2
ITALY (CONT.)																
112	Calabrians	Maida Catanzaro Province						(7.0)								
	Calabrians	Curinga Catanzaro Province						(9.7)								
	Calabrians	Staletti Catanzaro Province						(11.1)								
	Calabrians	Montauro Catanzaro Province						(7.7)								
	Calabrians	Badolato Catanzaro Province						(11.2)								
	Calabrians	Pizzo Calabro Catanzaro Province						(12.4)								
	Calabrians	Tropea Catanzaro Province						(7.1)								
	Calabrians	Strongoli Catanzaro Province						(13.1)								
	Calabrians	Sambiase Catanzaro Province						(2.8)								
	Total Examined	Catanzaro Province	7005					691 (9.9)								
484a	Italians	Lecce Province	275M	6 (2.2)												
636a	Italians	Lecce Province	992			69 (7.0)	2	65 (6.6)								1

REF.	POPULATION	PLACE	NUMBER TESTED	G6PD DEF.	SICKLE CELL	THALASSEMIA			HEMOGLOBIN TYPES							
						A_2	F	OSM. RES.			AG					
ITALY (CONT.)																
631	Italians	Salentino Salice District Lecce Province	743					84 (11.3)								
	Italians	Lecce Lecce Province	177					9 (5.1)								
	Italians	Muro District Lecce Province	348					37 (10.6)								
	Italians	Gallipoli Lecce Province	255					15 (5.9)								
	Italians	Matino Lecce Province	626					45 (7.2)								
87b	Italians	Town in Apulia	923			54	10 (6.8)	96 (10.4)								
637	Italians	Puglia and Basilicata Regions	652								1					
451a	Italians	Gargano Foggia Province	1290					56 (4.3)								
560	Italians	Ottaviano Naples Province	590					17 (2.9)								
	Italians	Pozzuoli Naples Province	509					33 (6.5)								
	Italians	Aversa Caserta Province	265					14 (5.3)								

REF.	POPULATION	PLACE	NUMBER TESTED	G6PD DEF.	SICKLE CELL	THALASSEMIA			HEMOGLOBIN TYPES							
						A_2	F	OSM. RES.		AD		AG				Barts
ITALY (CONT.)																
634	Italians	Naples Naples Province	914					16 (1.8)								
	Italians	Naples Province	754					18 (2.4)								
	Italians	Roma Roma Province	7595					125 (1.6)								
633	Italians (cord blood)	Roma Roma Province	3556													9 (0.3)
273	Italians	Fiano Romano Roma Province	220					18 (8.2)								
634	Italians	Ancona Ancona Province	787					13 (1.7)								
	Italians	Firenze Firenze Province	417					2 (0.5)								
	Italians	Ravenna Ravenna Province	216					8 (3.7)								
	Italians	Bologna Bologna Province	229					2 (0.9)								
593	Italian Newborn	Bologna Bologna Province	59M	0												
	Italian Newborn	Bologna Bologna Province	41F	0												
452	Italians	Po River Delta Region	1200							4 (0.3)		9 (0.8)				

REF.	POPULATION	PLACE	NUMBER TESTED	G6PD DEF.	SICKLE CELL	THALASSEMIA			HEMOGLOBIN TYPES							
						A_2	F	OSM. RES.								
ITALY (CONT.)																
120a	Italians	Perugia Umbria Province	1557	0												
634	Italians	Ferrara Ferrara Province	1718					127 (7.4)								
	Italians	Copparo Ferrara Province	626					78 (12.5)								
	Italians	Migliarino Ferrara Province	488					55 (11.3)								
	Italians	Massa Fiscaglia Ferrara Province	557					65 (11.7)								
	Italians	Comacchio Ferrara Province	279					23 (8.2)								
	Italians	Portomaggiore Ferrara Province	1301					151 (11.6)								
	Italians	San Giovanni Ferrara Province	228					14 (6.1)								
	Italians	Rovereto Ferrara Province	435					46 (10.6)								
	Italians	Gambalunga Ferrara Province	789					56 (7.1)								
	Italians	Codigoro Ferrara Province	3710					579 (15.6)								
	Italians	Mezzogoro Ferrara Province	1637					244 (14.9)								

REF.	POPULATION	PLACE	NUMBER TESTED	G6PD DEF.	SICKLE CELL	THALASSEMIA			HEMOGLOBIN TYPES							
						A_2	F	OSM. RES.								
ITALY (CONT.)																
634	Italians	Caprile Ferrara Province	1251					210 (16.8)								
	Italians	Pomposa Ferrara Province	513					93 (18.1)								
	Italians	Lagosanto Ferrara Province	2079					397 (19.1)								
	Italians	Mesola Ferrara Province	1048					203 (19.4)								
	Italians	Bosco Mesola Ferrara Province	341					63 (18.5)								
	Italians	Berra Ferrara Province	687					126 (18.3)								
	Italians	Serravalle Ferrara Province	576					104 (18.1)								
	Italians	Sant' Agostino Ferrara Province	697					23 (3.3)								
	Italians	Bondeno Ferrara Province	578					42 (7.3)								
	Italians	Cento Ferrara Province	383					24 (6.3)								
	Italians	Poggio Renatico Ferrara Province	623					33 (5.3)								
	Italians	Santa Maria Codifiume Ferrara Province	593					43 (7.3)								

REF.	POPULATION	PLACE	NUMBER TESTED	G6PD DEF.	SICKLE CELL	THALASSEMIA			HEMOGLOBIN TYPES							
						A_2	F	OSM. RES.								
ITALY (CONT.)																
634	Italians	Argenta Ferrara Province	438					41 (9.4)								
	Italians	Ambrogio Ferrara Province	1957					313 (16.0)								
	Italians	Formignana Ferrara Province	1508					156 (10.3)								
	Italians	Cologna Ferrara Province	1115					113 (10.1)								
	Italians	Ostellato Ferrara Province	441					65 (14.7)								
	Italians	Rovigo Rovigo Province	955					93 (9.7)								
	Italians	Porto Tolle Rovigo Province	367					65 (17.7)								
	Italians	Adria Rovigo Province	559					79 (14.1)								
	Italians	S. Martino di Venezze Rovigo Province	596					60 (10.1)								
	Italians	Lendinara Rovigo Province	303					36 (11.9)								
	Italians	Badia Polesine Rovigo Province	480					46 (9.6)								

REF.	POPULATION	PLACE	NUMBER TESTED	G6PD DEF.	SICKLE CELL	THALASSEMIA			HEMOGLOBIN TYPES							
						A_2	F	OSM. RES.								
ITALY (CONT.)																
634	Italians	Bergantino Rovigo Province	784					62 (7.9)								
	Italians	Castelmassa Rovigo Province	662					80 (12.1)								
	Italians	Ficarolo Rovigo Province	755					91 (12.1)								
	Italians	Fiesso Umbertiano Rovigo Province	704					82 (11.6)								
	Italians	Padova Padova Province	1082					22 (2.0)								
	Italians	Verona Province	2540					160 (6.3)								
152	Italians	Castagnaro Verona Province	77					12 (15.6)								
	Italians	Villabartolomea Verona Province	70					10 (14.3)								
	Italians	Legnago Verona Province	142					18 (12.7)								
	Italians	Cerea Verona Province	117					16 (13.7)								
	Italians	Sanguinetto Verona Province	35					3 (8.6)								

REF.	POPULATION	PLACE	NUMBER TESTED	G6PD DEF.	SICKLE CELL	THALASSEMIA			HEMOGLOBIN TYPES							
						A_2	F	OSM. RES.								
ITALY (CONT.)																
152	Italians	Nogara Verona Province	76					3 (3.9)								
	Italians	Minerbe Verona Province	54					7 (13.0)								
	Italians	Albaredo Verona Province	71					9 (12.7)								
	Italians	Ronco all'Adige Verona Province	40					5 (12.5)								
	Italians	Bovolone Verona Province	53					4 (7.5)								
	Italians	Erbe Verona Province	29					5 (17.2)								
	Italians	Verona Verona Province	813					36 (4.4)								
	Italians	Zevio Verona Province	56					3 (5.4)								
	Italians	S. Giovanni Lupatoto Verona Province	56					1 (1.8)								
	Italians	Isola della Scala Verona Province	67					4 (6.0)								
	Italians	S. Bonifacio Verona Province	72					4 (5.6)								

REF.	POPULATION	PLACE	NUMBER TESTED	G6PD DEF.	SICKLE CELL	THALASSEMIA			HEMOGLOBIN TYPES							
						A_2	F	OSM. RES.								
ITALY (CONT.)																
152	Italians	S. Martino B. A. Verona Province	31					1 (3.2)								
	Italians	Vigasio Verona Province	40					2 (5.0)								
	Italians	Villafranca Verona Province	62					3 (4.8)								
	Italians	Peschiera Verona Province	37					0								
	Italians	Garda Verona Province	43					3 (7.0)								
	Italians	Sommacampagna Verona Province	49					0								
	Italians	S. Giovanni Ilarione Verona Province	19					0								
	Italians	Tregnago Verona Province	43					2 (4.7)								
	Italians	Pescantina Verona Province	70					3 (4.3)								
	Italians	S. Pietro Inc. Verona Province	77					2 (2.6)								
	Italians	S. Anna Alf. Verona Province	59					2 (3.4)								

REF.	POPULATION	PLACE	NUMBER TESTED	G6PD DEF.	SICKLE CELL	THALASSEMIA			HEMOGLOBIN TYPES							
						A_2	F	OSM. RES.								
ITALY (CONT.)																
152	Italians	Caprino Verona Province	29					0								
	Italians	Dolce Verona Province	20					0								
	Italians	Grezzana Verona Province	31					1 (3.2)								
	Italians	Boscochiesanuova Verona Province	26					0								
	Italians	Rovere Verona Verona Province	16					0								
	Italians	Soave Verona Province	30					1 (3.3)								
634	Italians	Milano Milano Province	1072					15 (1.4)								
	Italians	Torino Torino Province	1174					11 (0.9)								
	Italians	Genova Genova Province	1156					18 (1.6)								
675	Italians	Genova Genova Province	1360	9 (0.7)												
598	Italians	Liguria	100	0												
675	Italians	(All Provinces Except Sardinia)	714	6 (0.8)												

REF.	POPULATION	PLACE	NUMBER TESTED	G6PD DEF.	SICKLE CELL	THALASSEMIA			HEMOGLOBIN TYPES							
						A_2	F	OSM. RES.								A
ITALY (CONT.)																
675	Italians	Sardinia	857	122 (14.2)												
598	Italians	Sardinia	61M	8 (13.1)												
	Italians	Sardinia	38F	4 (10.5)												
637	Italians	Sardinia	192													192
640a	Sardinians	Luras Sassari Province	100M	7 (7.0)												
	Sardinians	Luras Sassari Province	98					23 (23.5)								
	Sardinians	Usini Sassari Province	99M	6 (6.1)				14 (14.1)								
	Sardinians	Benetutti Sassari Province	100M	9 (9.0)												
149	Sardinians	Benetutti Sassari Province	250					25								
640a	Sardinians	Benetutti Sassari Province	100					12								
	Sardinians	Benetutti Sassari Province	350					37 (10.6)								
149	Sardinians	Sassari Sassari Province	234					49 (20.9)								

REF.	POPULATION	PLACE	NUMBER TESTED	G6PD DEF.	SICKLE CELL	THALASSEMIA			HEMOGLOBIN TYPES							
						A_2	F	OSM. RES.								
ITALY (CONT.)																
149	Sardinians	Bancali Sassari Province	65					13 (20.0)								
	Sardinians	P. Torres Sassari Province	137					20 (14.6)								
	Ligurians	Stintino Sassari Province	69					3 (4.3)								
	Italians	Canaglia Sassari Province	58					3 (5.2)								
	Sardinians	Castelsardo Sassari Province	300					64 (21.4)								
	Sardinians	Codaruina Sassari Province	100					16 (16.0)								
	Sardinians	Tempio Sassari Province	294					40 (13.6)								
	Sardinians	Trinita Sassari Province	113					17 (15.0)								
	Sardinians	S. Teresa Sassari Province	91					12 (13.2)								
	Sardinians	Calangianus Sassari Province	110					15 (13.6)								
	Sardinians	Palau Sassari Province	100					13 (13.0)								
	Sardinians	Monti Sassari Province	100					22 (22.0)								

REF.	POPULATION	PLACE	NUMBER TESTED	G6PD DEF.	SICKLE CELL	THALASSEMIA			HEMOGLOBIN TYPES							
						A_2	F	OSM. RES.								
ITALY (CONT.)																
149	Sardinians	La Maddelena Sassari Province	119					8 (6.7)								
	Sardinians	Ozieri Sassari Province	224					34 (15.2)								
	Catalans	Alghero Sassari Province	150					6 (4.0)								
640a	Sardinians	Ala Dei Sardi Sassari Province	80M	18 (22.5)				16 (20.0)								
149	Sardinians	Sorso, Sennori, Tissi, Ossi, and Ittiri Sassari Province	180					31 (17.2)								
640a	Sardinians	Lode Nuoro Province	820M	231 (28.2)				226 (27.6)								
	Sardinians	Siniscola Nuoro Province	195M	22 (11.3)												
	Sardinians	Siniscola Nuoro Province	97					24 (24.7)								
	Sardinians	Suni Nuoro Province	98M	14 (14.3)												
	Sardinians	Suni Nuoro Province	100					25 (25.0)								
	Sardinians	Isili Nuoro Province	100M	9 (9.0)				17 (17.0)								

REF.	POPULATION	PLACE	NUMBER TESTED	G6PD DEF.	SICKLE CELL	THALASSEMIA			HEMOGLOBIN TYPES							
						A_2	F	OSM. RES.								
ITALY (CONT.)																
640a	Sardinians	Orosei Nuoro Province	180M	23 (13.0)												
149	Sardinians	Orosei Nuoro Province	1047					255								
640a	Sardinians	Orosei Nuoro Province	308					58								
	Sardinians	Orosei Nuoro Province	1355					313 (23.1)								
640a	Sardinians	Galtelli Nuoro Province	175M	21 (12.0)												
640a	Sardinians	Galtelli Nuoro Province	235					50								
149	Sardinians	Galtelli Nuoro Province	854					213								
	Sardinians	Galtelli Nuoro Province	1089					263 (24.2)								
640a	Sardinians	Fonni Nuoro Province	100M	3 (3.0)												
149	Sardinians	Fonni Nuoro Province	250					14 (5.6)								
640a	Sardinians	Desulo Nuoro Province	313M	9 (2.9)												

REF.	POPULATION	PLACE	NUMBER TESTED	G6PD DEF.	SICKLE CELL	THALASSEMIA A_2	THALASSEMIA F	THALASSEMIA OSM. RES.	HEMOGLOBIN TYPES
ITALY (CONT.)									
640a	Sardinians	Desulo Nuoro Province	320					12	
149	Sardinians	Desulo Nuoro Province	639					26	
	Sardinians	Desulo Nuoro	959					38 (4.0)	
640a	Sardinians	Tonara Nuoro Province	148M	6 (4.1)					
640a	Sardinians	Tonara Nuoro Province	102					5	
149	Sardinians	Tonara Nuoro Province	408					22	
	Sardinians	Tonara Nuoro Province	510					27 (5.3)	
640a	Sardinians	Lanusei Nuoro Province	100M	4 (4.0)					
149	Sardinians	Lanusei Nuoro Province	200					20 (10.0)	
640a	Sardinians	Tortoli Nuoro Province	50M	8 (16.0)					
149	Sardinians	Tortoli Nuoro Province	360					91 (25.3)	
	Sardinians	Ilbono Nuoro Province	150					12 (8.0)	

REF.	POPULATION	PLACE	NUMBER TESTED	G6PD DEF.	SICKLE CELL	THALASSEMIA A_2	THALASSEMIA F	THALASSEMIA OSM. RES.	HEMOGLOBIN TYPES							
ITALY (CONT.)																
149	Sardinians	Aritzo Nuoro Province	315					13 (4.1)								
	Sardinians	Girasole Nuoro Province	190					47 (24.7)								
	Sardinians	Arzana Nuoro Province	200					15 (7.5)								
	Sardinians	Arbatax Nuoro Province	220					46 (20.9)								
	Sardinians	Loculi Nuoro Province	80					20 (25.0)								
	Sardinians	Onifai Nuoro Province	91					26 (28.6)								
640a	Sardinians	Irgoli Nuoro Province	100M	15 (15.0)												
149	Sardinians	Irgoli Nuoro Province	120					30								
640a	Sardinians	Irgoli Nuoro Province	100					32								
	Sardinians	Irgoli Nuoro Province	220					62 (28.2)								
640a	Sardinians	Torpe Nuoro Province	100M	22 (22.0)				38 (38.0)								
	Sardinians	Barisardo Nuoro Province	98M	15 (15.3)				18 (18.4)								

REF.	POPULATION	PLACE	NUMBER TESTED	G6PD DEF.	SICKLE CELL	THALASSEMIA			HEMOGLOBIN TYPES							
						A_2	F	OSM. RES.								
ITALY (CONT.)																
640a	Sardinians	Ottana Nuoro Province	72M	6 (8.3)				20 (27.8)								
	Sardinians	Tresnuraghes Nuoro Province	86M	11 (12.8)				27 (31.4)								
	Sardinians	Dualchi Nuoro Province	75M	16 (21.3)												
	Sardinians	Dualchi Nuoro Province	100					18 (18.0)								
	Sardinians	Borore Nuoro Province	100M	9 (9.0)												
	Sardinians	Borore Nuoro Province	99					33 (33.3)								
	Sardinians	Bolotana Nuoro Province	93M	11 (11.8)				20 (21.5)								
	Sardinians	Lula Nuoro Province	100M	7 (7.0)				19 (19.0)								
	Sardinians	Bitti Nuoro Province	193M	10 (5.2)				24 (12.4)								
	Sardinians	Orune Nuoro Province	97M	6 (6.2)				14 (14.4)								
	Sardinians	Gavoi Nuoro Province	98M	3 (3.1)				10 (10.2)								
149	Sardinians	Dorgali Nuoro Province	462					38 (8.2)								

REF.	POPULATION	PLACE	NUMBER TESTED	G6PD DEF.	SICKLE CELL	THALASSEMIA			HEMOGLOBIN TYPES							
						A_2	F	OSM. RES.								
ITALY (CONT.)																
149	Sardinians	Bortigali Nuoro Province	142					16 (11.3)								
	Sardinians	Bosa Nuoro Province	260					26 (10.0)								
	Sardinians	Nuoro Nuoro Province	239					44 (18.4)								
640a	Sardinians	Cabras Cagliari Province	200M	70 (35.0)												
	Sardinians	Cabras Cagliari Province	100					28 (28.0)								
	Sardinians	Gergei Cagliari Province	92M	17 (18.5)				12 (13.0)								
	Sardinians	S. Giusta Cagliari Province	42M	13 (31.0)												
	Sardinians	Terralba Cagliari Province	100M	30 (30.0)												
	Sardinians	Teulada Cagliari Province	101M	17 (16.8)												
	Sardinians	Teulada Cagliari Province	100					25 (25.0)								
	Sardinians	Gonnosfanadiga Cagliari Province	49M	12 (24.5)												
149	Sardinians	Gonnosfanadiga Cagliari Province	301					36 (12.0)								

REF.	POPULATION	PLACE	NUMBER TESTED	G6PD DEF.	SICKLE CELL	THALASSEMIA A_2	THALASSEMIA F	THALASSEMIA OSM. RES.	HEMOGLOBIN TYPES
ITALY (CONT.)									
641	Sardinians	Cagliari Cagliari Province		(25.0)					
149	Sardinians	Cagliari Cagliari Province	450					90	
632	Sardinians	Cagliari Cagliari Province	1374					302	
	Sardinians	Cagliari Cagliari Province	1824					392 (21.3)	
149	Sardinians	Arborea Cagliari Province	359					58	
632	Sardinians	Arborea Cagliari Province	251					43	
	Sardinians	Arborea Cagliari Province	610					101 (16.6)	
149	Sardinians	Oristano Cagliari Province	300					63	
632	Sardinians	Oristano Cagliari Province	125					28	
	Sardinians	Oristano Cagliari Province	425					91 (21.4)	
149	Sardinians	Iglesias Cagliari Province	200					50 (25.0)	

REF.	POPULATION	PLACE	NUMBER TESTED	G6PD DEF.	SICKLE CELL	THALASSEMIA			HEMOGLOBIN TYPES							
						A_2	F	OSM. RES.								
ITALY (CONT.)																
149	Sardinians	Sestu Cagliari Province	350					46 (13.1)								
632	Sardinians	Quartu S Elena Cagliari Province	33					7 (21.2)								
	Sardinians	Planusanguini Cagliari Province	89					11 (12.4)								
	Sardinians	S. Gregorio Cagliari Province	86					21 (24.4)								
	Sardinians	Milis Cagliari Province	19					5 (26.3)								
640a	Sardinians	Guspini Cagliari Province	99M	28 (28.3)				31								
632	Sardinians	Guspini Cagliari Province	110					23								
	Sardinians	Guspini Cagliari Province	209					54 (25.8)								
632	Sardinians	Fontanazza Cagliari Province	198					52 (26.3)								
	Sardinians	Sant'Angelo Cagliari Province	103					20 (19.4)								
	Sardinians	Portopaglietta Cagliari Province	306					79 (25.8)								

REF.	POPULATION	PLACE	NUMBER TESTED	G6PD DEF.	SICKLE CELL	THALASSEMIA A_2	THALASSEMIA F	THALASSEMIA OSM. RES.	HEMOGLOBIN TYPES							
ITALY (CONT.)																
632	Sardinians	Portoscuso Cagliari Province	245					82 (33.5)								
	Sardinians	Porto Pino Cagliari Province	201					54 (26.9)								
640a	Sardinians	Carloforte Cagliari Province	99M	5 (5.1)				5								
632	Sardinians	Carloforte Cagliari Province	388					117								
	Sardinians	Carloforte Cagliari Province	487					122 (25.1)								
632	Sardinians	Calasetta Cagliari Province	275					61 (22.2)								
640a	Sardinians	Assemini Cagliari Province	108M	22 (20.4)				12 (11.1)								
	Sardinians	Marrubiu Cagliari Province	98M	32 (32.7)				28 (28.6)								
	Sardinians	Decimomannu Cagliari Province	100M	26 (26.0)				25 (25.0)								
	Sardinians	Pula Cagliari Province	100M	15 (15.0)				16 (16.0)								
	Sardinians	S. Gavino Cagliari Province	100M	26 (26.0)												
	Sardinians	Capoterra Cagliari Province	92M	15 (16.3)				19 (20.7)								

REF.	POPULATION	PLACE	NUMBER TESTED	G6PD DEF.	SICKLE CELL	THALASSEMIA A$_2$	THALASSEMIA F	THALASSEMIA OSM. RES.	HEMOGLOBIN TYPES							
ITALY (CONT.)																
640a	Sardinians	Siligua Cagliari Province	100M	26 (26.0)				22 (22.0)								
	Sardinians	Vallermosa Cagliari Province	86M	18 (20.9)				18 (20.9)								
	Sardinians	Monastir Cagliari Province	94M	22 (23.4)				20 (21.3)								
	Sardinians	Nuraminis Cagliari Province	100M	25 (25.0)				17 (17.0)								
	Sardinians	Villamar Cagliari Province	100M	23 (23.0)				18 (18.0)								
	Sardinians	Domusnovas Cagliari Province	100M	22 (22.0)				19 (19.0)								
	Sardinians	Senorbi Cagliari Province	101M	25 (24.8)				14 (13.9)								
	Sardinians	Sedilo Cagliari Province	100M	22 (22.0)												
	Sardinians	Sedilo Cagliari Province	96					18 (18.8)								
	Sardinians	Serrenti Cagliari Province	100M	21 (21.0)				25 (25.0)								
	Sardinians	Arbus Cagliari Province	95M	34 (35.8)				31 (32.6)								
	Sardinians	Abbasanta Cagliari Province	97M	18 (18.6)												

REF.	POPULATION	PLACE	NUMBER TESTED	G6PD DEF.	SICKLE CELL	THALASSEMIA			HEMOGLOBIN TYPES							
						A_2	F	OSM. RES.		S		AJ				A
ITALY (CONT.)																
640a	Sardinians	Abbasanta Cagliari Province	92					21 (22.8)								
PORTUGAL																
689a	Portuguese	Lisbon	3042							3 (0.1)						
188	Portuguese	Lisbon	4142			4	17 (0.6)	23 (0.6)								
302	Portuguese	Madeira	458M	4 (0.9)												
359	Portuguese	Hawaii	222													222
66	Portuguese	Curacao	1499		0											
CZECHOSLOVAKIA																
694	Slovaks	Trnava Slovakia	171													171
	Gypsies	Trnava Slovakia	63													63
SWEDEN																
65	Gypsies	Stockholm	116													116
64a	Swedes	Uppsala	411									1				

REF.	POPULATION	PLACE	NUMBER TESTED	G6PD DEF.	SICKLE CELL	THALASSEMIA A_2	THALASSEMIA F	THALASSEMIA OSM. RES.	HEMOGLOBIN TYPES AE	A Koln		AM				B_2
WEST GERMANY																
78	Germans	Freiburg	2245			3 (0.1)			1	1		4 (0.2)				2
SWITZERLAND																
463	Swiss Recruits	Tessin	965			2 (0.2)	2									
	Swiss Recruits	Wallis	1130			0										
	Swiss Recruits	Graubunden	750			0										
	Swiss Recruits	Basel and Umgeburg	404			0										
NETHERLANDS																
580a	Dutch		250M	0												
527	Dutch Soldiers		100M	1 (1.0)												
385	Dutch Kindred	Sloten West Amsterdam	547	56 (10.2)												
GREAT BRITAIN																
238	British and Irish		116M	0												

REF.	POPULATION	PLACE	NUMBER TESTED	G6PD DEF.	SICKLE CELL	THALASSEMIA			HEMOGLOBIN TYPES							
						A_2	F	OSM. RES.	S	AS	SC	AC	AD	AG	AJ	AE
GREAT BRITAIN (CONT.)																
238	British and Irish		88F	0												
335	English	Norfolk	1000										1	1		
425a	English	Oxford and Peterborough	1971												1	
472a	British	Rhondda Fach South Wales	340M	4 (1.2)												
763	Scotch	Glasgow Scotland	404M	0												
249	British Soldiers	Nigeria	568		0											
707	British Soldiers	Malaya	4153												1	4
125a	Pregnant Women of West Indian, West African and Mediterranean Ancestry	London	518						2	56 (11.4)	1	28 (5.6)				
EUROPE																
621	Ashkenazim Jews from Europe	Israel	819M	3 (0.4)												

REF.	POPULATION	PLACE	NUMBER TESTED	G6PD DEF.	SICKLE CELL	THALASSEMIA			HEMOGLOBIN TYPES							
						A_2	F	OSM. RES.								Barts
EUROPE (CONT.)																
700	Europeans	Malaya	16			0										
701	Europeans	Malaya	76M	0												
707	European (cord blood)	Malaya	142													1 (0.7)

REF.	POPULATION	PLACE	NUMBER TESTED	G6PD DEF.	SICKLE CELL	THALASSEMIA			HEMOGLOBIN TYPES							
						A_2	F	OSM. RES.								
EGYPT																
235	Egyptians	Cairo	5000		8 (0.2)											
	Northern Sudanese	Cairo	82		0											
370	Egyptians	Cairo	350			1	1 (0.3)									
621	Jews from Egypt	Israel	112M	4 (3.6)												
560a	Egyptians	Alexandria	27M	5 (18.5)												
	Egyptians	Port Said	18M	1 (5.6)												
	Egyptians	Cairo	49M	9 (18.4)												
	Egyptians	Beheira District Lower Egypt	30M	7 (23.3)												
	Egyptians	Sharkiya District Lower Egypt	56M	14 (25.0)												
	Egyptians	Ismailia and Suez Districts Lower Egypt	6M	2 (33.3)												
	Egyptians	Kafrel Sheikh Dist., Lower Egypt	21M	10 (47.6)												

REF.	POPULATION	PLACE	NUMBER TESTED	G6PD DEF.	SICKLE CELL	THALASSEMIA A_2	THALASSEMIA F	THALASSEMIA OSM. RES.	HEMOGLOBIN TYPES							
EGYPT (CONT.)																
560a	Egyptians	Dakahlia District Lower Egypt	23M	11 (47.8)												
	Egyptians	Menofia District Lower Egypt	27M	7 (25.9)												
	Egyptians	Gharbia District Lower Egypt	15M	5 (33.3)												
	Egyptians	Kalyoubia Dist. Lower Egypt	24M	8 (33.3)												
	Egyptians	Arish District Lower Egypt	3M	0												
	Egyptians	Guiza District Upper Egypt	16M	3 (18.8)												
	Egyptians	Benisuef Dist. Upper Egypt	36M	12 (33.3)												
	Egyptians	Menya District Upper Egypt	19M	4 (21.0)												
	Egyptians	Assiut District Upper Egypt	15M	4 (26.7)												
	Egyptians	Girga District Upper Egypt	20M	6 (30.0)												
	Egyptians	Aswan District Upper Egypt	12M	3 (25.0)												
	Egyptians		83M	21 (25.3)												

REF.	POPULATION	PLACE	NUMBER TESTED	G6PD DEF.	SICKLE CELL	THALASSEMIA			HEMOGLOBIN TYPES							
						A_2	F	OSM. RES.		AS		AC				A
EGYPT (CONT.)																
48	Nubians	Konouz village North Nubia	115													115
	Nubians	Fedikyaees vill. South Nubia	121													121
	Arabs	Nubia	120													120
LIBYA																
487	Libyans	Tripolitania	600		5 (0.8)											
486	Libyans	Tripolitania	1540							14 (0.9)						
485	Libyans	Tauorga Oasis Misurata Province	260		27 (10.4)											
621	Jews from Libya	Israel	219M	2 (0.9)												
TUNISIA																
139	Tunisians		275							9 (3.3)		1 (0.4)				
205	Tunisians	Tunis	820		16 (2.0)											

REF.	POPULATION	PLACE	NUMBER TESTED	G6PD DEF.	SICKLE CELL	THALASSEMIA			HEMOGLOBIN TYPES							
						A_2	F	OSM. RES.		AS		AC				A
TUNISIA (CONT.)																
556	Tunisians		457					30 (6.6)								
621	Jews from Djerba	Israel	52M	0												
MOROCCO																
621	Jews from Morocco	Israel	219M	1 (0.5)												
	Jews from Atlas Mts.	Israel	23M	1 (4.3)												
561	Jews from Morocco	Israel	147			2 (2.7)	2									
534	Berbers	Ouarzazate, Atlas Mountains	48									2 (4.2)				
139	Berbers		197							1 (0.5)						
	Riffian Berbers		91													91
	Shluh Berbers		156							1 (0.6)		3 (1.9)				
	Arabs		297							6 (2.0)		1 (0.3)				
	Arabo-Berbers		28													28

REF.	POPULATION	PLACE	NUMBER TESTED	G6PD DEF.	SICKLE CELL	THALASSEMIA			HEMOGLOBIN TYPES							
						A_2	F	OSM. RES.		AS		AC	AJ			A
MOROCCO (CONT.)																
139	Saharans and Sudanese		18													18
137	Europeans		300							1 (0.3)		2 (0.7)				
139	Moroccans		65													65
294a	Moroccans with cancer		50			8	7 (24.0)					2 (4.0)				
137	Moroccans	Tindouf, Algeria	14										1			
ALGERIA																
137	Reguibat Moors	Tindouf	384									1 (0.3)				
	Tadjacan Moors	Tindouf	69													69
	Arabo-Berbers	Tindouf	27													27
	M'Sirda Berbers	Nemours, Oran	134													134
367	Europeans	Algiers	748		0											
	Arabs	Algiers	252		2 (0.8)											
21	Berbers	Algiers	180		1 (0.6)											

REF.	POPULATION	PLACE	NUMBER TESTED	G6PD DEF.	SICKLE CELL	THALASSEMIA A_2	THALASSEMIA F	THALASSEMIA OSM. RES.	HEMOGLOBIN TYPES S	AS	SC	AC	C	AD	AK	A	AI	AJ
ALGERIA (CONT.)																		
139	Arabo-Berbers	Algiers	15564						13	67 (0.6)	11	65 (0.5)	7	39	3		5	2
141	Arabo-Berbers	Algiers	8120					125 (1.5)										
	Arabo-Berbers	Rural Algeria	5886					62 (1.1)	7	113 (2.1)	2	105 (1.9)	2	8	19		2	
139	Arabo-Berbers	Constantine	430						1	7 (2.3)	2	4 (2.1)	3		2			1
141	Arabo-Berbers	Constantine	356					55 (15.5)										
720a	Algerians	Constantine	13	0														
139	Europeans	Algiers	274													274		
141	Europeans	Algiers	230					20 (8.7)										
139	Jews	Algiers	176													176		
141	Jews	Algiers	159					4 (2.5)										
720a	Algerians	Algiers	95	2 (2.1)														
	Algerians	Medea	20	0														
	Algerians	Setif	26	1 (3.8)														

REF.	POPULATION	PLACE	NUMBER TESTED	G6PD DEF.	SICKLE CELL	THALASSEMIA			HEMOGLOBIN TYPES							
						A_2	F	OSM. RES.	S	AS	SC	AC	C	AD	AK	A
ALGERIA (CONT.)																
141	Arabo-Berbers	Dahra Cherchell	240					20 (8.3)	1	3 (3.3)	4	10 (7.1)	3			
139	Arabo-Berbers	Oran	120									1 (0.8)				
	Arabo-Berbers	LeKouif	78													78
720a	Algerians	Grand Kabylie	290	10 (3.4)												
21	Kabyle Berbers	Tizi Ouzou	105		0											
141	Kabyle Berbers	Grand Kabylie	272					48 (17.6)								272
	Kabyle Berbers	Petite Kabylie	235					38 (16.2)		3 (1.3)		2 (0.9)		3	19 (8.1)	
720a	Algerians	Azazga Arrondissement	24	1 (4.2)												
	Algerians	Bouiba Arrondissement	27	1 (3.7)												
	Algerians	Bordj Menaiel Arrondissement	34	4 (11.8)												
	Algerians	Tizi Ouzou Arrondissement	54	1 (1.9)												
141	Shawia Berbers	Aures Mountains	58					6 (10.3)								58

REF.	POPULATION	PLACE	NUMBER TESTED	G6PD DEF.	SICKLE CELL	THALASSEMIA			HEMOGLOBIN TYPES							
						A_2	F	OSM. RES.	S	AS	C	AC		AK		A
ALGERIA (CONT.)																
141	Berbers	Mzab Oasis	69									1 (1.4)				
139	Jews	Mzab Oasis	49													49
	Chaambas	In Salah Oasis	469							14 (3.0)		2 (0.4)		1		
136	Algerians	El Golea Oasis	58						1	5 (10.3)	1	1 (3.4)		3 (5.2)		
139	Touareg Nobles	Hoggar	7													7
	Touareg Vassals	Hoggar	19									2				
	Touareg	Hoggar	**26**							**2**		—		1		
	Touareg	Hoggar	52							2 (3.8)		2 (3.8)				
	Haratin,Slaves and Sudanese	Hoggar	156						1	8 (5.8)	1	5 (3.8)		8 (5.1)		
	Arabs	Hoggar	24							1				1		
MAURETANIA																
137	Fulani(Peul)		14							2				1		
	Wolof		5							1				1		

REF.	POPULATION	PLACE	NUMBER TESTED	G6PD DEF.	SICKLE CELL	THALASSEMIA			HEMOGLOBIN TYPES						
						A_2	F	OSM. RES.		AS	SC	AC		AK	
MAURETANIA (CONT.)															
137	Sarakole		26							1 (3.8)				2 (7.7)	
	Tukulor		95							11 (12.6)	1	1 (2.1)		3 (3.2)	
530	Moors		24		0										
508	Moors		10		1					1		1			
137	Moors		44		6					6		1		2	
	Moors		78		7 (9.0)					7		2 (3.7)		2 (3.7)	
CAPE VERDE ISLANDS															
540	Cape Verdeans	Santo Antao Island	2063		70 (3.4)										
540	Cape Verdeans	Brava Island	437		6										
687	Cape Verdeans	Brava Island	198		12					12					
	Cape Verdeans	Brava Island	635		18 (2.8)										
687	Cape Verdeans	Sao Tiago Island	453		33 (7.3)										
	Cape Verdeans	Todas Island	897		47 (5.2)										
689b	Cape Verdeans	St. Vincent and St. James Islands	1682							74 (4.4)					

REF.	POPULATION	PLACE	NUMBER TESTED	G6PD DEF.	SICKLE CELL	THALASSEMIA A_2	THALASSEMIA F	THALASSEMIA OSM. RES.	HEMOGLOBIN TYPES	AS		AC	C		AK	
SENEGAL																
137	Serer		176							24 (13.6)		1 (0.6)			2 (1.1)	
508	Serer		303		12					12						
435	Serer		1212		38											
	Serer		1515		50 (3.3)											
137	Wolof		116							18 (15.5)		1 (0.9)			5 (4.3)	
435	Wolof		1995		124											
508	Wolof		282		27					27		2 (0.7)	1			
	Wolof		2277		151 (6.6)											
435	Bambara		214		18											
508	Bambara		48		9					9		3 (6.3)				
	Bambara		262		27 (10.3)											
435	Fulani(Fula)		146		15											
508	Fulani(Fula)		21		4					4						
	Fulani(Fula)		167		19 (11.4)											

REF.	POPULATION	PLACE	NUMBER TESTED	G6PD DEF.	SICKLE CELL	THALASSEMIA			HEMOGLOBIN TYPES							
						A_2	F	OSM. RES.		AS		AC				A
SENEGAL (CONT.)																
435	Lebu		493		29											
508	Lebu		29		2					2						
	Lebu		522		31 (5.9)											
435	Sarakole		182		14											
508	Sarakole		14		4					4						
	Sarakole		196		18 (9.2)											
435	Soce		70		11 (15.7)											
435	Lobe		49		0											
508	Lobe		14		0											14
	Lobe		63													
530	Susu		27		9											
508	Susu		18		6					6		1 (5.6)				
	Susu		45		15 (33.3)											
508	Mandingo		33		0											33
530	Mandingo		38		8											
	Mandingo		71		8 (11.3)											

REF.	POPULATION	PLACE	NUMBER TESTED	G6PD DEF.	SICKLE CELL	THALASSEMIA			HEMOGLOBIN TYPES							
						A_2	F	OSM. RES.	S	AS		AC	AG		AK	A
	SENEGAL (CONT.)															
435	Fulani(Peul)		257		23											
508	Fulani(Peul)		42		4					4						
137	Fulani(Peul)		100		22					22		3 (3.0)	1		2 (2.0)	
	Fulani(Peul)		399		49 (12.3)											
435	Tukulor		555		40											
508	Tukulor		79		20				1	19		3				
137	Tukulor		197		24					24		3	1		5	
	Tukulor		831		84 (10.1)							6 (2.2)			5 (1.8)	
508	Dyola		6		0											6
435	Mandiago		54		0											
530	Dyola, Manyak and Mancagne		50		3											
	Casamance Tribes		110		3 (2.7)											
436	Africans	Dakar	242	16 (6.6)												
572a	Africans	Dakar	91M	7 (7.7)												
277	Coniagui		22							1 (4.5)						

REF.	POPULATION	PLACE	NUMBER TESTED	G6PD DEF.	SICKLE CELL	THALASSEMIA			HEMOGLOBIN TYPES							
						A_2	F	OSM. RES.	S	AS						
SENEGAL (CONT.)																
277	Bassari		87							12 (13.8)						
	Bassari		9				6									
	Bedik		79			1	7 (10.1)		1	7 (10.1)						
GUINEA																
95	Coniagui	Ourous Youkounkoun District	149		20 (13.4)											
	Bassari	Ourous and Koudiang Youkounkoun District	72		7 (9.7)											
	Baga Fore	Monchon Boffa District	137		26 (19.0)											
	Susu	Negueah Dubreka District	141		30 (21.3)											
	Mandingo	Negueah Dubreka District	18		6 (33.3)											
	Fulani (Fula)	Negueah Dubreka District	7		6											
	Mandingo	Sitakoto Mamou District	165		54 (32.7)											
	Mandingo	Houre-Kaba Mamou District	142		48 (33.8)											

REF.	POPULATION	PLACE	NUMBER TESTED	G6PD DEF.	SICKLE CELL	THALASSEMIA			HEMOGLOBIN TYPES							
						A_2	F	OSM. RES.		AS		AC	AN		AK	
GUINEA (CONT.)																
95	Susu	Houre-Kaba Mamou District	8		0											
	Fulani (Fula)	Soumbalako Mamou District	179		42 (23.5)											
	Mandingo	Soumbalako Mamou District	3		0											
	Mandingo	Kenenkou Dabola District	123		23 (18.7)											
	Dialonke	Dantilia Faranah District	110		18 (16.4)											
	Kuranko	Banian Faranah District	105		18 (17.1)											
PORTUGUESE GUINEA																
591	Tenda (Pajadinca)		358		66											
689	Tenda (Pajadinca)		300		48					48			2		1	
	Tenda (Pajadinca)		658		114 (17.3)											
689	Fulani (Fula)		1553							248 (16.0)		6 (0.4)	4		2	
591	Fulani (Fula)	Futa Djalon	515		90 (17.5)											
	Fulani (Fula Forro)		500		115 (23.0)											

REF.	POPULATION	PLACE	NUMBER TESTED	G6PD DEF.	SICKLE CELL	THALASSEMIA			HEMOGLOBIN TYPES							
						A_2	F	OSM. RES.		AS		AC	AN		AK	
PORTUGUESE GUINEA (CONT.)																
591	Fulani (Fula Preto)		430		108 (25.1)											
591	Mandingo		500		75											
689	Mandingo		895		115					115		10 (1.1)			1	
	Mandingo		1395		190 (13.6)											
591	Sarakole		286		24											
689	Sarakole		268		44					44		4 (1.5)				
	Sarakole		654		68 (10.4)											
591	Biafada		505		77											
689	Biafada		797		103					103		1	1		1	
	Biafada		1302		180 (13.8)											
689	Banyun (Banhun)		63							10 (15.9)						
	Kassanga (Cassanga)		144							34 (23.6)						
	Jacanca		43							4 (9.3)						

REF.	POPULATION	PLACE	NUMBER TESTED	G6PD DEF.	SICKLE CELL	THALASSEMIA A_2	THALASSEMIA F	THALASSEMIA OSM. RES.
PORTUGUESE GUINEA (CONT.)								
591	Balante (Balanta)		500		25			
689	Balante (Balanta)		776		7			
	Balante (Balanta)		1276		32 (2.5)			
591	Nalu		501		14			
689	Nalu		100		6			
	Nalu		601		20 (3.3)			
591	Bayot (Baiote)		473		6			
689	Bayot (Baiote)		342		1			
	Bayot (Baiote)		815		7 (0.9)			
591	Felup (Felupe)		466		8			
689	Felup (Felupe)		641		36			
	Felup (Felupe)		1107		44 (4.0)			
591	Mandyako (Manjaca)		500		16			
689	Mandyako (Manjaco)		758		16			
	Mandyako		1258		32 (2.5)			

REF.	POPULATION	HEMOGLOBIN TYPES	AS			AN		AK	
591	Balante (Balanta)								
689	Balante (Balanta)		7			1		1	
	Balante (Balanta)								
591	Nalu								
689	Nalu		6						
	Nalu								
591	Bayot (Baiote)								
689	Bayot (Baiote)		1						
	Bayot (Baiote)								
591	Felup (Felupe)								
689	Felup (Felupe)		36						
	Felup (Felupe)								
591	Mandyako (Manjaca)								
689	Mandyako (Manjaco)		16			3		1	
	Mandyako								

REF.	POPULATION	PLACE	NUMBER TESTED	G6PD DEF.	SICKLE CELL	THALASSEMIA			HEMOGLOBIN TYPES							
						A_2	F	OSM. RES.		AS		AC	AN		AK	
PORTUGUESE GUINEA (CONT.)																
689	Susu(Sosso)		94							3 (3.2)			2			
	Mankanya (Mancanha)		534							1 (0.2)			1		2	
	Pepel(Papel)		1244							16 (1.3)						
690	Pepel(Papel)	Quinhamel Bissau Island	368		12 (3.3)											
	Pepel(Papel)	Bucomil Bissau Island	80		2 (2.5)											
	Pepel(Papel)	Prabis Bissau Island	52		1 (1.9)											
689	Bijogo(Bijago)		632							2 (0.3)					1	
	Other Tribes		40							5 (12.5)					1	
GAMBIA																
242	Gambian Soldiers		67		19 (28.4)											
	Gambian Villagers		69		13 (18.8)											
24	Mandingo	Keneba Central Division	240							15 (6.3)		3 (1.3)				

REF.	POPULATION	PLACE	NUMBER TESTED	G6PD DEF.	SICKLE CELL	THALASSEMIA			HEMOGLOBIN TYPES							
						A_2	F	OSM. RES.	S	AS		AC				
GAMBIA (CONT.)																
30	Mandingo	Keneba Central Division	103M	16												
387	Mandingo	Keneba Central Division	289M	24												
	Mandingo	Keneba Central Division	392M	40 (10.2)												
24	Mandingo	Jali Central Division	115							7 (6.1)		2 (1.7)				
	Mandingo	Manduar Central Division	59							10 (16.9)		1 (1.7)				
	Mandingo	Tankular Central Division	132							32 (24.2)		2 (1.5)				
	Mandingo	Western Division	167							18 (10.8)		2 (1.2)				
	Dyola(Jola)	Western Division	416						1	68 (16.6)		9 (2.2)				
	Fulani(Fula)	Western Division	196						1	36 (18.9)		4 (2.0)				
	Wolof(Jolloff)	Western Division	152							27 (17.8)		2 (1.3)				
	Sarakole (Serahuli)	Bwiam and Sibanor Western Division	96							8 (8.3)		2 (2.1)				
	Banyun (Bainunka)	Jarol and Joram Western Division	90							15 (16.7)		2 (2.2)				

REF.	POPULATION	PLACE	NUMBER TESTED	G6PD DEF.	SICKLE CELL	THALASSEMIA			HEMOGLOBIN TYPES							
						A_2	F	OSM. RES.	S	AS		AC		AN		
SIERRA LEONE																
288	Africans	Freetown	1038		280 (27.0)											
24	Creoles	Freetown	42							10 (23.8)		3 (7.1)				
	Timne	Freetown	52							15 (28.8)		2 (3.8)				
	Mende	Freetown	124							36 (29.0)		5 (4.0)				
581	Mende	Segbwema	1000		306 (30.6)											
LIBERIA																
443	Mende		110		18 (16.4)											
509	Mende		61							11						
	Mende		19			0										
	Mende		42				0									
543	Gola		100		19											
443	Gola		268		31											
	Gola		368		50 (13.6)											
509	Gola		158						1	16		1 (0.6)		1		

REF.	POPULATION	PLACE	NUMBER TESTED	G6PD DEF.	SICKLE CELL	THALASSEMIA			HEMOGLOBIN TYPES							
						A_2	F	OSM. RES.	S	AS		AC	C			
LIBERIA (CONT.)																
509	Gola		10			0										
	Gola		125				7 (5.6)									
443	Vai		114		17 (14.9)											
509	Vai		57							4						
	Vai		8			0										
	Vai		40				0									
443	Kissi	Tamba Taylor Chiefdom	459		99 (21.6)											
509	Kissi		141							28						
	Kissi		22			1 (4.5)										
	Kissi		91				0									
443	Gbandi	Boymah Jollah Chiefdom	421		62 (14.7)											
509	Gbandi		155						1	19		1 (1.3)	1			
	Gbandi		17			1 (5.9)										
	Gbandi		117				4 (3.4)									

REF.	POPULATION	PLACE	NUMBER TESTED	G6PD DEF.	SICKLE CELL	THALASSEMIA			HEMOGLOBIN TYPES							
						A_2	F	OSM. RES.	S	AS		AC		AN		
LIBERIA (CONT.)																
442	Belle		29		3 (10.3)											
509	Belle		13							2						
	Belle		3			0										
	Belle		6				0									
443	Loma	Guzeh Chiefdom	143		16 (11.2)											
	Loma	Tellewoyan Chiefdom	62		7 (11.3)											
509	Loma		330						1	41		5 (1.5)		2		
	Loma		144			1 (0.7)										
	Loma		255				0									
443	Kpelle	Gleh Chiefdom	59		8 (13.6)											
	Kpelle	Kpangbai Chiefdom	344		63 (18.3)											
	Kpelle	Tarkono Chiefdom	76		12 (15.8)											
	Kpelle	Fahn Gwilly Chiefdom	53		1 (1.9)											

REF.	POPULATION	PLACE	NUMBER TESTED	G6PD DEF.	SICKLE CELL	THALASSEMIA			HEMOGLOBIN TYPES							
						A_2	F	OSM. RES.	S	AS		AC	AK		AN	
LIBERIA (CONT.)																
443	Kpelle	Steven Giddings Chiefdom	82		16 (19.5)											
	Kpelle	Kole Gwee Chiefdom	43		5 (11.6)											
	Kpelle	Wea Wea Chiefdom	66		4 (6.1)											
	Kpelle	Swar Gbanyah Chiefdom	65		5 (7.7)											
	Kpelle	Doloken Paye Chiefdom	123		3 (2.4)											
	Kpelle	Lango Lipaye Chiefdom	37		7 (18.9)											
	Kpelle	Southwest Chiefdoms	20		4 (20.0)											
	Kpelle	Bassa Chiefdoms	20		2 (10.0)											
509	Kpelle		399						1	37		6 (1.5)	1		5	
	Kpelle		127			7 (5.5)										
	Kpelle		241				0									
443	Bassa	Menyongar Chiefdom	32		5 (15.6)											

REF.	POPULATION	PLACE	NUMBER TESTED	G6PD DEF.	SICKLE CELL	THALASSEMIA			HEMOGLOBIN TYPES							
						A_2	F	OSM. RES.	S	AS			AK			
LIBERIA (CONT.)																
443	Bassa	Northern Chiefdoms	40		10 (25.0)											
	Bassa	Garbudu Chiefdom	48		7 (14.6)											
	Bassa	Mamba Chiefdom	76		6 (7.9)											
	Bassa	Buchanan and Vicinity	23		6 (26.1)											
	Bassa	Frank Yarsee Chiefdom	42		2 (4.8)											
	Bassa	Central Chiefdoms	50		1 (2.0)											
	Bassa	Southern Chiefdoms	53		0											
509	Bassa		283						1	23			1			
	Bassa		61			0										
	Bassa		132				4 (3.0)									
443	Mano	Bona Sua Chiefdom	199		3 (1.5)											
	Mano	Yennigen Chiefdom	102		0											

REF.	POPULATION	PLACE	NUMBER TESTED	G6PD DEF.	SICKLE CELL	THALASSEMIA A_2	THALASSEMIA F	THALASSEMIA OSM. RES.	HEMOGLOBIN TYPES							
										AS		AC	AD		AN	A
LIBERIA (CONT.)																
509	Mano		116							2		1 (0.9)	1		1	
	Mano		10			0										
	Mano		82				1 (1.2)									
443	Gio		522		9 (1.7)											
509	Gio		105							3					1	
	Gio		23			2 (8.7)										
	Gio		63				1 (1.6)									
443	Dei		54		2 (3.7)											
509	Dei		37													37
	Dei		36				1 (2.8)									
443	Kru		196		1 (0.5)											
509	Kru		140							1						
	Kru		12			0										
	Kru		109				3 (2.8)									

REF.	POPULATION	PLACE	NUMBER TESTED	G6PD DEF.	SICKLE CELL	THALASSEMIA			HEMOGLOBIN TYPES							
						A_2	F	OSM. RES.		AS						A
LIBERIA (CONT.)																
443	Krahn		186		1 (0.5)											
509	Krahn		88													88
	Krahn		13			0										
	Krahn		51				2 (3.9)									
443	Grebo		123		1 (0.8)											
509	Grebo		104							1						
	Grebo		28			0										
	Grebo		99				2 (2.0)									
443	Webbo		178		1 (0.6)											
509	Webbo		180							1						
	Webbo		46			0										
	Webbo		182				6 (3.3)									
443	Americo-Liberians		110		17 (15.5)											
509	Americo-Liberians		16							5						

REF.	POPULATION	PLACE	NUMBER TESTED	G6PD DEF.	SICKLE CELL	THALASSEMIA			HEMOGLOBIN TYPES							
						A_2	F	OSM. RES.		AS		AC				A
LIBERIA (CONT.)																
509	Americo-Liberians		2			0										
	Americo-Liberians		13				0									
	Mandingo		55							16 (29.1)		2 (3.6)				
	Mandingo		25			0										
	Mandingo		52				0									
	Other Tribes		15							3		1				
	Other Tribes		11				0									
448	Fanti	Marshall	60		20 (33.3)											
IVORY COAST																
509	Kru		36				0									36
	Bakwi, Oubi, and Ouanbi		11							1 (9.1)		1 (9.1)				
	Bakwi, Oubi, and Ouanbi		12				0									
	Wobe and Guere		51									1 (2.0)				
	Wobe and Guere		40				0									

REF.	POPULATION	PLACE	NUMBER TESTED	G6PD DEF.	SICKLE CELL	THALASSEMIA			HEMOGLOBIN TYPES							
						A_2	F	OSM. RES.	S	AS		AC			A?	
IVORY COAST (CONT.)																
509	Bete, Dida, Godye, and Neyo		34							1 (2.9)		1 (2.9)				
	Bete, Dida, Godye, and Neyo		26				0									
	Lagoon Tribes		46							2 (4.3)		1 (2.2)				
	Lagoon Tribes		35				0									
530	Agni and Baule		14		3											
509	Agni and Baule		<u>35</u>		<u>3</u>					3		1 (2.9)				
	Agni and Baule		49		6 (12.2)											
509	Agni and Baule		34				0									
	Mandingo and Dyula		30							2 (6.7)						
	Mandingo and Dyula		12				0									
74a	Ivory Coast Tribes	Abidjan	177						6	19 (14.1)		4 (2.3)			4	
	Upper Volta Tribes	Abidjan	35							5 (14.2)		4 (11.4)			1	

REF.	POPULATION	PLACE	NUMBER TESTED	G6PD DEF.	SICKLE CELL	THALASSEMIA			HEMOGLOBIN TYPES							
						A_2	F	OSM. RES.	S	AS	SC	AC	C	AG	AK	A
UPPER VOLTA																
596	Senufo	N'Gorlani	113						1	11 (12.4)	2	22 (25.7)	5			
	Senufo	Sillorla	88							4 (4.5)		13 (15.9)	1			
	Senufo	Sana	6													6
	Senufo	Banakoro	87							6 (6.9)		17 (19.5)				
	Senufo	Karna	200							17 (9.0)	1	29 (16.5)	3		2 (1.0)	
	Senufo	Sarakadiala	96						1	21 (28.1)	5	30 (40.6)	4		3 (3.1)	
	Senufo	Foloni	38							2 (5.3)		3 (13.2)	2		1 (2.6)	
	Senufo	Oueleni	108							5 (8.3)	4	7 (12.0)	2		4 (3.7)	
	Tusyan (Toussian)	Kourignon	277							18 (6.5)		52 (20.6)	5	3	2 (0.7)	
	Tusyan (Toussian)	Banzon	100							10 (10.0)		15 (15.0)				
	Vigye (Vigue)	Karankasso	350							25 (8.9)	6	50 (17.4)	5		5 (1.4)	
	Bobo Fing	Longofourso	135						2	12 (10.4)		18 (14.8)	2			

REF.	POPULATION	PLACE	NUMBER TESTED	G6PD DEF.	SICKLE CELL	THALASSEMIA			HEMOGLOBIN TYPES						
						A_2	F	OSM. RES.	S	AS	SC	AC	C		AK
UPPER VOLTA (CONT.)															
596	Bobo Fing	Sagassamassio	200						1	6 (4.0)	1	21 (11.5)	1		
	Bobo Fing	Leguema	99							2 (2.0)		26 (26.3)			
	Bobo Fing	Ouolonkoto	119						1	3 (3.4)		18 (17.6)	3		
	Bobo Fing	Padema	161									31 (19.9)	1		
	Bobo Nienige (Nieniegue)	Kouimbia	173						2	9 (6.4)		23 (15.0)	3		2 (1.2)
	Bobo Nienige (Nieniegue)	Ouakuy	247							3 (1.6)	1	32 (15.4)	5		1 (0.4)
	Bobo Nienige (Nieniegue)	Doumin and Duho	42							2 (4.8)		9 (21.4)			1 (2.4)
	Bobo Nienige (Nieniegue)	Tiere	200						2	11 (6.5)		25 (15.0)	5		5 (2.5)
	Bobo Dyula (Dioula)	Satri	156						1	12 (8.3)		30 (19.9)	1		
	Bobo Dyula (Dioula)	Pandamasso	374						2	13 (4.5)	2	97 (27.0)	2		
	Sembla Dyula (Dioula)	Diefourma	98							8 (8.2)		26 (27.6)	1		1 (1.0)
564a	Bobo Fing	Sinorosso	96		15 (15.6)										

REF.	POPULATION	PLACE	NUMBER TESTED	G6PD DEF.	SICKLE CELL	THALASSEMIA			HEMOGLOBIN TYPES							
						A_2	F	OSM. RES.	S	AS		AC	C			
UPPER VOLTA (CONT.)																
564a	Bobo Fing	Borodougou	121		41 (33.8)											
528	Samoro (Samogo)	Tougan	115		8 (7.0)											
	Gurma (Gourma)	Fada N'Gourma	30		3 (10.0)											
	Songhai (Sonrai)	Tigre	100		11 (11.0)											
	Fulani (Peul)	Tigre	152		22 (14.5)											
	Mossi	Yako-Koudougou	100		13 (13.0)											
509	Mossi		71							6 (8.5)		9 (15.5)	2			
	Mossi		56				0									
	Other Tribes		71						1	7 (11.3)		10 (14.1)				
	Other Tribes		48				1 (2.1)									
GHANA																
177	Frafra	Yorugu	680		66 (9.7)											

REF.	POPULATION	PLACE	NUMBER TESTED	G6PD DEF.	SICKLE CELL	THALASSEMIA			HEMOGLOBIN TYPES				
						A_2	F	OSM. RES.	AS	SC	AC	C	AK
GHANA (CONT.)													
228	Dagomba	Yendi District	1046						89 (9.8)	14	190 (21.5)	21	3 (0.3)
230	Dagomba		71						3 (4.2)		19 (28.2)	1	
	Dagari (Dagarti)		97						9 (11.3)	2	14 (16.5)		
	Mossi (Moshie)		115						5 (4.3)		24 (21.7)	1	
24	Zerma (Zabrama)		63						13 (22.2)	1	6 (11.1)		
	Other Tribes	Northern Territories	276						38 (14.3)	1	43 (16.3)	1	
178	Fanti	Kwansakrom	255		57 (22.4)								
448	Fanti	Marshall, Liberia	60		20 (33.3)								
230	Fanti		29						9		4		
24	Fanti		156						32	1	16	1	
	Fanti		185						41 (22.7)	1	20 (11.9)	1	
155	Akyem (Akim)		64M	16 (25.0)									
30	Ga		32M	7 (21.9)									

REF.	POPULATION	PLACE	NUMBER TESTED	G6PD DEF.	SICKLE CELL	THALASSEMIA A$_2$	THALASSEMIA F	THALASSEMIA OSM. RES.	HEMOGLOBIN TYPES S	AS	SC	AC	C		AG	
	GHANA (CONT.)															
230	Ga		108							15	1	6			1	
24	Ga		174							34	1	15			—	
	Ga		282							49 (18.1)	2	21 (8.2)			1	
230	Ewe		46							10		6				
24	Ewe		167						1	39		15	1			
	Ewe		213						1	49 (23.5)		21 (10.3)	1			
24	Ashanti		102						1	22		9				
229	Ashanti		3						—	—		1				
	Ashanti		105						1	22 (21.9)		10 (9.5)				
24	Twi		104							21	1	10				
229	Twi		7							2	—	1				
	Twi		111							23 (21.6)	1	11 (10.8)				
229	Other Tribes		32						1	8	1	8	1			
358	Ghanaian Children		79M	16 (20.3)												
	Ghanaian Children		74F	5 (6.8)												

REF.	POPULATION	PLACE	NUMBER TESTED	G6PD DEF.	SICKLE CELL	THALASSEMIA			HEMOGLOBIN TYPES							
						A_2	F	OSM. RES.	S	AS	SC	AC	C			
GHANA (CONT.)																
177	Ghanaians	Accra	1015		173 (17.0)											
226	Ghanaians (Pregnant)	Accra	413		75 (18.2)											
672	Ghanaian Policemen	Accra	278							52 (20.1)	4	30 (13.3)	3			
	Ghanaian Policemen's Children	Accra	840						4	123 (16.5)	12	101 (14.3)	7			
309	Ghanaians (Pregnant)	Accra	1222							202 (17.1)	7	80 (7.4)	3			
TOGO																
83	Kabre	Lama-Kara	735		80 (10.9)											
	Losso	Niamtougou	369		29 (7.9)											
DAHOMEY																
530	Fon, Mina, and Nago		48		6 (12.5)											
509	Dahomey and Togo Tribes		34							5 (14.7)		1 (2.9)				
	Dahomey and Togo Tribes		7				0									

REF.	POPULATION	PLACE	NUMBER TESTED	G6PD DEF.	SICKLE CELL	THALASSEMIA			HEMOGLOBIN TYPES							
						A_2	F	OSM. RES.	S	AS	SC	AC	C			
NIGER																
52	Tuareg	Agades	93		5 (5.4)											
529	Kanembu	N'Guigmi	76		17 (22.4)											
	Manga (Mangawa)	Maine and Soroa	58		12 (20.7)											
	Sugurti	Tiokoudjani	37		6 (16.2)											
	Mober	Tiokoudjani	273		49 (17.9)											
NIGERIA																
730	Nigerian Children	Sokoto Province	620		68 (11.0)											
227	Fulani	Katsina Province	343						1	64 (19.0)		3 (0.9)				
	Kado	Katsina Province	785						3	175 (23.1)	3	7 (1.3)				
	Busu	Katsina Province	101							23 (22.8)		1 (1.0)				
356	Karekare (Kerikeri)	Potiskum	159		17 (10.7)											
	Fulani	Potiskum	184		33 (17.9)											

REF.	POPULATION	PLACE	NUMBER TESTED	G6PD DEF.	SICKLE CELL	THALASSEMIA			HEMOGLOBIN TYPES							
						A_2	F	OSM. RES.		AS	SC	AC				
NIGERIA (CONT.)																
356	Hausa	Potiskum	316		48 (15.2)											
578	Kanuri	Bornu Province	294							82 (27.9)		2 (0.7)				
	Bede (Bedduwai)	Bornu Province	92							30 (32.6)						
30	Hausa	Northern Nigeria	136M	28 (20.6)												
4	Hausa	Northern Nigeria	200		35											
24	Hausa	Northern Nigeria	92		18					18		4				
227	Hausa	Northern Nigeria	216		45					45		—				
	Hausa	Northern Nigeria	508		98 (19.3)					63		4 (1.3)				
332	Northern Nigerian Soldiers		418		58 (13.9)											
	Western Nigerian Soldiers		283		56 (19.8)											
227	Beni		321							74 (23.0)		2 (0.7)				
576	Yoruba	Ilora	461							113 (25.4)	4	34 (8.5)				

REF.	POPULATION	PLACE	NUMBER TESTED	G6PD DEF.	SICKLE CELL	THALASSEMIA A$_2$	THALASSEMIA F	THALASSEMIA OSM. RES.	HEMOGLOBIN TYPES S	AS	SC	AC	C		SG	
NIGERIA (CONT.)																
576	Yoruba	Imesi	267						4	50 (20.6)	1	8 (3.4)				
	Yoruba	Ilesha	178						1	44 (25.3)		5 (2.8)				
146	Yoruba (Pregnant)	Ilesha	306		30 (9.8)											
280a	Yoruba	Akufo	179M	32 (17.9)												
	Yoruba	Akufo	183F	20 (10.9)												
	Yoruba	Akufo	894						4	214 (25.6)	11	63 (8.4)	1			
731	Yoruba	Ilobi	940						3	224 (25.1)	9	58 (7.1)				
489	Yoruba	Igbile	48							10 (20.8)		1 (2.1)				
489a	Yoruba	Isheri	129							25 (20.2)	1	3 (3.1)				
730	Yoruba	Agege	827		231 (27.9)											
282	Yoruba	Ibadan	65M	11 (17.0)												
227	Yoruba	Ibadan	12387						29	2923 (24.4)	69	595 (5.6)	30		1	

REF.	POPULATION	PLACE	NUMBER TESTED	G6PD DEF.	SICKLE CELL	THALASSEMIA			HEMOGLOBIN TYPES							
						A_2	F	OSM. RES.	S	AS	SC	AC	C	S ?		B_2
NIGERIA (CONT.)																
106	Yoruba Children	Ibadan	50			0										
269	Yoruba Children	Ibadan	305							76 (25.6)	1	19 (6.6)		1		
281	Yoruba		691	132 (19.1)												
24	Yoruba		104							25 (24.0)		6 (5.8)				
105	Yoruba		76													3 (3.9)
232	Nigerians	Ibadan	100M	20 (20.0)												
	Nigerians	Ibadan	100F	5 (5.0)												
231a	Nigerians	Ibadan	100					23 (23.0)								
116	Nigerian Postmortems	Ibadan	2435						33	455 (22.0)	48	122 (7.2)	5			
147	Nigerian Newborns		93M	19 (20.4)												
	Nigerian Newborns		103F	11 (10.7)												
734	Nigerian Sickle Cell Trait Carriers		9618				4		3							

REF.	POPULATION	PLACE	NUMBER TESTED	G6PD DEF.	SICKLE CELL	THALASSEMIA A_2	THALASSEMIA F	THALASSEMIA OSM. RES.	HEMOGLOBIN TYPES AS	HEMOGLOBIN TYPES AC	HEMOGLOBIN TYPES AG	HEMOGLOBIN TYPES Barts
NIGERIA (CONT.)												
314	Nigerians		69					8 (11.6)				
315	Nigerian Newborns		140									15 (10.7)
643	Nigerian Child Postmortems	Lagos	500		24 (4.8)							
249	Syrians		188		0							
	British Soldiers		568		0							
332	Eastern Nigerian Soldiers		138		27 (19.6)							
731	Igalla		155						28 (18.1)			
24	Ibo		51						11	3		
411	Ibo		257						64	2	1	
227	Ibo		489						119	1	—	
	Ibo		797						194 (24.3)	6 (0.8)	1	
227	Ibo (Lepers)	Uzuakoli	138						30 (21.7)			
	Ibo	Enugu	305						63 (20.7)			

REF.	POPULATION	PLACE	NUMBER TESTED	G6PD DEF.	SICKLE CELL	THALASSEMIA			HEMOGLOBIN TYPES							
						A_2	F	OSM. RES.		AS						
NIGERIA (CONT.)																
282	Ibo (Lepers)	Uzuakoli	139M	9 (6.5)												
281	Ibo		290	59 (20.3)												
308	Southern Ibo		153M	32 (20.9)												
	Ogoni		179M	49 (27.4)												
281	Ogoni		346	71 (20.5)												
308	Abua		81M	18 (22.2)												
281	Abua		175	45 (25.7)												
	Ikwere		116	19 (16.4)												
	Degema		108	16 (14.8)												
308	Kalabari		56M	6 (10.7)												
227	Ijaw	Niger Delta	276							67 (24.3)						

REF.	POPULATION	PLACE	NUMBER TESTED	G6PD DEF.	SICKLE CELL	THALASSEMIA			HEMOGLOBIN TYPES							
						A_2	F	OSM. RES.	S	AS		AC				
CHAD																
142	Teda (Nomads)	Tibesti Mountains	88							8 (9.1)						
	Daza	Tibesti Oases	28							5 (17.9)						
	Teda-Daza	Tibesti Oases	28							2 (7.1)						
	Kamadja	Tibesti Oases	18							5 (27.8)						
CAMEROONS																
242	Cameroonian Soldiers		138		21 (15.2)											
279	Southern Cameroonians		1030		15 (1.5)											
63	Bamileke		543		45 (8.3)											
401	Bantu Tribes	Southern Cameroons	225						2	52 (24.0)		1 (0.4)				
266	Fang (Eton)	Yaounde	436							123 (28.2)						
	Fang (Ewondo)	Yaounde	337						3	70 (21.7)						
402	Bantu (Beti, Basa, Duala, Maka, Djem, Bakundu, Fang)		1200		219 (18.3)											

REF.	POPULATION	PLACE	NUMBER TESTED	G6PD DEF.	SICKLE CELL	THALASSEMIA			HEMOGLOBIN TYPES							
						A_2	F	OSM. RES.								
CAMEROONS (CONT.)																
402	Bamileke, Bamun, Tikar, Kaka, and Bakun		432		51 (11.8)											
	Babinga (Pygmies)		350		42 (12.0)											
	Fulani (Foulbe)	Maroua	100		4 (4.0)											
	Fulani (Foulbe)	Bogo	100		6 (6.0)											
	Fulani (Foulbe)	Mindif	100		9 (9.0)											
	Mundang		180		14 (7.8)											
	Tuburi		200		15 (7.5)											
	Musgu		200		16 (8.0)											
	Gisiga		200		17 (8.5)											
	Mofu		100		8 (8.0)											
	Masa		200		4 (2.0)											
	Mandara		50		5 (10.0)											

REF.	POPULATION	PLACE	NUMBER TESTED	G6PD DEF.	SICKLE CELL	THALASSEMIA			HEMOGLOBIN TYPES							
						A_2	F	OSM. RES.		AS		AC	AD		AK	
CAMEROONS (CONT.)																
578	Shuwa Arabs	North Cameroons	312							65 (20.8)		1 (0.3)				
	Wakura	Gwoza, North Cameroons	182							36 (19.8)		10 (5.5)				
	Hidkala	Gwoza, North Cameroons	129							17 (13.2)		6 (4.7)				
SAO TOME AND PRINCIPE ISLANDS																
687	Africans	Sao Tome	422							60 (14.2)		13 (3.1)			2	
	Africans	Principe	380							84 (22.1)		4 (1.1)				
	Africans	Sao Tome and Principe	802										5			
CENTRAL AFRICAN REPUBLIC																
190	N'Zakara	Bangassou	149		15 (10.1)											
	N'Zakara	Villaggi	184		39 (21.2)											
151b	Babinga (Pygmies)		71M	2 (2.8)												
	Babinga (Pygmies)		23F	3 (13.0)												
	Babinga		110			1 (0.9)										

REF.	POPULATION	PLACE	NUMBER TESTED	G6PD DEF.	SICKLE CELL	THALASSEMIA			HEMOGLOBIN TYPES							
						A_2	F	OSM. RES.	S	AS						
CENTRAL AFRICAN REPUBLIC (CONT.)																
151b	Babinga (Pygmies)		95							16 (16.8)						
CONGO (BRAZZAVILLE)																
569	Babinga (Pygmies)	Likouala	537		37 (6.9)											
	Bondjo	Likouala	221		56 (25.3)											
137	Congolese	Brazzaville	53						1	12 (24.5)						
GABON																
38	Fang	Mitzic District	600		81 (13.5)											
	Fang (Lepers)	Mitzic District	549		45 (8.2)											
394	Fang		522		69 (13.2)											
	Mpongwe		160		13 (8.1)											
	Bakota, Bapunu, and Bambamba		158		28 (17.7)											
	Bandjabi and Aduma		130		25 (19.2)											
	Other Tribes		42		6 (14.3)											

REF.	POPULATION	PLACE	NUMBER TESTED	G6PD DEF.	SICKLE CELL	THALASSEMIA			HEMOGLOBIN TYPES							
						A_2	F	OSM. RES.				AE				
CONGO (KINSHASA)																
19	Mongo	Befale	3366		765 (22.7)											
199	Mongo	Coquihatville	11321		2729 (24.1)											
321	Lia	Lac Leopold II	213		35 (16.4)											
	Twa	Lac Leopold II	104		14 (13.5)											
494	Bwaka		49M	2 (4.1)												
	Bwaka		57		6 (10.5)											
494	Congolese	Kinshasa	379M	72												
646	Congolese	Kinshasa	522M	112												
	Congolese	Kinshasa	901M	184 (20.4)												
494	Congolese	Kinshasa	248		56											
646	Congolese	Kinshasa	151		33											
699	Congolese	Kinshasa	2160		568											
	Congolese	Kinshasa	2459		627 (25.5)											
699	Congolese	Kinshasa	?									1				

REF.	POPULATION	PLACE	NUMBER TESTED	G6PD DEF.	SICKLE CELL	THALASSEMIA			HEMOGLOBIN TYPES							
						A_2	F	OSM. RES.								
CONGO (KINSHASA) (CONT.)																
780	Yaka	Kabamba Kwango Province	91M	15 (16.5)	10 (11.0)											
	Yaka	Kialala Kwango Province	100M	23 (23.0)	17 (17.0)											
	Yaka	Lusanga Kwango Province	76M	11 (14.5)	12 (15.8)											
	Yaka	Kisoma Kwango Province	120M	33 (27.5)	39 (32.5)											
	Yaka	Mukoko Kwango Province	100M	29 (29.0)	19 (19.0)											
	Yaka	Mutayi Kwango Province	100M	27 (27.0)	19 (19.0)											
134	Bayanzi	Itakenene Saio District	256		77 (30.1)											
	Bayanzi	Mokubi Saio District	110		35 (31.8)											
	Bayanzi	Bankene Saio District	168		64 (38.1)											
	Bayanzi	Nsala Saio District	140		43 (30.7)											
	Bayanzi	Ndu Saio District	60		25 (41.7)											
	Bayanzi	Nti Saio District	41		18 (43.9)											

REF.	POPULATION	PLACE	NUMBER TESTED	G6PD DEF.	SICKLE CELL	THALASSEMIA			HEMOGLOBIN TYPES							
						A_2	F	OSM. RES.								
CONGO (KINSHASA) (CONT.)																
134	Bayanzi	Luwone-Turu Saio District	338		117 (34.6)											
	Bayanzi	Opoyengo Saio District	100		36 (36.0)											
	Bayanzi	Mokutu Saio District	306		120 (39.2)											
	Bayanzi	Mowaka Saio District	213		47 (22.1)											
	Bayanzi	Malita Saio District	246		66 (26.8)											
	Bayanzi	Ngelemalita Saio District	115		47 (40.9)											
	Bayanzi	Pana Saio District	181		43 (23.8)											
	Bayanzi	Baba Saio District	160		63 (39.4)											
	Bayanzi-Bambala	Ntsaka Saio District	115		37 (32.2)											
	Bayanzi-Bambala	Lareme Saio District	384		112 (29.2)											
	Bayanzi-Bambala	Kenene Saio District	291		104 (35.7)											
	Bayanzi-Bambala	Mbene Saio District	163		42 (25.8)											

REF.	POPULATION	PLACE	NUMBER TESTED	G6PD DEF.	SICKLE CELL	THALASSEMIA			HEMOGLOBIN TYPES							
						A_2	F	OSM. RES.								
CONGO (KINSHASA) (CONT.)																
134	Bayanzi-Bambala	Tope Saio District	240		48 (20.0)											
	Bayanzi-Bambala	Kindambury Saio District	204		58 (28.4)											
	Bayanzi	Motorensiene Tshimbane District	241		64 (26.6)											
	Bayanzi	Buba Tshimbane District	146		49 (33.6)											
	Bayanzi	Pana Moke Tshimbane District	114		23 (20.2)											
	Bayanzi	Baya Ndi Tshimbane District	181		66 (36.5)											
	Bayanzi	Pana Tshimbane District	227		74 (32.6)											
	Bayanzi	Kwaya Tshimbane District	294		106 (36.1)											
	Bayanzi	Ngela Tshimbane District	166		77 (46.4)											
	Bayanzi	Emia Tshimbane District	297		71 (23.9)											
	Bayanzi	Bukwebe Tshimbane District	187		59 (31.6)											
	Bayanzi	Gomina Tshimbane District	360		107 (29.7)											

REF.	POPULATION	PLACE	NUMBER TESTED	G6PD DEF.	SICKLE CELL	THALASSEMIA			HEMOGLOBIN TYPES							
						A_2	F	OSM. RES.								
CONGO (KINSHASA) (CONT.)																
134	Bayanzi	Nteta Tshimbane District	46		14 (30.4)											
	Bayanzi	Gambila Tshimbane District	127		42 (33.1)											
	Bayanzi	Milundu Tshimbane District	161		49 (30.4)											
	Bayanzi	Kimbanda Tshimbane District	90		26 (28.9)											
	Bayanzi	Kingwo Tshimbane District	277		112 (40.4)											
	Bambala	Kimboko Tshimbane District	233		59 (25.3)											
	Bambala	Nto Tshimbane District	110		25 (22.7)											
	Bambala	Paku Tshimbane District	183		58 (31.7)											
	Bambala	Lukweye Tshimbane District	482		146 (30.3)											
	Bambala	Bimi Tshimbane District	122		39 (32.0)											
	Bayanzi-Bambala	Wubu Tshimbane District	467		163 (34.9)											
	Bayanzi-Bambala	Luano Tshimbane District	255		60 (23.5)											

REF.	POPULATION	PLACE	NUMBER TESTED	G6PD DEF.	SICKLE CELL	THALASSEMIA			HEMOGLOBIN TYPES						
						A_2	F	OSM. RES.							
CONGO (KINSHASA) (CONT.)															
134	Bayanzi-Bambala	Webe Tshimbane District	374		88 (23.5)										
	Bayanzi-Bambala	Pwonga Tshimbane District	212		55 (25.9)										
	Bayanzi-Bambala	Pita Tshimbane District	247		70 (28.3)										
	Bayanzi-Bambala	Peni Tshimbane District	50		14 (28.0)										
	Bayanzi-Bambala	Buwulu Tshimbane District	152		51 (33.6)										
	Bayanzi-Bambala	Kibeye Tshimbane District	293		107 (36.5)										
	Bayanzi-Bambala	Kwebimi Tshimbane District	234		64 (27.4)										
	Bayanzi-Bambala	Kwo Tshimbane District	145		54 (37.2)										
	Bayanzi	Manie Bilili-Kiamfu District	362		89 (24.6)										
	Bayanzi	Bwatundu Bilili-Kiamfu District	829		252 (30.4)										
	Bayanzi	Modjiki Bilili-Kiamfu District	886		225 (25.4)										

REF.	POPULATION	PLACE	NUMBER TESTED	G6PD DEF.	SICKLE CELL	THALASSEMIA			HEMOGLOBIN TYPES							
						A_2	F	OSM. RES.								
CONGO (KINSHASA) (CONT.)																
134	Bayanzi	Mokaya Bilili-Kiamfu District	440		133 (30.2)											
	Bayanzi	Kimolo Bilili-Kiamfu District	532		158 (29.7)											
	Bayanzi	Bilili Bilili-Kiamfu District	452		122 (27.0)											
	Bayanzi	Mokamo Bilili-Kiamfu District	335		101 (30.1)											
	Bayanzi	Kikuku Bilili-Kiamfu District	375		67 (17.9)											
	Bayanzi	Kibwari Bilili-Kiamfu District	196		58 (29.6)											
	Bayanzi	Kingombe Bilili-Kiamfu District	299		73 (24.4)											
	Bayanzi	Bawime Bilili-Kiamfu District	151		47 (31.1)											
	Bayanzi	Kimburi Bilili-Kiamfu District	320		96 (30.0)											

REF.	POPULATION	PLACE	NUMBER TESTED	G6PD DEF.	SICKLE CELL	THALASSEMIA			HEMOGLOBIN TYPES							
						A_2	F	OSM. RES.								
CONGO (KINSHASA) (CONT.)																
134	Bayanzi	Moseke Bilili-Kiamfu District	701		209 (29.8)											
	Bayanzi	Ntete Bilili-Kiamfu District	83		38 (45.8)											
	Bayanzi	Lubolo Bilili-Kiamfu District	191		69 (36.1)											
	Bayanzi	Pupu Bilili-Kiamfu District	416		111 (26.7)											
	Bayanzi	Kingonzi Bilili-Kiamfu District	98		42 (42.9)											
	Bayanzi	Nsamba-Nseke Bilili-Kiamfu District	355		91 (25.6)											
	Bayanzi	Lukala Bilili-Kiamfu District	257		105 (40.9)											
	Bambala	Dunga Bilili-Kiamfu District	371		73 (19.7)											
	Bambala	Kikwiti Bilili-Kiamfu District	149		20 (13.4)											

REF.	POPULATION	PLACE	NUMBER TESTED	G6PD DEF.	SICKLE CELL	THALASSEMIA			HEMOGLOBIN TYPES							
						A_2	F	OSM. RES.								
CONGO (KINSHASA) (CONT.)																
134	Bambala	Tumusabu Bilili-Kiamfu District	412		100 (24.3)											
	Bambala	Mutoy-Mukoko Bilili-Kiamfu District	299		106 (35.5)											
	Bambala	Kiamfu Bilili-Kiamfu District	797		205 (25.7)											
	Bambala	Mawa Bilili-Kiamfu District	169		45 (26.6)											
	Bambala	Mundele-Mundondo Bilili-Kiamfu District	256		71 (27.7)											
	Bambala	Galangi-Bulangungu Bilili-Kiamfu District	332		97 (29.2)											
	Bambala	Kinzamba Bilili-Kiamfu District	105		15 (14.3)											
	Bambala	Pinzi Bilili-Kiamfu District	670		244 (36.4)											

REF.	POPULATION	PLACE	NUMBER TESTED	G6PD DEF.	SICKLE CELL	THALASSEMIA			HEMOGLOBIN TYPES							
						A_2	F	OSM. RES.								
CONGO (KINSHASA) (CONT.)																
134	Bahungana	Bwatundu Bilili-Kiamfu District	164		30 (18.3)											
	Bahungana-Bambala	Pukusu Bilili-Kiamfu District	879		242 (27.5)											
	Bayanzi	Bukanga Kitoy District	171		64 (37.4)											
	Bayanzi	Kitoy Kitoy District	395		104 (26.3)											
	Bayanzi	Bondo-Kongo Kitoy District	252		80 (31.7)											
	Bayanzi	Kim.-Gomvuka Kitoy District	160		41 (25.6)											
	Bayanzi	Kisala Kitoy District	174		34 (19.5)											
	Bayanzi	Kambumba Kitoy District	183		50 (27.3)											
	Bayanzi	Kim.-Tabwala Kitoy District	149		48 (32.2)											
	Bayanzi	Kibaya Kitoy District	279		92 (33.0)											
	Bayanzi	Kim.-Twala Kitoy District	193		61 (31.6)											

REF.	POPULATION	PLACE	NUMBER TESTED	G6PD DEF.	SICKLE CELL	THALASSEMIA			HEMOGLOBIN TYPES							
						A_2	F	OSM. RES.								
CONGO (KINSHASA) (CONT.)																
134	Bayanzi	Malele Kitoy District	211		55 (26.1)											
	Bayanzi	Kiputu Kitoy District	99		44 (44.4)											
	Bayanzi	Kimbi-Sayala Kitoy District	312		106 (34.0)											
	Bayanzi-Bambala	Lulau Kitoy District	343		102 (29.7)											
	Bayanzi-Bambala	Bende Kitoy District	324		90 (27.8)											
	Bambala	Misele Kitoy District	99		33 (33.3)											
	Bambala	Mosango Kitoy District	125		27 (21.6)											
	Bambala	Bumba Kitoy District	177		36 (20.3)											
	Bambala	Misimbiri Kitoy District	333		88 (26.4)											
	Bambala	Kindambi Kitoy District	128		30 (23.4)											
	Bambala	Pombo Kitoy District	137		27 (19.7)											
	Bambala	Kindundu Kitoy District	215		46 (21.4)											

REF.	POPULATION	PLACE	NUMBER TESTED	G6PD DEF.	SICKLE CELL	THALASSEMIA			HEMOGLOBIN TYPES							
						A_2	F	OSM. RES.								
CONGO (KINSHASA) (CONT.)																
134	Bambala	Bulangungu Kitoy District	106		18 (17.0)											
	Bahungana	Kingangu Kitoy District	149		28 (18.8)											
	Bahungana	Kinkwe-Ngilu Kitoy District	136		45 (33.1)											
	Bangongo	Banza Wanba Nseke Kitoy District	103		29 (28.2)											
	Bayanzi	Kinkama Dunda-Bonga District	344		79 (23.0)											
	Bayanzi	Kimuilu Kuba Dunda-Bonga District	339		98 (28.9)											
	Bayanzi	Tebe Dunda-Bonga District	167		30 (18.0)											
	Bayanzi	Kisomo Kayeye Dunda-Bonga District	138		37 (26.8)											
	Bayanzi	Kindia Dunda-Bonga District	241		95 (39.4)											
	Bayanzi	Kimuilu-Mabanda Dunda-Bonga District	365		94 (25.8)											

REF.	POPULATION	PLACE	NUMBER TESTED	G6PD DEF.	SICKLE CELL	THALASSEMIA			HEMOGLOBIN TYPES							
						A_2	F	OSM. RES.								
CONGO (KINSHASA) (CONT.)																
134	Bayanzi	Kinkwe Zey Dunda-Bonga District	80		22 (27.5)											
	Bambala	Mianzi Galala Dunda-Bonga District	454		121 (26.7)											
	Bambala	Muwele Dunda-Bonga District	123		29 (23.6)											
	Bambala	Kina Kaboba Dunda-Bonga District	300		98 (32.7)											
	Bambala	Mundondo Venge Dunda-Bonga District	101		26 (25.7)											
	Bambala	Kina Gulututu Dunda-Bonga District	143		23 (16.1)											
	Bambala	Bonga Kapuka Dunda-Bonga District	321		57 (17.8)											
	Bambala	Kitumba Dunda-Bonga	150		35 (23.3)											
	Bangongo	Kimbata Dunda-Bonga District	195		59 (30.3)											

REF.	POPULATION	PLACE	NUMBER TESTED	G6PD DEF.	SICKLE CELL	THALASSEMIA			HEMOGLOBIN TYPES							
						A_2	F	OSM. RES.								
CONGO (KINSHASA) (CONT.)																
134	Bangongo	Kisomi-Dunda Dunda-Bonga District	118		29 (24.6)											
	Bambala-Bayanzi	Kilembe Dunda-Bonga District	471		112 (23.8)											
	Bambala-Bayanzi	Mbaya Dunda-Bonga District	373		64 (17.2)											
	Bambala-Bayanzi	Mundondo Dunda-Bonga District	166		73 (44.0)											
	Bambala-Bayanzi	Makala Dunda-Bonga District	136		42 (30.9)											
	Bayanzi-Bahungana	Mumbanda Dunda-Bonga District	455		143 (31.4)											
	Bayanzi-Bahungana	Manie-Miboti Dunda-Bonga District	153		40 (26.1)											
	Bayanzi-Basuku	Kim. Putub. Dunda-Bonga District	267		57 (21.3)											
	Bayanzi-Bangongo	Kisala Dunda-Bonga District	202		83 (41.1)											

REF.	POPULATION	PLACE	NUMBER TESTED	G6PD DEF.	SICKLE CELL	THALASSEMIA			HEMOGLOBIN TYPES							
						A_2	F	OSM. RES.		AS						
CONGO (KINSHASA) (CONT.)																
134	Bambala-Bangongo	Kindambi Dunda-Bonga District	184		43 (23.4)											
	Bangongo-Basuku	Kitsoko Dunda-Bonga District	165		44 (26.7)											
675a	Basuku and Baluba		655		93 (14.2)											
419	Basuku Infants	Feshi	464		62 (13.4)											
321	Bushong	Mushenge	388		83 (21.4)											
	Twa (Kuba)	Bushole, Kembi, and Lukombe	295		56 (19.0)											
698	Baluba	Luluabourg	500							148 (29.6)						
71	Baluba	Kanda-Kanda	1020		205 (20.1)											
321	Baluba	Lualaba River (Bukama to Mwanza)	280		43 (15.4)											
531	Congolese	Jadotville Katanga	1004		305 (30.4)											

REF.	POPULATION	PLACE	NUMBER TESTED	G6PD DEF.	SICKLE CELL	THALASSEMIA			HEMOGLOBIN TYPES							
						A_2	F	OSM. RES.		AS	AD	AP				
CONGO (KINSHASA) (CONT.)																
699	Congolese	Lumumbashi	515		128											
71	Congolese	Lumumbashi	78		12											
	Congolese	Lumumbashi	593		140 (23.6)											
494	Congolese	Kisangani	98M	14 (14.3)												
	Congolese	Kisangani	96		28 (29.2)											
697	Congolese	Kisangani	1000							278 (27.8)	3	2				
71	Bakumu and Barumbi	Angumu	552		31 (5.6)											
319	Warega	Kamituga	81		11 (13.6)											
319	Warega	Kitutu	150		18											
320	Warega	Kitutu	300		68											
	Warega	Kitutu	450		86 (19.1)											
321a	Forest Bira		223		30 (13.5)											
	Savannah Bira		298		52 (17.4)											

REF.	POPULATION	PLACE	NUMBER TESTED	G6PD DEF.	SICKLE CELL	THALASSEMIA			HEMOGLOBIN TYPES							
						A_2	F	OSM. RES.		AS						
CONGO (KINSHASA) (CONT.)																
71	Mamvu	Epulu	217		48 (22.1)											
	Efe Pygmies	Epulu and Gombari	456		118 (25.9)											
780	Efe Pygmies		125M	5 (4.0)												
	Efe Pygmies		126M							39 (31.0)						
320	Fulero		300		55 (18.3)											
	Havu	Putu, Tchagala and Kalehe	300		15 (5.0)											
	Hunde	Kirotshe to Bweremana	300		13 (4.3)											
	Swaga	Butembo to Lubero	300		23 (7.7)											
	Shu	Mumole and Vuhovi	300		27 (9.0)											
	Mbuba	Matemora and Bwanandeke	300		108 (36.0)											
	Nyanga	Mutongo and Pinga	300		22 (7.3)											
	Tembo	Tshabunda	300		16 (5.3)											

REF.	POPULATION	PLACE	NUMBER TESTED	G6PD DEF.	SICKLE CELL	THALASSEMIA			HEMOGLOBIN TYPES							
						A_2	F	OSM. RES.		AS						
CONGO (KINSHASA) (CONT.)																
508	Shi		301							12 (4.0)						
320	Shi		375		16											
494	Shi		92		6											
	Shi		467		22 (4.7)											
494	Shi		116M	16 (13.8)												
319	Banande		291		33 (11.3)											
	Bamate		25		3 (12.0)											
	Batangi		16		2 (12.5)											
	Bahera		25		1 (4.0)											
	Bakira		20		3 (15.0)											
	Congo Bahutu (Rutshuru)		100		2 (2.0)											
320	Humu		273		99 (36.3)											
321	Tutsi	Itombwe Plateau	191		2 (1.0)											

REF.	POPULATION	PLACE	NUMBER TESTED	G6PD DEF.	SICKLE CELL	THALASSEMIA			HEMOGLOBIN TYPES							
						A_2	F	OSM. RES.		AS						
RWANDA AND BURUNDI																
319	Batwa	Rwanda and Burundi	141		4 (2.8)											
508	Tutsi	Rwanda and Burundi	306							2 (0.7)						
494	Tutsi	Rwanda and Burundi	90		0											
	Tutsi	Rwanda and Burundi	90M	2 (2.2)												
	Hutu	Rwanda and Burundi	99		5 (5.1)											
	Hutu	Rwanda and Burundi	99M	6 (6.1)												
319	Hutu	Rwanda	403		21 (5.2)											
71	Hutu and Tutsi	Astrida, Rwanda	1000		25 (2.5)											
319	Tutsi	Rwanda	294		4 (1.4)											
	Hutu	Burundi	395		47 (11.9)											
320	Tutsi	Burundi	264		4 (1.5)											

REF.	POPULATION	PLACE	NUMBER TESTED	G6PD DEF.	SICKLE CELL	THALASSEMIA			HEMOGLOBIN TYPES							
						A_2	F	OSM. RES.		AS						
RWANDA AND BURUNDI (CONT.)																
319	Bamosso	Malagarasi River Burundi	478		124 (25.9)											
508	Imbo	Ruzizi River Burundi	328							62 (18.9)						
412	Hutu from Rwanda	Uganda	496		40 (8.1)											
	Hutu from Burundi	Uganda	108		21 (19.4)											
386	Hutu from Rwanda	Uganda	17M	2 (11.8)												
453	Rwandans	Uganda	133M	4 (3.0)												
690a	Rwandans	Uganda	271		12 (4.4)											
ANGOLA																
590	Bushmen	Southeast Angola	249		0											
686	Koroka Bushmen	Southwest Angola	27		1 (3.7)											
	Kwise Bushmen	Southwest Angola	70		7 (10.0)											
	Twa		41		2 (4.9)											

REF.	POPULATION	PLACE	NUMBER TESTED	G6PD DEF.	SICKLE CELL	THALASSEMIA			HEMOGLOBIN TYPES							
						A_2	F	OSM. RES.								
	ANGOLA (CONT.)															
686	Kwando		43		2 (4.7)											
	Bantu		36		3 (8.3)											
670	Bantu	Luanda	186		52 (28.0)											
605	Mbundu	Benguela and Nova Lisboa	216		18 (8.3)											
	Other Bantu	Benguela and Nova Lisboa	202		17 (8.4)											
652	Mbundu	Bie and Camacupa	1676		386 (23.0)											
	Luimbi	Bie and Camacupa	232		26 (11.2)											
	Chokwe	Bie and Camacupa	112		16 (14.3)											
	Songo	Bie and Camacupa	20		5 (25.0)											
599	Luimbi	Lunda and Songo Districts	72		13 (18.1)											
	Caconga	Lunda and Songo Districts	135		33 (24.4)											
	Mataba	Lunda and Songo Districts	61		17 (27.9)											

REF.	POPULATION	PLACE	NUMBER TESTED	G6PD DEF.	SICKLE CELL	THALASSEMIA			HEMOGLOBIN TYPES							
						A_2	F	OSM. RES.		AS	AK					
ANGOLA (CONT.)																
599	Others	Lunda and Songo Districts	53		8 (15.1)											
497	Chokwe	Chitato Concelho	459		93 (20.3)											
	Lunda	Chitato Concelho	213		51 (23.9)											
	Lunda-Chokwe	Chitato Concelho	328		69 (21.0)											
599	Lunda	Lunda District	605		116											
600	Lunda	Lunda District	600		109					109	1					
	Lunda	Lunda District	1205		225 (18.7)											
599	Chokwe	Lunda District	1709		290											
	Chokwe	Lunda District	600		105					105	1					
	Chokwe	Lunda District	2309		395 (17.1)											
599	Songo	Songo District	542		134											
600	Songo	Songo District	600		160					160						
	Songo	Songo District	1142		294 (25.7)											

REF.	POPULATION	PLACE	NUMBER TESTED	G6PD DEF.	SICKLE CELL	THALASSEMIA			HEMOGLOBIN TYPES							
						A_2	F	OSM. RES.		AS	AK					
ANGOLA (CONT.)																
599	Minungo	Lunda and Songo Districts	280		58											
600	Minungo	Lunda and Songo Districts	485		88					88	1					
	Minungo	Lunda and Songo Districts	765		146 (19.1)											
599	Luvale	Lunda and Songo Districts	88		10 (11.4)											
	Bangala	Lunda and Songo Districts	98		43											
600	Bangala	Lunda and Songo Districts	600		213					213						
	Bangala	Lunda and Songo Districts	698		256 (36.7)											
601	Bangala	Lunda and Songo Districts	147M	40 (27.2)												
599	Xinge	Lunda and Songo Districts	290		62											
600	Xinge	Lunda and Songo Districts	600		153					153						
	Xinge	Lunda and Songo Districts	890		215 (24.2)											
601	Xinge	Lunda and Songo Districts	96M	16 (16.7)												

REF.	POPULATION	PLACE	NUMBER TESTED	G6PD DEF.	SICKLE CELL	THALASSEMIA			HEMOGLOBIN TYPES							
						A_2	F	OSM. RES.		AS		AD				A
ANGOLA (CONT.)																
601	Bangala and Xinge	Lunda and Songo Districts	400							137 (34.3)		4 (1.0)				
BOTSWANA																
118	!Kung Bushmen	Okavango River	500		0											
675a	!Kung Bushmen		79		0											
	River Bushmen	Okavango River	58		0											
291	Bushmen	Okavango River	60		0											
	Bushmen	Barakwenga Caprivi Strip	58		0											
156	Bushmen	Northern Kalahari	13M	0												
	Bushmen	Northern Kalahari	10F	0												
	Bushmen	Central Kalahari	16M	1 (6.3)												
	Bushmen	Central Kalahari	31F	1												
751	Bushmen	Central Kalahari	232		0											
675a	Bushmen	South and Central Kalahari	110													110
751	Hottentot	South and Central Kalahari	210		0											

REF.	POPULATION	PLACE	NUMBER TESTED	G6PD DEF.	SICKLE CELL	THALASSEMIA			HEMOGLOBIN TYPES							
						A_2	F	OSM. RES.		AC						A
BOTSWANA (CONT.)																
675a	Kgalakadi Bantu	South and Central Kalahari	60													60
291	Mpukushu Bantu	Okavango River	119		0											
292	Bechuana	Francistown to Maun	252		5 (2.0)											
74	Bechuana		85M	6 (7.1)												
SOUTH AFRICA																
240	Cape Coloured	Capetown	1555		9 (0.6)											
111	Cape Coloured	Capetown	219							2 (0.9)						
504	Indians	Natal	1000		10 (1.0)											
74	Cape Coloured	Capetown	208M	3												
156	Cape Coloured	Capetown	13M	1												
	Cape Coloured	Capetown	221M	4 (1.8)												

REF.	POPULATION	PLACE	NUMBER TESTED	G6PD DEF.	SICKLE CELL	THALASSEMIA			HEMOGLOBIN TYPES							
						A_2	F	OSM. RES.								
SOUTH AFRICA (CONT.)																
74	Indians		200M	2												
156	Indians		100M	0												
	Indians		300M	2 (0.7)												
74	Cape Malays		51M	1												
156	Cape Malays		53M	2												
	Cape Malays		104M	3 (2.9)												
74	European South Africaners		250M	0												
34	Bantu		403		1 (0.2)											
127	Nguni	Ciskei and Fort Hare	76		0											
74	Xhosa		184M	7												
156	Xhosa		43M	1												
	Xhosa		227M	8 (3.5)												
74	Pondo		44M	0												

REF.	POPULATION	PLACE	NUMBER TESTED	G6PD DEF.	SICKLE CELL	THALASSEMIA			HEMOGLOBIN TYPES							
						A_2	F	OSM. RES.								
SOUTH AFRICA (CONT.)																
74	Baca		30M	0												
	Hlubi		17M	1												
	Baca-Hlubi		47M	1 (2.1)												
74	Msutu		85M	4												
156	Msutu		74M	2												
	Msutu		159M	6 (3.8)												
127	Sotho-Tswana		12		0											
156	Tswana		25M	2 (8.0)												
292	Zulu	North of Eshowe	421		0											
74	Zulu		116M	5												
156	Zulu		73M	1												
	Zulu		189M	6 (3.2)												
74	Pedi		45M	3												
156	Pedi		11M	0												
	Pedi		56M	3 (5.4)												

REF.	POPULATION	PLACE	NUMBER TESTED	G6PD DEF.	SICKLE CELL	THALASSEMIA			HEMOGLOBIN TYPES							
						A_2	F	OSM. RES.								A
SOUTH AFRICA (CONT.)																
675a	Pedi		40													40
156	Swazi		8M	1												
74	Venda		9M	1												
74	Ndebele		12M	1												
	Transvaal Shangaan		81M	8												
156	Shangaan		18M	1												
	Shangaan		99M	9 (9.1)												
292	Bantu	Rustenburg to Waterburg Transvaal	56		0											
	Bantu	Waterburg to Potgietersrust Transvaal	56		0											
	Bantu	West of Beit Bridge, Transvaal	76		1 (1.3)											
	Bantu	Beit Bridge to Pafuri, Transvaal	59		0											
	Bantu	Shwingdzi to Barberton, Transvaal	107		2 (1.9)											

REF.	POPULATION	PLACE	NUMBER TESTED	G6PD DEF.	SICKLE CELL	THALASSEMIA			HEMOGLOBIN TYPES							
						A_2	F	OSM. RES.								
SOUTH AFRICA (CONT.)																
74	Other Bantu		49M	1												
156	Other Bantu		38M	0												
	Other Bantu		87M	1 (1.1)												
292	Bantu Mineworkers		1741		2 (0.1)											
MOZAMBIQUE																
422	Ndebele (Landins)		188		1 (0.5)											
259	Tongas		100		1 (1.0)											
	Rongas		100		1 (1.0)											
	Shangaan		150		3 (2.0)											
	Ngoni (Mungones)	Chibuto and Joao Bello	50		1 (2.0)											
	Chopi (Muchopes)	Inhambane and Villanculos	100		2 (2.0)											
	Tswa (Vatswas)	Villanculos	100		2 (2.0)											

REF.	POPULATION	PLACE	NUMBER TESTED	G6PD DEF.	SICKLE CELL	THALASSEMIA			HEMOGLOBIN TYPES							
						A_2	F	OSM. RES.		AS						
MOZAMBIQUE (CONT.)																
678	Bantu	South and Central Mozambique	61							6 (9.8)						
259	Sena	Beira, Zambesia	50		1 (2.0)											
	Ngoni (Angonis)	Tete, Lourenco Marques	50		0											
	Chuabo		100		3 (3.0)											
	Maravi	Nampula	25		0											
	Eratis	Nampula, Milange	25		0											
	Tachanas	Milange, Inhambane, Panda	50		1 (2.0)											
	Manhaua	Milange, Chinde, Namacurra	50		2 (4.0)											
259	Lomwe	Milange, Namacurra,Quilimane, Murrambala	100		4											
109	Lomwe		101		0											
	Lomwe		201		4 (2.0)											
259	Makonde	North Coast	100		40 (40.0)											

REF.	POPULATION	PLACE	NUMBER TESTED	G6PD DEF.	SICKLE CELL	THALASSEMIA			HEMOGLOBIN TYPES							
						A_2	F	OSM. RES.		AS						A
MOZAMBIQUE (CONT.)																
259	Makua	Nampula	110		42 (38.2)											
678	Makua	North Coast	387							14 (3.6)						
260	Makonde	Porto Amelia	100		40 (40.0)											
	Makonde	Vipinco	50		2 (4.0)											
RHODESIA, ZAMBIA, MALAWI																
274	Shona	Salisbury Rhodesia	120													120
	Shona	Salisbury Rhodesia	60			0	0									
109	Shangaan		136		0											
	Karanga		956		6 (0.6)											
	Ndau		318		11 (3.5)											
109	Sena		142		9											
259	Sena		50		1											
	Sena		192		10 (5.2)											

REF.	POPULATION	PLACE	NUMBER TESTED	G6PD DEF.	SICKLE CELL	THALASSEMIA A_2	THALASSEMIA F	THALASSEMIA OSM. RES.	HEMOGLOBIN TYPES							
RHODESIA, ZAMBIA, MALAWI (CONT.)																
109	Nyanja		118		4 (3.4)											
	Yao		189		6 (3.2)											
	Kunda (Cikunda)		54		7 (13.0)											
109	Chewa		275		26											
68	Chewa		522		65											
	Chewa		797		91 (11.4)											
109	Ngoni (Angoni)		226		14											
68	Ngoni		359		33											
	Ngoni		585		47 (8.0)											
68	Tumbuka		50		6 (12.0)											
	"Coloureds"	Fort Jameson Zambia	83		4 (4.8)											
	Senga (Nsenga)		169		32 (18.9)											
156	Nyasa		7M	1 (14.2)												

REF.	POPULATION	PLACE	NUMBER TESTED	G6PD DEF.	SICKLE CELL	THALASSEMIA			HEMOGLOBIN TYPES							
						A_2	F	OSM. RES.		AS		AC				
RHODESIA, ZAMBIA, MALAWI (CONT.)																
109	Nyakyusa		108		20 (18.5)											
	Bemba-Bisa		37		10 (27.0)											
	Senga		82		18 (22.0)											
69	Lala	Serenje District Zambia	308		42 (13.6)											
357	Nambya	Wankie District Rhodesia	571		12 (2.1)											
675a	Plateau Tonga	Wankie District Rhodesia	84		5 (6.0)											
357	Valley Tonga	Wankie District Rhodesia	401		0											
675a	Valley Tonga	Wankie District Rhodesia	253		10											
	Valley Tonga	Wankie District Rhodesia	654		10 (1.5)											
	Valley Tonga	Wankie District Rhodesia	85							?		1 (1.2)				
357	Dombe	Wankie District Rhodesia	60		7 (11.7)											
	Lozi		298		18 (6.0)											

REF.	POPULATION	PLACE	NUMBER TESTED	G6PD DEF.	SICKLE CELL	THALASSEMIA			HEMOGLOBIN TYPES							
						A_2	F	OSM. RES.	S	AS						
RHODESIA, ZAMBIA, MALAWI (CONT.)																
67	Kaounde Lunda	Boma, Balovale District, Zambia	349		47 (13.5)											
	Kaounde Lunda	Southeast of Boma	38		5 (13.2)											
	Kaounde Lunda	Manyinga River	140		18 (12.9)											
	Kaounde Lunda	North of Boma	94		15 (16.0)											
	Lovale	West of Zambezi River, Zambia	94		6 (6.4)											
	Lovale	East of Zambezi River, Zambia	120		20 (16.7)											
	Lovale From Angola		44		5 (11.4)											
	Other Bantu	Balovale District Zambia	41		6 (14.6)											
237	Bantu Mineworkers	Zambia	717		128 (17.9)											
73	Bantu Tribes	Rhodesia	1200M	(5–23)												
TANZANIA																
464	Masai	Ulanga District	8							1						
	Bantu	Ulanga District	1109						2	222 (20.2)						

REF.	POPULATION	PLACE	NUMBER TESTED	G6PD DEF.	SICKLE CELL	THALASSEMIA			HEMOGLOBIN TYPES								
						A_2	F	OSM. RES.		AS							
TANZANIA (CONT.)																	
464	Bantu	Ulanga District	409M	59 (14.4)													
	Bantu	Ulanga District	701F	70 (10.0)													
	Bantu	Ifakara Valley Ulanga District	404							89 (22.0)							
	Bantu	Ifakara Valley Ulanga District	109M	20 (18.3)													
	Bantu	Mountain Villages Ulanga District	173							18 (10.4)							
	Bantu	Mountain Villages Ulanga District	59M	5 (8.5)													
22	Kuria	Busigire Musoma District	102		28 (27.5)												
	Kwaya	Busigire Musoma District	107		33 (30.8)												
	Simbiti	Kanesi Musoma District	126		51 (40.5)												
	Jita	Ukerewe Musoma District	124		36 (29.0)												
	Zanaki	Busegwe Musoma District	104		37 (35.6)												

REF.	POPULATION	PLACE	NUMBER TESTED	G6PD DEF.	SICKLE CELL	THALASSEMIA			HEMOGLOBIN TYPES							
						A_2	F	OSM. RES.	S	AS						
	TANZANIA (CONT.)															
22	Kizu	Ikizu Musoma District	52		15 (28.8)											
24	Bantu	Musoma District	654						5	249 (38.8)						
22	Sukuma	Mwanza	175		47 (26.9)											
	Kerewe	Ukerewe Island	92		29 (31.5)											
	Kara	Ukerewe Island	52		15 (28.8)											
	Iraqw	Mbulu	102		2 (2.0)											
	Chaga	Old Moshi	130		0											
260	Chaga	Kibo	75		0											
22	Arusha	Arusha	126		1 (0.8)											
408	Bantu	Dar Es Salaam	104							12 (11.5)						
307	Bantu	Dar Es Salaam	156	16 (10.3)												
22	Sambaa	Amani Tanga District	103		9 (8.7)											

REF.	POPULATION	PLACE	NUMBER TESTED	G6PD DEF.	SICKLE CELL	THALASSEMIA			HEMOGLOBIN TYPES							
						A_2	F	OSM. RES.								
TANZANIA (CONT.)																
26	Sambaa	Tanga District	29M	6 (20.7)												
	Sambaa	Tanga District	33F	5 (15.2)												
22	Zigua	Tanga District	57		8 (14.0)											
26	Zigua	Tanga District	26M	6 (23.1)												
	Zigua	Tanga District	29F	4 (13.8)												
22	Bondei	Tanga District	81		23 (28.4)											
26	Bondei	Muheza	121M	33												
31	Bondei	Tanga District	424M	105												
	Bondei		545M	138 (25.3)												
26	Bondei	Muheza	124F	24												
31	Bondei	Tanga District	452F	121												
	Bondei		576F	145 (25.2)												

REF.	POPULATION	PLACE	NUMBER TESTED	G6PD DEF.	SICKLE CELL	THALASSEMIA			HEMOGLOBIN TYPES							
						A_2	F	OSM. RES.								
TANZANIA (CONT.)																
260	Digo (Nyika)	Msambweni	50		11											
22	Digo (Nyika)	Tanga District	66		18											
	Digo (Nyika)		116		29 (25.0)											
26	Digo (Nyika)	Tanga District	26M	6 (23.1)												
	Digo (Nyika)	Tanga District	33F	6 (18.2)												
260	Duruma (Nyika)	Msambweni	68		7											
491	Duruma (Nyika)	Msambweni	302		31											
	Duruma (Nyika)	Msambweni	370		38 (10.3)											
22	Pare	Same	54		4 (7.4)											
KENYA																
260	Pare	Taveta	40		2 (5.0)											
	Taveta	Taveta	154		37 (24.0)											

REF.	POPULATION	PLACE	NUMBER TESTED	G6PD DEF.	SICKLE CELL	THALASSEMIA			HEMOGLOBIN TYPES							
						A_2	F	OSM. RES.		AS						
KENYA (CONT.)																
225	Taveta Infants	Taveta	52							10 (19.2)						
260	Teita	Wesu Teita Hills	127		0											
260	Kambe (Nyika)	Ribe	78		27											
491	Kambe (Nyika)	Ribe	220		75											
	Kambe (Nyika)	Ribe	298		102 (34.2)											
260	Ribe (Nyika)	Ribe	50		13 (26.0)											
	Rabai (Nyika)	Rabai	48		5 (10.4)											
	Jibana (Nyika)	Kaloleni	119		16 (13.4)											
	Chonyi (Nyika)	Kaloleni	90		23 (25.6)											
	Giryama and Kauma (Nyika)	Ganda, Kilifi, Jarabuni	39		4 (10.3)											
	Giryama	Malindi	150		16 (10.7)											

REF.	POPULATION	PLACE	NUMBER TESTED	G6PD DEF.	SICKLE CELL	THALASSEMIA			HEMOGLOBIN TYPES							
						A_2	F	OSM. RES.								
KENYA (CONT.)																
26	Giryama	Malindi	101M	17 (16.8)												
	Giryama	Malindi	65F	10 (15.4)												
260	Pokomo (Ngatana)	Garsen	102		27 (26.5)											
	Galla	Garsen	30		0											
	Boni	Bargoni	81		0											
	Sanye	Witu	61		0											
	Sanye	Adu	68		8 (11.8)											
	Bajun	Lamu	45		1 (2.2)											
	Swahili	Ganda	50		2 (4.0)											
	Swahili	Kakunyi	50		5 (10.0)											
	Arabs	Malindi	61		1 (1.6)											
	Boran	Sakuya	6		0											
	Turkana	North Kenya	50		0											

REF.	POPULATION	PLACE	NUMBER TESTED	G6PD DEF.	SICKLE CELL	THALASSEMIA			HEMOGLOBIN TYPES							
						A_2	F	OSM. RES.								
KENYA (CONT.)																
22	Kamba	Machakos	213		0											
260	Kamba	Machakos	134		2											
	Kamba	Machakos	347		2 (0.6)											
22	Kikiyu	Nairobi	227		1											
260	Kikiyu	Nairobi	67		1											
	Kikiyu	Nairobi	294		2 (0.7)											
26	Kikiyu	Nairobi and Naivasha	70M	2 (2.9)												
	Kikiyu	Nairobi and Naivasha	73F	2 (2.7)												
260	Masai	Kajiado	100		0											
26	Masai	Kajiado	59M	1 (1.7)												
	Masai	Kajiado	12F	0												
260	Masai	Narok	82		0											
22	Masai	Magadi	104		0											

REF.	POPULATION	PLACE	NUMBER TESTED	G6PD DEF.	SICKLE CELL	THALASSEMIA			HEMOGLOBIN TYPES							
						A_2	F	OSM. RES.								
KENYA (CONT.)																
260	Kipsigi	Kericho	100		2 (2.0)											
22	Kipsigi	Letain	75		0											
260	Gusii	Kericho	100		3 (3.0)											
22	Gusii	Chemagal	160		7 (4.4)											
260	Wanga	Mumias Kavirondo District	96		19 (19.8)											
	Marama	Buteri Kavirondo District	100		10 (10.0)											
	Kakamega	Kakamega Kavirondo District	96		6 (6.3)											
	Kitosh	Bungoma Kavirondo District	100		21 (21.0)											
	Nyangori	Kapsengeri Kavirondo District	44		2 (4.5)											
	Nyoro	Kimba Kavirondo District	100		6 (6.0)											
	Maragoli	Majengo Kavirondo District	100		9 (9.0)											
22	Suba	Rusinga Island	173		48 (27.8)											

REF.	POPULATION	PLACE	NUMBER TESTED	G6PD DEF.	SICKLE CELL	THALASSEMIA			HEMOGLOBIN TYPES							
						A_2	F	OSM. RES.								
KENYA (CONT.)																
260	Luo	South Kavirondo District	100		28											
22	Luo	Kisumu	288		74											
	Luo		388		102 (26.3)											
26	Luo	Nairobi and Kisumu District	50M	14 (28.0)												
	Luo	Nairobi and Kisumu District	27F	4 (14.8)												
UGANDA																
690a	Luo		490		101											
412	Luo		130		37											
	Luo		620		138 (22.3)											
453	Luo		45M	3												
386	Luo		19M	2												
	Luo		64M	5 (7.8)												
386	Luo (Padhola)		48M	14 (29.2)												
412	Gisu (Bagishu)		207		62 (30.0)											

REF.	POPULATION	PLACE	NUMBER TESTED	G6PD DEF.	SICKLE CELL	THALASSEMIA			HEMOGLOBIN TYPES							
						A_2	F	OSM. RES.								
UGANDA (CONT.)																
386	Gisu		25M	4 (16.0)												
346	Soga	Senda Tororo Province	339		69 (20.3)											
412	Soga (Basoga)		241		70 (29.0)											
386	Soga, Nyuli, Gwere, Kenyi		43M	7												
580	Soga		4M	1												
453	Soga		14M	1												
	Soga		61M	9 (14.7)												
412	Kenyi (Bakenyi)		88		23 (26.1)											
690a	Ganda		1711		288											
412	Ganda (Baganda)		740		141											
22	Ganda (Baganda)	Kampala	334		65											
	Ganda		2785		494 (17.7)											

REF.	POPULATION	PLACE	NUMBER TESTED	G6PD DEF.	SICKLE CELL	THALASSEMIA A_2	THALASSEMIA F	THALASSEMIA OSM. RES.	HEMOGLOBIN TYPES S	HEMOGLOBIN TYPES AS	HEMOGLOBIN TYPES AD	HEMOGLOBIN TYPES AJ				
UGANDA (CONT.)																
453	Ganda		424M	53												
26	Ganda	Kampala	40M	6												
386	Ganda		39M	6												
	Ganda		503M	65 (12.9)												
26	Ganda	Kampala	46F	5 (10.9)												
386	Ugandans		164F	0												
345	Ganda	Kampala	3362						3	542 (16.2)						
567	Indians	Kampala	500								4	1				
386	Bantu Ugandans		14M	2												
22	Hutu	Kisoro	135		4 (3.0)											
	Twa	Kisoro	33		0											
	Chiga	Kabale	206		2 (1.0)											
350	Chiga	Kayonza District Kigezi	843		34 (4.0)											

REF.	POPULATION	PLACE	NUMBER TESTED	G6PD DEF.	SICKLE CELL	THALASSEMIA			HEMOGLOBIN TYPES							
						A_2	F	OSM. RES.								
UGANDA (CONT.)																
453	Kiga		54M	1												
386	Kiga		11M	0												
	Kiga		65M	1 (1.5)												
22	Iru	Mbarara	127		7											
412	Iru		139		3											
	Iru		266		10 (3.8)											
22	Hima	West Ankole	134		3											
412	Hima		166		4											
	Hima		300		7 (2.3)											
386	Nkole		10M	0												
453	Nkole		63M	2												
	Nkole		73M	2 (2.7)												
22	Konjo	Kichwamba and Kisomoro	124		12											
412	Konjo		102		18											
	Konjo		226		30 (13.3)											

REF.	POPULATION	PLACE	NUMBER TESTED	G6PD DEF.	SICKLE CELL	THALASSEMIA			HEMOGLOBIN TYPES							
						A_2	F	OSM. RES.								
UGANDA (CONT.)																
22	Amba	Bundibugyo	220		86											
412	Amba		140		63											
413	Amba		503		191											
	Amba		863		340 (39.4)											
412	Toro		120		15 (12.5)											
453	Toro		35M	3												
386	Toro		8M	1												
	Toro		43M	4 (8.9)												
412	Nyoro		91		11 (12.1)											
453	Nyoro		18M	2 (11.1)												
412	Lango		278		75 (27.0)											
260	Lango	Torit	30		1 (3.3)											
386	Lango		36M	5 (13.9)												

REF.	POPULATION	PLACE	NUMBER TESTED	G6PD DEF.	SICKLE CELL	THALASSEMIA			HEMOGLOBIN TYPES							
						A_2	F	OSM. RES.		AS		AG				
UGANDA (CONT.)																
22	Teso	Kampala	81		12 (14.8)											
412	Teso		416		74 (17.8)											
453	Teso		21M	2												
386	Teso		<u>142M</u>	<u>28</u>												
	Teso		163M	30 (18.4)												
386	Kuman		19M	3 (15.8)												
412	Sebei		124		1 (0.8)											
	Suk		128		5 (3.9)											
20	Karamojong	Moroto	53			0	0					1				
412	Karamojong		156		5 (3.2)											
406	Karamojong	Lutomi Kraal	53		46 (86.8)											
349	Karamojong		637		12 (1.9)											
20	Labwor		14			0	0			3 (21.4)						

REF.	POPULATION	PLACE	NUMBER TESTED	G6PD DEF.	SICKLE CELL	THALASSEMIA			HEMOGLOBIN TYPES							
						A_2	F	OSM. RES.		AS						
UGANDA (CONT.)																
386	Karamajong, Sebei, Nandi		24M	2 (8.3)												
20	Other Tribes	Northeast Uganda	42			0	0			3 (7.1)						
412	Acholi		141		38 (27.0)											
260	Acholi	Torit	54		6 (11.1)											
351	Northern Acholi	Gulu to Sudan Border	380		58 (15.3)											
453	Acholi		23M	2												
386	Acholi		<u>10M</u>	<u>1</u>												
	Acholi		33M	3 (9.1)												
412	Alur		114		29 (25.4)											
	Jonam		109		28 (25.7)											
22	Madi	Kampala	62		14 (22.6)											
412	Madi		109		3 (2.8)											

REF.	POPULATION	PLACE	NUMBER TESTED	G6PD DEF.	SICKLE CELL	THALASSEMIA			HEMOGLOBIN TYPES							
						A_2	F	OSM. RES.								
UGANDA (CONT.)																
22	Lugbara	Kampala	76		18 (23.7)											
412	Lugbara		120		25 (20.8)											
352	Lugbara	Aringa District	473		9 (1.9)											
386	Lugbara, Madi, Alur		13M	1 (7.7)												
412	Kakwa		101		25 (24.8)											
SUDAN																
260	Madi	Opari	71		13 (18.3)											
	Kakwa	Yei	76		6 (7.9)											
1	Azande		100		18											
260	Azande	Juba	28		3											
	Azande		128		21 (16.4)											
260	Longarim	Walthit Forest	73		1 (1.4)											
	Logir	Walthit Forest	38		0											

REF.	POPULATION	PLACE	NUMBER TESTED	G6PD DEF.	SICKLE CELL	THALASSEMIA			HEMOGLOBIN TYPES							
						A_2	F	OSM. RES.								
SUDAN (CONT.)																
260	Lokoya	Liria	98		5 (5.1)											
	Dongotono	Isoke	70		0											
	Lotuko	Lambalua	72		0											
	Moru	Juba	71		2 (2.8)											
	Mundu	Yei	80		13 (16.3)											
	Baka	Yei	105		9 (8.6)											
	Kuku	Yei	39		3 (7.7)											
	Fadjulu (Pojulu)	Lainya	100		9 (9.0)											
	Bari	Rejaf	100		7 (7.0)											
	Anuak	Lafon	96		8 (8.3)											
	Mandari	Terakeka	105		18 (17.1)											
	Mandari	Tali Post	98		7 (7.1)											

REF.	POPULATION	PLACE	NUMBER TESTED	G6PD DEF.	SICKLE CELL	THALASSEMIA			HEMOGLOBIN TYPES							
						A_2	F	OSM. RES.								A
SUDAN (CONT.)																
260	Nuer	Adok and Ler	100		1											
577	Nuer		100		0											
	Nuer		200		1 (0.5)											
260	Shilluk	Tonga	110		0											
	Shilluk	Malakal	56		0											
577	Shilluk		271		0											
	Mabaan		34		0											
	Mabaan		4													4
	Dinka-Shilluk-Nuer		14		0											
	Dinka-Shilluk-Nuer		7		0											7
	Northern Dinka		320		0											
	Northern Dinka		64													64
260	Dinka	Malek	87		0											
	Dinka	Bor	77		2 (2.6)											
	Dinka	Duk	22		0											

REF.	POPULATION	PLACE	NUMBER TESTED	G6PD DEF.	SICKLE CELL	THALASSEMIA			HEMOGLOBIN TYPES							
						A_2	F	OSM. RES.								
SUDAN (CONT.)																
260	Dinka	Melut	20		0											
	Dinka	Toich	38		0											
710	Nubans (Nubawi)	El Fasher, Darfur	24		0											
712a	Nubans (Nubawi)	Omdurman	57		0											
	Nubans (Nubawi)	Khartoum North	51		2											
	Nubans (Nubawi)		132		2 (1.5)											
710	Dinka	El Fasher, Darfur	42		1											
712a	Dinka	Omdurman	21		0											
	Dinka	Khartoum North	50		1											
	Dinka		113		2 (1.8)											
710	Zaghawa (Zagawi)	El Fasher, Darfur	296		7 (2.4)											
	Tama (Tamawi)	El Fasher, Darfur	30		1 (3.3)											
	Bartawi	El Fasher, Darfur	172		7 (4.1)											
	Kababish (Hawwari)	El Fasher, Darfur	64		3 (4.7)											
	Midobi	El Fasher, Darfur	43		2 (4.7)											

REF.	POPULATION	PLACE	NUMBER TESTED	G6PD DEF.	SICKLE CELL	THALASSEMIA			HEMOGLOBIN TYPES							
						A_2	F	OSM. RES.								
SUDAN (CONT.)																
710	Kinani	El Fasher,Darfur	21		1 (4.8)											
710	Shaigi	El Fasher,Darfur	29		1											
712a	Shaigi	Omdurman	104		1											
	Shaigi	Khartoum North	104		0											
	Shaigi		237		2 (0.8)											
710	Mahasi	El Fasher,Darfur	27		1											
712a	Mahasi	Omdurman	75		0											
	Mahasi	Khartoum North	84		0											
	Mahasi		186		1 (0.5)											
710	Gamai	El Fasher,Darfur	70		3											
712a	Gamai	Omdurman	39		1											
	Gamai		109		4 (3.7)											
710	Fur(Furawi)	El Fasher,Darfur	146		8											
712a	Fur(Furawi)	Omdurman	17		1											
	Fur(Furawi)	Khartoum North	14		0											
	Fur(Furawi)		177		9 (5.1)											

REF.	POPULATION	PLACE	NUMBER TESTED	G6PD DEF.	SICKLE CELL	THALASSEMIA			HEMOGLOBIN TYPES							
						A_2	F	OSM. RES.								
SUDAN (CONT.)																
710	Gaaliin(Gaali)	El Fasher,Darfur	84		6											
712a	Gaaliin(Gaali)	Omdurman	255		2											
	Gaaliin(Gaali)	Khartoum North	152		0											
	Gaaliin(Gaali)		491		8 (1.6)											
710	Tungur (Tungurawi)	El Fasher,Darfur	141		11 (7.8)											
	Sharifi	El Fasher,Darfur	44		4 (9.1)											
	Darooki	El Fasher,Darfur	31		3 (9.7)											
	Fezara(Zaiada)	El Fasher,Darfur	31		3 (9.7)											
710	Bederia (Bideri)	El Fasher,Darfur	25		2											
712a	Bederia (Bideri)	Omdurman	24		1											
	Bederia (Bideri)	Khartoum North	7		0											
	Bederia (Bideri)		56		3 (5.4)											

REF.	POPULATION	PLACE	NUMBER TESTED	G6PD DEF.	SICKLE CELL	THALASSEMIA			HEMOGLOBIN TYPES							
						A_2	F	OSM. RES.								
SUDAN (CONT.)																
710	Dongolans (Dongolawi)	El Fasher, Darfur	33		3											
712a	Dongolans (Dongolawi)	Omdurman	122		2											
	Dongolans (Dongolawi)	Khartoum North	50		0											
	Dongolans (Dongolawi)		205		5 (2.4)											
710	Mograbi	El Fasher, Darfur	20		2											
712a	Mograbi	Omdurman	19		0											
	Mograbi	Khartoum North	21		0											
	Mograbi		60		2 (3.3)											
712a	Other Tribes	Omdurman	653		14 (2.1)											
	Other Tribes	Khartoum North	527		15 (2.8)											
710	Rayafi	El Fasher, Darfur	27		3 (11.1)											
	Bargawi	El Fasher, Darfur	73		10 (13.7)											
	Habbania (Rizejgi)	El Fasher, Darfur	63		9 (14.3)											

REF.	POPULATION	PLACE	NUMBER TESTED	G6PD DEF.	SICKLE CELL	THALASSEMIA			HEMOGLOBIN TYPES							
						A_2	F	OSM. RES.								
SUDAN (CONT.)																
710	Mimi (Mimawi)	El Fasher, Darfur	42		6 (14.3)											
	Falati	El Fasher, Darfur	92		14 (15.2)											
	Habbania (Hilbawi)	El Fasher, Darfur	32		5 (15.6)											
	Barnawi	El Fasher, Darfur	22		4 (18.2)											
	Kimr (Gimrawi)	El Fasher, Darfur	36		7 (19.4)											
	Habbania (Taaishi)	El Fasher, Darfur	29		6 (20.7)											
	Masalit (Masalati)	El Fasher, Darfur	46		10 (21.7)											
	Issirawi	El Fasher, Darfur	15		4 (26.7)											
	Habbania (Habbani)	El Fasher, Darfur	33		9 (27.3)											
	Messiria (Miseiri)	El Fasher, Darfur	23		7 (30.4)											
	Other Tribes	El Fasher, Darfur	519		31 (6.0)											
708	All Tribes	Wau, Bahr el Ghazal	1252		75 (6.0)											

REF.	POPULATION	PLACE	NUMBER TESTED	G6PD DEF.	SICKLE CELL	THALASSEMIA			HEMOGLOBIN TYPES							
						A_2	F	OSM. RES.	S	AS	AO					Barts
SUDAN (CONT.)																
708	Dinka	Wau, Bahr el Ghazal			(2)											
	Jur, Kreish (Kresh), and Ndogo (Golo)	Wau, Bahr el Ghazal			(2-5)											
	Ndogo, Bongo, and Ndogo (Shere)	Wau, Bahr el Ghazal			(5-7)											
	Ndogo (Bai, and Belanda)	Wau, Bahr el Ghazal			(7-12)											
711	Sudanese (cord blood)		64													6 (9.4)
	Sudanese	Khartoum	200			12 (6.0)										
715	Sudanese (cord blood)	Khartoum	41M	3 (7.3)												
	Sudanese	Khartoum	148M	12 (8.1)												
711	Sudanese	Khartoum	2230						8	42	1					
712c	Sudanese	Khartoum	9100		182 (2.0)											
	Sudanese	Khartoum	9300							?	11					
711	Sudanese Children		4500					1350 (30.0)								

REF.	POPULATION	PLACE	NUMBER TESTED	G6PD DEF.	SICKLE CELL	THALASSEMIA			HEMOGLOBIN TYPES							
						A_2	F	OSM. RES.								
SUDAN (CONT.)																
711	Sudanese	Kurmuk, Blue Nile	200					17 (8.5)								
	Sudanese Soldiers		300					71 (23.7)								
714	Greek and Greek Cypriots	Khartoum	553					159 (28.8)								
716	Egyptiams	Khartoum	1416					331 (23.4)								
	Egyptian Arabs	Khartoum	362					101 (27.9)								
705	Syrians	Khartoum	85					10 (11.8)								
	Armenians	Khartoum	59					16 (27.1)								
	Italians	Khartoum	31					5 (16.1)								
	Indians	Khartoum	31					10 (32.3)								
	Ethiopians	Khartoum	12					4 (33.3)								
	Others	Khartoum	99					20 (20.2)								

REF.	POPULATION	PLACE	NUMBER TESTED	G6PD DEF.	SICKLE CELL	THALASSEMIA			HEMOGLOBIN TYPES							
						A_2	F	OSM. RES.								A
ETHIOPIA																
574	Ethiopians	Addis Ababa	154		0											
2	Guraghe	Atat, Shoa Province	108M	0												
414	Guraghe	Atat, Shoa Province	108				0									108
2	Galla	Shamshamane, Arusi Province	110M	0												
414	Galla	Shamshamane, Arusi Province	110													110
	Galla	Shamshamane, Arusi Province	90				0									
2	Amhara	Gondar Province	125M	0												
414	Amhara	Gondar Province	115													115
	Amhara	Gondar Province	94				0									
2	Southern Falasha	Gondar Province	147M	0												
414	Southern Falasha	Gondar Province	109				0									109
2	Northern Falasha	Enda Selassie, Eritrea	78M	0												
414	Northern Falasha	Enda Selassie, Eritrea	58													58

REF.	POPULATION	PLACE	NUMBER TESTED	G6PD DEF.	SICKLE CELL	THALASSEMIA			HEMOGLOBIN TYPES							
						A_2	F	OSM. RES.								A
ETHIOPIA (CONT.)																
414	Northern Falasha	Enda Selassie, Eritrea	44				0									
2	Billen	Keren, Eritrea	110M	0												
414	Billen	Keren,Eritrea	116													116
	Billen	Keren, Eritrea	97				0									
2	Tigre	Asmara and Enda Selassie,Eritrea	146M	0												
414	Tigre	Asmara and Enda Selassie,Eritrea	164													164
	Tigre	Asmara and Enda Selassie,Eritrea	127				0									
685a	Ethiopians	Asmara,Eritrea	1000					129 (12.9)								
SOMALIA																
407	Somalis		50		0											
260	Ajuran Somali		14		0											
	Digodia Somali		20		0											
	Ogadein Somali		16		0											
SOCOTRA																
440b	Bedouin	Inland Socotra	99													99

REF.	POPULATION	PLACE	NUMBER TESTED	G6PD DEF.	SICKLE CELL	THALASSEMIA			HEMOGLOBIN TYPES							
						A_2	F	OSM. RES.		AS						A
SEYCHELLES																
647	Seychelles Islanders		5587		82 (1.5)											
258	Seychelles Islanders	Mahe	2376		(2.0)											
COMORO ISLANDS																
131	Comoro Islanders		2		0											2
640	Comoro Islanders		126		6											
	Comoro Islanders		128		6 (4.7)											
MADAGASCAR																
153	St.Mary's Islanders		247		26 (10.5)											
640	Merina		1004		33											
131	Merina		81		3					3						
607	Merina		775		27											
	Merina		1860		61 (3.3)											
208	Merina		81M	8 (9.9)												

REF.	POPULATION	PLACE	NUMBER TESTED	G6PD DEF.	SICKLE CELL	THALASSEMIA			HEMOGLOBIN TYPES							
						A_2	F	OSM. RES.		AS						A
MADAGASCAR (CONT.)																
131	Tsimihety		19		0											19
640	Tsimihety		43		7											
	Tsimihety		62		7 (11.3)											
208	Tsimihety		22M	6 (27.3)												
131	Sianaka		7		0											7
640	Sianaka		45		3											
	Sianaka		52		3 (5.8)											
131	Antaimoro		13		4					4						
640	Antaimoro		13		0											
290	Antaimoro		148		27											
	Antaimoro		174		31 (17.8)											
208	Antaimoro		9M	0												
607	Antaimoro	Vohipeno	230		47 (20.4)											
	Antaimoro	Manakara	185		43 (23.2)											
	Others	Manakara	290		58 (20.0)											

REF.	POPULATION	PLACE	NUMBER TESTED	G6PD DEF.	SICKLE CELL	THALASSEMIA A_2	THALASSEMIA F	THALASSEMIA OSM. RES.	HEMOGLOBIN TYPES	AS						A
MADAGASCAR (CONT.)																
607	Antaimoro	Manamjary	64		14 (21.9)											
	Others	Manamjary	324		31 (9.5)											
290	Antambohoaka		122		21											
131	Antambohoaka		1		0											1
	Antambohoaka		123		21 (17.1)											
290	Antaitsimatra		100		16 (16.0)											
131	Betsimisaraka		34		6					6						
640	Betsimisaraka		47		3											
290	Betsimisaraka		147		17											
	Betsimisaraka		228		26 (11.4)											
208	Betsimisaraka		44M	8 (18.2)												
131	Tanala		6		0											6
640	Tanala		7		3											
290	Tanala		258		28											
	Tanala		271		31 (11.4)											

REF.	POPULATION	PLACE	NUMBER TESTED	G6PD DEF.	SICKLE CELL	THALASSEMIA A_2	THALASSEMIA F	THALASSEMIA OSM. RES.	HEMOGLOBIN TYPES							
										AS						A
MADAGASCAR (CONT.)																
208	Tanala		9M	3 (33.3)												
290	Betsileo		39		4											
131	Betsileo		14		1					1						
640	Betsileo		130		6											
607	Betsileo		272		14											
	Betsileo		455		25 (5.5)											
208	Betsileo		43M	10 (23.3)												
131	Bezanozano		4		0											4
640	Bezanozano		19		1											
	Bezanozano		23		1 (4.3)											
131	Sakalava		10		1					1						
640	Sakalava		90		10											
	Sakalava		100		11 (11.0)											
208	Sakalava and Vezo		32M	2 (6.3)												
272	Masikoro (Coastal Sakalava)		60		3 (5.0)											

REF.	POPULATION	PLACE	NUMBER TESTED	G6PD DEF.	SICKLE CELL	THALASSEMIA			HEMOGLOBIN TYPES							
						A_2	F	OSM. RES.		AS						
MADAGASCAR (CONT.)																
272	Vezo (Inland Sakalava)		70		2 (2.9)											
607	Sakalava	Morondava	601		70 (11.6)											
	Others	Morondava	624		48 (7.7)											
	Sakalava	Maintirano	59		7 (11.9)											
	Makoa	Maintirano	229		5 (2.2)											
131	Bara		58		9					9						
640	Bara		37		4											
290	Bara		22		3											
	Bara		117		16 (13.7)											
272	Bara	Tulear	108		8 (7.4)											
607	Bara	Betroka	184		41 (22.3)											
	Others	Betroka	35		4 (11.4)											
	Mahafaly	Ampanihy	80		6 (7.5)											

REF.	POPULATION	PLACE	NUMBER TESTED	G6PD DEF.	SICKLE CELL	THALASSEMIA			HEMOGLOBIN TYPES							
						A_2	F	OSM. RES.		AS						A
MADAGASCAR (CONT.)																
131	Antandroy		13		0											13
640	Antandroy		22		0											
607	Antandroy	Ambovombe	91		0											
208	Antandroy		7M	1 (7.3)												
607	Others	Ambovombe	10		2											
131	Antanosy		2		1					1						
640	Antanosy		11		1											
	Antanosy		13		2 (15.4)											
607	Antanosy	Fort Dauphin	48		3 (6.3)											
208	Antanosy		7M	0												
607	Others	Fort Dauphin	151		12 (7.9)											
131	Antaisaka		11		5					5						
640	Antaisaka		14		2											
290	Antaisaka		36		3											
	Antaisaka		61		10 (16.4)											

REF.	POPULATION	PLACE	NUMBER TESTED	G6PD DEF.	SICKLE CELL	THALASSEMIA			HEMOGLOBIN TYPES							
						A_2	F	OSM. RES.								A
MADAGASCAR (CONT.)																
208	Antaisaka		16M	5 (31.3)												
607	Antaisaka	Vangaindrano and Farafangana	333		71 (21.3)											
290	Antaifasy		15		1 (6.7)											
131	Antankarana		4		0											4
640	Vakinankaraka		26		0											
	Other Madagascans		38		3 (7.9)											
290	Other Madagascans		22		0											
208	Other Madagascans		9M	1 (11.1)												

REF.	POPULATION	PLACE	NUMBER TESTED	G6PD DEF.	SICKLE CELL	THALASSEMIA			HEMOGLOBIN TYPES							
						A_2	F	OSM. RES.	S	AS		AK		AC	AD	A
CANADA																
265a	Chipewyan	Wollaston Lake Saskatchewan	45	0												45
712b	Canadians (Patients)	Saskatoon Saskatchewan	6300				2		1	1		1				
	Canadians	Saskatoon Saskatchewan	5400									21 (0.4)		2		
	Canadians	Regina Saskatchewan	650									4 (0.6)				
	Canadians (Patients)	Regina Saskatchewan	1100													1100
UNITED STATES																
615	Eskimos	Alaska	708													708
	Aleuts	Alaska	200													200
	Indians	Central Alaska	44													44
97	Athabascan Indians	Fort Yukon Alaska	92													92
	Athabascan Indians	Brooks Range Alaska	77													77
494	Negroes	Seattle Washington	658M	67 (10.2)												
283	Shoshone and Arapaho	Wyoming and Montana	338												2 (0.6)	

REF.	POPULATION	PLACE	NUMBER TESTED	G6PD DEF.	SICKLE CELL	THALASSEMIA			HEMOGLOBIN TYPES							
						A_2	F	OSM. RES.								A
UNITED STATES (CONT.)																
150	Whites	Chicago Illinois	307		1 (0.3)											
623	Whites	Chicago Illinois	215	2 (0.9)												
79	Whites	Chicago Illinois	32	0												
150	Negroes	Chicago Illinois	1263		119 (9.4)											
94b	Negroes (Pregnant)	Chicago Illinois	6360		528 (8.3)											
36	Negroes	Chicago Illinois	130M	16 (12.3)												
79	Negroes	Chicago Illinois	121	6 (5.0)												
201a	Negroes (Schizophrenic)	Illinois	177M	21 (11.9)												
	Negroes (Schizophrenic)	Illinois	174F	32 (18.4)												
	Negroes	Illinois	260M	34 (13.1)												
	Negroes	Illinois	359F	62 (17.3)												
507	Caucasians	Detroit Michigan	72													72

REF.	POPULATION	PLACE	NUMBER TESTED	G6PD DEF.	SICKLE CELL	THALASSEMIA			HEMOGLOBIN TYPES							
						A_2	F	OSM. RES.		AS		AC		AI		A
UNITED STATES (CONT.)																
507	Negroes	Detroit Michigan	209							?		3 (1.4)				
185	Negroes	Detroit	400		30 (7.5)											
506	Negroes	Detroit and Ann Arbor, Michigan	1000		91 (9.1)											
117	Negroes (Schizophrenic)	Michigan	165M	19 (11.5)												
	Negroes (Schizophrenic)	Michigan	148F	25 (16.9)												
	Negroes	Michigan	541M	59 (10.9)												
	Negroes	Michigan	133F	29 (21.8)												
741a	Negroes	Cleveland Ohio	988		79 (8.0)											
519	Americans	Northern Vermont	615											1 (0.2)		
780	Senecas	Western New York	327			0										327
	Senecas	Western New York	105M	0												
	Senecas	Western New York	157F	0												
769	Negro Children	Albany New York	83M	5 (6.0)												

REF.	POPULATION	PLACE	NUMBER TESTED	G6PD DEF.	SICKLE CELL	THALASSEMIA			HEMOGLOBIN TYPES								
						A_2	F	OSM. RES.									
UNITED STATES (CONT.)																	
769	Negro Children	Albany New York	52F	4 (7.7)													
294	Caucasians	New York New York	118	2 (1.7)													
	Negroes	New York New York	109	11 (10.1)													
746	Negroes	New York New York	150		13 (8.7)												
210	Negroes (TB Patients)	New York New York	77		4 (5.2)												
582	Negroes (TB Patients)	Brooklyn New York	200		16 (8.0)												
423	Negroes	New Rochelle New York	213		12 (5.6)												
733	Negroes	Long Island New York	226		18 (8.0)												
64	Negroes	Philadelphia Pennsylvania	100		13												
459	Negroes	Philadelphia Pennsylvania	1000		72												
	Negroes	Philadelphia Pennsylvania	1100		85 (7.7)												

REF.	POPULATION	PLACE	NUMBER TESTED	G6PD DEF.	SICKLE CELL	THALASSEMIA A_2	THALASSEMIA F	THALASSEMIA OSM. RES.	HEMOGLOBIN TYPES S	AS	SC	AC	C	AD		A	Barts
UNITED STATES (CONT.)																	
526	Negroes	Philadelphia Pennsylvania	1000				1										
499	Negroes	Philadelphia Pennsylvania	1000				3		3	74 (7.9)	2	23 (2.5)		1			
	Negroes	Philadelphia Pennsylvania	2000				4 (0.2)										
739	Negroes (TB Patients)	Philadelphia Pennsylvania	150		19 (12.6)												
	Negroes	Philadelphia Pennsylvania	150		8 (5.3)												
644	Whites	Baltimore Maryland	500													500	
168	Greeks	Baltimore Maryland	75	8 (10.7)													
736	Caucasians (Cord Blood)	Baltimore Maryland	180														4 (2.2)
366	Negroes	Baltimore Maryland	250		16 (6.4)												
644	Negroes	Baltimore Maryland	500						5	36 (8.4)	1	9 (2.0)					
168	Negroes	Baltimore Maryland	144M	21 (14.6)													
	Negroes	Baltimore Maryland	184F	4 (2.2)													

REF.	POPULATION	PLACE	NUMBER TESTED	G6PD DEF.	SICKLE CELL	THALASSEMIA			HEMOGLOBIN TYPES								
						A_2	F	OSM. RES.	S	AS	SC	AC	C	AD	G	B_2	Barts
UNITED STATES (CONT.)																	
458	Negroes	Baltimore Maryland	400 HbAS											4			
108	Negroes	Baltimore Maryland	2200				7										
183	Negroes	Baltimore Maryland	5000				5										
	Negroes	Baltimore Maryland	7200				12 (0.2)										
736	Negroes (Cord Blood)	Baltimore Maryland	900						1	67 (7.6)		26 (3.2)	3		2	2	15 (2.1)
105	Negroes	Maryland	681							44 (6.5)		12 (1.8)				15 (2.2)	
554	Negroes	Maryland	238M	15 (6.3)													
584	Wesorts	Charles and Prince George Counties, Maryland	2578						20	496 (20.2)	4	5 (0.3)					
585	Wesorts	Charles and Prince George Counties, Maryland	34M	2 (5.9)													
	Wesorts	Charles and Prince George Counties, Maryland	45F	2 (4.4)													
584	Negroes	Charles County Maryland	191			1 (0.5)				10 (5.2)		4 (2.1)				2 (1.0)	

REF.	POPULATION	PLACE	NUMBER TESTED	G6PD DEF.	SICKLE CELL	THALASSEMIA			HEMOGLOBIN TYPES								
						A_2	F	OSM. RES.	S	AS		AC		AD		B_2	Barts
UNITED STATES (CONT.)																	
588	Negroes (Pregnant)	Washington District of Columbia	3000		201 (6.7)												
356a	Negroes (Pregnant)	Washington District of Columbia	828						1	36 (4.5)		18 (2.2)					
588	Negroes (TB Patients)	Washington District of Columbia	330							28 (8.5)		4 (1.2)					
676	Negroes	Montgomery West Virginia	275		18 (6,5)												
484	Whites	Missouri	100		0												
479	Caucasians (Cord Blood)	St. Louis Missouri	90														1 (1.1)
484	Negroes	St. Louis Missouri	300		19 (6.3)												
162	Negroes	St. Louis Missouri	1000							94 (9.4)		26 (2.6)		4 (0.4)			
285	Negroes	St. Louis Missouri	500			4 (0.8)				43 (8.6)		12 (2.4)				6 (1.2)	
479	Negroes (Cord Blood)	St. Louis	449							47 (10.5)		9 (2.0)		2			32 (7.1)
206	Whites	Memphis Tennessee	309		0												

REF.	POPULATION	PLACE	NUMBER TESTED	G6PD DEF.	SICKLE CELL	THALASSEMIA			HEMOGLOBIN TYPES								
						A_2	F	OSM. RES.	S	AS	SC	AC	C	AD	AG	A	AL
UNITED STATES (CONT.)																	
388	Caucasians	Memphis Tennessee	92M	3 (3.3)												92	
206	Negroes	Memphis Tennessee	2539		211 (8.3)												
3a	Negroes (Pregnant)	Memphis Tennessee	2011		159 (7.9)												
388	Negroes	Memphis Tennessee	157M	22 (14.0)													
	Negroes	Memphis Tennessee	69F	4 (5.8)													
470	Negroes	West Tennessee	2800						19	254 (9.9)	4	60 (2.3)	1	1	1		1
	Whites	West Tennessee	1250													1250	
547	Melungeons	Sneedville Tennessee	78													78	
166	Non-Negroes	Durham North Carolina	734							1 (0.1)				1 (0.1)			
305	Whites	Durham North Carolina	25		0												
545	Cherokees	North Carolina	534													534	
	Lumbees	Robson County North Carolina	1332							23 (1.7)		23 (1.7)		1			

REF.	POPULATION	PLACE	NUMBER TESTED	G6PD DEF.	SICKLE CELL	THALASSEMIA A$_2$	THALASSEMIA F	THALASSEMIA OSM. RES.	HEMOGLOBIN TYPES S	AS	SJ	AC	C	AJ	AD	B$_2$
UNITED STATES (CONT.)																
546	Tri-racial Isolate (Indian Section)	Northeast North Carolina	232							4 (1.7)		13 (5.6)				
	Tri-racial Isolate (Non-Indian Section)	Northeast North Carolina	145							1 (0.7)		19 (13.1)				
305	Negroes	Durham North Carolina	100		7 (7.0)											
166	Negroes	Durham North Carolina	390				2		1	33 (9.0)	1	13 (3.3)		1	1	
547	Tri-racial Isolate	Walterboro South Carolina	74							9 (12.2)						
360	Negroes	South Carolina	719		57 (7.9)											
666	Negroes	Charleston South Carolina	1000		140 (14.0)											
665	Negroes	Sea Island South Carolina	2378		337 (14.2)											
547	Negroes	James Island South Carolina	276			9 (3.3)				57 (20.6)		2 (0.7)		1		3 (1.1)
544	Gullah Negroes	Coastal South Carolina	483						2	73 (15.5)		14 (3.1)	1			
186	Whites	Evans County Georgia	91	0												

REF.	POPULATION	PLACE	NUMBER TESTED	G6PD DEF.	SICKLE CELL	THALASSEMIA A_2	THALASSEMIA F	THALASSEMIA OSM. RES.	HEMOGLOBIN TYPES S	AS		AC				B_2
UNITED STATES (CONT.)																
186	Negroes	Evans and Bullock Counties, Georgia	247			6	2 (2.4)		2	19 (8.5)		4 (1.6)				
	Negroes	Evans and Bullock Counties, Georgia	76M	9 (11.8)												
	Negroes	Evans and Bullock Counties, Georgia	97F	10 (10.3)												
667	Whites	Augusta, Georgia	1000		0											
	Negroes	Augusta, Georgia	1800		101 (5.6)											
327	Negroes	Georgia	?													(2-3)
547	Seminoles	Hollywood Florida	374							36 (9.6)						
	Seminoles	Hollywood Florida	372	0												
206	Negroes	Gainesville Florida	674		65 (9.6)											
188a	Negroes (Pregnant)	Gainesville Florida	944						1	65 (7.0)		9 (1.0)				
289	Negroes	Birmingham Alabama	1500		122 (8.1)											
102b	Negroes	Tuskegee Alabama	332M	39 (11.7)												
	Negroes (Schizophrenic)	Tuskegee Alabama	783M	99 (12.6)												

REF.	POPULATION	PLACE	NUMBER TESTED	G6PD DEF.	SICKLE CELL	THALASSEMIA			HEMOGLOBIN TYPES								
						A_2	F	OSM. RES.	S	AS	SC	AC	C	AD		B_2	Barts
UNITED STATES (CONT.)																	
674	Whites	Mississippi	1045			8	3 (1.1)		1							1	
	Americans (Cord Blood)	Mississippi	429							7		7					13 (3.0)
	Negroes	Mississippi	1310			11	15 (2.0)		37	114 (11.8)	4	38 (3.7)	7	14		27 (2.1)	
674a	Negroes	Mississippi	12000				12 (0.1)										
521	Whites	New Orleans Louisiana	910		0												
488	Whites	New Orleans, Pineville, and Independence Louisiana	140							1 (0.7)							
	Negroes	New Orleans, Pineville, Independence Louisiana	564						18	47 (12.2)	4	10 (2.5)					
189	Negroes (TB Patients)	New Orleans Louisiana	220						1	15 (7.3)		9 (4.1)					
60a	Negroes (Pregnant)	New Orleans Louisiana	1200		100 (8.3)												

REF.	POPULATION	PLACE	NUMBER TESTED	G6PD DEF.	SICKLE CELL	THALASSEMIA A_2	THALASSEMIA F	THALASSEMIA OSM. RES.	HEMOGLOBIN TYPES S	AS	SC	AC	C			A	Barts
UNITED STATES (CONT.)																	
645	Negroes	Louisiana	100		5												
521	Negroes	Louisiana	692		45												
	Negroes	Louisiana	792		50 (6.3)												
609	Negroes	Galveston Texas	505							57		15					
610	Negroes	Galveston Texas	1550						6	139	1	35					
	Negroes	Galveston Texas	2055						6	196 (9.9)	1	50 (2.5)					
611	Negroes (Cord Blood)	Galveston Texas	1192														3 (0.3)
609	Whites	Galveston Texas	60													60	
611	Whites (Cord Blood)	Galveston Texas	361														1 (0.3)
310	Whites	Houston Texas	350													350	
114	Negroes	Houston Texas	150		10 (6.7)												
310	Negroes	Houston Texas	400						5	36 (10.5)	1	6 (2.0)	1				
379	Whites	Dallas Texas	322		0												

REF.	POPULATION	PLACE	NUMBER TESTED	G6PD DEF.	SICKLE CELL	THALASSEMIA			HEMOGLOBIN TYPES							
						A_2	F	OSM. RES.	S	AS		AC		A?		A
UNITED STATES (CONT.)																
728	Mexicans	Dallas Texas	239		0											
379	Negroes	Dallas Texas	1205		65 (5.4)											
450	Negroes	Dallas Texas	1165						7	78 (6.7)		40 (3.1)		1		
	Negroes	Dallas Texas	1276M	170 (13.3)												
741a	Negroes (Pregnant)	Dallas Texas	13835		1138 (8.2)											
583	Cherokees	Oklahoma	87							1 (1.1)						
	Muskhogean	Oklahoma	76							1 (1.3)						
	Caddoans	Oklahoma	12							1 (8.3)						
	Siouan Tribes	Oklahoma	9													9
	South Athabascans	Oklahoma	9													9
	Uto-Aztecans	Oklahoma	45													45
	Algonquins	Oklahoma	10													10
	Other Indians	Oklahoma	11													11

REF.	POPULATION	PLACE	NUMBER TESTED	G6PD DEF.	SICKLE CELL	THALASSEMIA			HEMOGLOBIN TYPES							
						A_2	F	OSM. RES.				AJ				A
MEXICO																
438	Tarahumara	Chihuahua	99													99
35	Tarahumara	Chihuahua	79M	0												
	Tarahumara	Chihuahua	20F	0												
439	Yaqui	Sonora	111													111
35	Yaqui	Sonora	66M	0												
	Yaqui	Sonora	4F	0												
438	Tarasco	Michoacan	133													133
35	Tarasco	Michoacan	55M	0												
	Tarasco	Michoacan	78F	0												
440a	Nahua	Puebla	356									2 (0.6)				
	Nahua	Puebla	303M	4 (1.3)												
35	Nahua	Puebla	43F	0												
372	Mazatecans	Papaloapan River Valley	123													123
440a	Mazatecans		138M	0								1 (0.7)				
661	Totonacans	Vera Cruz	18													18
440a	Totonacans	Vera Cruz	86M	0												86

REF.	POPULATION	PLACE	NUMBER TESTED	G6PD DEF.	SICKLE CELL	THALASSEMIA			HEMOGLOBIN TYPES							
						A_2	F	OSM. RES.		AS						A
MEXICO (CONT.)																
440a	Huastecans		77													77
	Huastecans		72M	0												
	Huastecans	San Luis	235M	3 (1.3)												
	Mixe		32M	0												32
468	Mixe		31													31
440a	Coras	Nayarit	101M	0						1 (1.0)						
440	Mexicans	Cuajinicuilapa Guerrero	418M	26 (6.2)						42 (10.0)						
	Mexicans	Ometepec Guerrero	406M							17 (4.2)						
	Mexicans	Ometepec Guerrero	405M	9 (2.2)												
	Mexicans	San Pedro Mixetepec, Oaxaca	335M	6 (1.8)						9 (2.7)						
	Mexicans	Pochutla Oaxaca	346M	1 (0.3)												346
369	Mexicans	Boquilla, Jamiltepec, Oaxaca	16M	0						1 (6.3)						
	Mexicans	Pedra Ancha, Jamiltepec, Oaxaca	15M	1 (6.7)						1 (6.7)						
	Mexicans	Pedra Ancha, Jamiltepec, Oaxaca	9F	1												9

REF.	POPULATION	PLACE	NUMBER TESTED	G6PD DEF.	SICKLE CELL	THALASSEMIA			HEMOGLOBIN TYPES							
						A_2	F	OSM. RES.								A
MEXICO (CONT.)																
438	Mixtecans	Mountain Regions Oaxaca	50													50
35	Mixtecans	Mountain Regions Oaxaca	48M	0												
	Mixtecans	Mountain Regions Oaxaca	2F	0												
438	Mixtecans	Coastal Regions Oaxaca	64													64
35	Mixtecans	Coastal Regions Oaxaca	56M	2 (3.6)												
	Mixtecans	Coastal Regions Oaxaca	8F	0												
661	Zapotecans	Oaxaca	16													16
440a	Zapotecans	Oaxaca	111M	0												111
	Chinantecans		21M	0												21
468	Chinantecans		49													49
440a	Popolocans		17M	0												17
468	Zoque		31													31
438	Yucatan Mayans		266													266
35	Yucatan Mayans		20M	0												
	Yucatan Mayans		26F	0												

REF.	POPULATION	PLACE	NUMBER TESTED	G6PD DEF.	SICKLE CELL	THALASSEMIA			HEMOGLOBIN TYPES							
						A_2	F	OSM. RES.		AS		AG				A
MEXICO (CONT.)																
661	Itza Mayans		67													67
	Tzeltal Mayans	Chiapas	57													57
	Tzotzil Mayans	Chiapas	11													11
468	Tzotzil Mayans	Chiapas	52													52
438	Tzeltal and Tzotzil Mayans	Chiapas	163													163
35	Tzeltal and Tzotzil Mayans	Chiapas	14M	0												
	Tzeltal and Tzotzil Mayans	Chiapas	18F	0												
661	Lacandon Mayans	Chiapas	34													34
468	Lacandon Mayans	Chiapas	55													55
661	Chol Mayans	Chiapas	13													13
440a	Chol Mayans	Chiapas	152M	0								1 (0.7)				
661	Mam Mayans	Chiapas	6													6
440a	Chontol	Chiapas	99M	2 (2.0)						2 (2.0)						

REF.	POPULATION	PLACE	NUMBER TESTED	G6PD DEF.	SICKLE CELL	THALASSEMIA A_2	THALASSEMIA F	THALASSEMIA OSM. RES.	HEMOGLOBIN TYPES	AS	SC	AC		AN		A
MEXICO (CONT.)																
661	Chiapanecans	Chiapas	6													6
468	Chiapanecans	Chiapas	39				1			1				2		
	Chiapanecans	Chiapas	45				1 (2.2)			1 (2.2)				2 (4.4)		
438	Mestizos		218									1 (0.5)				
35	Mestizos		82M	0												
	Mestizos		58F	0												
GUATEMALA																
661	Quiche Maya		39													39
468	Mam Maya		50													50
	Cakchiquel Maya		45													45
	Kekchi		50													50
BRITISH HONDURAS																
469	Maya	San Antonio	149													149
	Kekchi	Crique Sarco	111													111
250	Black Caribs	Stann Creek	454							100 (22.2)	1	13 (3.1)				

REF.	POPULATION	PLACE	NUMBER TESTED	G6PD DEF.	SICKLE CELL	THALASSEMIA A_2	THALASSEMIA F	THALASSEMIA OSM. RES.	HEMOGLOBIN TYPES	AS		AC				A
BRITISH HONDURAS (CONT.)																
250	Black Caribs	Seine Bight	211							49 (23.2)		5 (2.4)				
	Black Caribs	Hopkins	59							15 (25.4)						
HONDURAS																
472	Black Caribs	San Juan	300		24 (8.0)											
468	Jicaque		49													49
	Lenca		45													45
	Paya		47													47
EL SALVADOR																
96	Salvadoreans	Zacatecoluca	136							2 (1.5)						
	Salvadoreans	San Miguel	92							1 (1.1)						
NICARAGUA																
468	Chorotega		66													66
	Rama		40													40
	Subtiaba		28													28

REF.	POPULATION	PLACE	NUMBER TESTED	G6PD DEF.	SICKLE CELL	THALASSEMIA			HEMOGLOBIN TYPES							
						A_2	F	OSM. RES.	S	AS						A
NICARAGUA (CONT.)																
468	Sumo		50													50
	Miskito		117													117
313	Miskito (Mixed)	Puerto Cabezas	174M	33 (19.0)												
	Creoles	Puerto Cabezas	313M	57 (18.2)												
COSTA RICA																
469	Bribri	Salitre	78													78
	Cabecar	Ujarras	46													46
	Terrabas	Terraba	67							2 (3.0)						
	Boruca	Curres	73													73
PANAMA																
469	Guaymi	Cerro Iglesia	101						1	5 (5.9)						
	Guaymi-Cricamola	Almirante and Changuinola	52													52
	Choco	Rio Tuira	80													80
	San Blas Cuna	Ustupu	152													152

REF.	POPULATION	PLACE	NUMBER TESTED	G6PD DEF.	SICKLE CELL	THALASSEMIA			HEMOGLOBIN TYPES							
						A_2	F	OSM. RES.		AS						A
PANAMA (CONT.)																
469	San Blas Cuna	Ailigandi	198							2						
234	San Blas Cuna	Ailigandi	98							—						98
	San Blas Cuna	Ailigandi	296							2 (0.7)						
677	Panamanians	New San Juan Chagres River	154		8 (5.2)											
	Panamanians	Gatuncillo Chagres River	38		2 (5.3)											
	Panamanians	Los Guacos Chagres River	9		0											
	Panamanians	Agua Clara Chagres River	34		2 (5.9)											
	Panamanians	Santa Rosa Chagres River	39		8 (20.5)											
	Panamanians	Guayabalito Chagres River	48		5 (10.4)											
	Panamanians	La Laguna Chagres River	86		0											
	Panamanians	Mendoza Chagres River	146		4 (2.7)											
	Panamanians	Camaron Chagres River	74		12 (16.2)											
145	Whites		105		0											

REF.	POPULATION	PLACE	NUMBER TESTED	G6PD DEF.	SICKLE CELL	THALASSEMIA			HEMOGLOBIN TYPES							
						A_2	F	OSM. RES.		AS		AC				
PANAMA (CONT.)																
145	Mestizos		395		3 (0.8)											
	Mulattos		106		13 (12.3)											
	Negroes		264		38 (14.4)											
677	Mestizos and Negroes		777		59 (7.6)											
	Mestizos from the West Indies		998		96 (9.6)											
	Mestizos from Colombia		66		6 (9.1)											
	Mestizos from British Honduras		11		4											
	Mestizos from El Salvador		16		0											
	Mestizos from Elsewhere		504		48 (9.5)											
CUBA																
161	Cubans (Colored)	Havana	57		3 (5.3)											
187	Cubans (Colored)	Havana	200							13 (6.5)		1 (0.5)				

REF.	POPULATION	PLACE	NUMBER TESTED	G6PD DEF.	SICKLE CELL	THALASSEMIA			HEMOGLOBIN TYPES							
						A_2	F	OSM. RES.	S	AS	SC	AC		AD		
HAITI																
421	Haitians	Port-au-Prince	602		62 (10.3)											
276	Haitians	Port-au-Prince	381							44 (11.5)		7 (1.8)				
	Haitians	Tortuga	965		119 (12.3)											
70	Haitians	Tortuga	350		24 (6.9)											
DOMINICAN REPUBLIC																
317	Creoles		138		8 (5.8)											
JAMAICA																
740	Jamaicans		1018						2	106 (10.8)	2	30 (3.1)				
741	Jamaicans		153			6 (3.9)										
478	Rural Jamaicans (Negroid)		550							?		?		11 (2.0)		
354	Maroons	Accompong	167		6 (3.6)											
	Jamaicans	Goshen	260		10 (3.8)											

REF.	POPULATION	PLACE	NUMBER TESTED	G6PD DEF.	SICKLE CELL	THALASSEMIA			HEMOGLOBIN TYPES							
						A_2	F	OSM. RES.	S	AS	SC	AC	C			
JAMAICA (CONT.)																
354	East Indians	Cockburn Pen	152		1 (0.7)											
	Chinese	Kingston	100		0											
	Germans	Seaford Town	100		0											
	Caucasians	Kingston	70		0											
	Jamaicans	Kingston	1267		71 (5.6)											
PUERTO RICO																
552	Puerto Ricans		388		9 (2.3)											
475	Puerto Ricans	San Juan	500						1	8 (2.2)	2	2 (0.8)				
683	Puerto Ricans (Whites)		263		2 (0.8)											
	Puerto Ricans (Mulattos)		167		14 (8.4)											
	Puerto Ricans (Negroes)		188		10 (5.3)											
654	Puerto Ricans (Negroes)		602						2	29 (5.5)	2	7 (1.7)	1			
655	Puerto Ricans		1047	38 (3.6)												

REF.	POPULATION	PLACE	NUMBER TESTED	G6PD DEF.	SICKLE CELL	THALASSEMIA A_2	THALASSEMIA F	THALASSEMIA OSM. RES.	HEMOGLOBIN TYPES S	AS		AC		AD		
PUERTO RICO (CONT.)																
655	Caucasians		163	0												
	Negroes		199	7 (3.5)												
LESSER ANTILLES																
399	Negroes	Guadeloupe	3000		240 (8.0)											
87a	Guadeloupeans	Guadeloupe	1000						5	92 (9.7)		27 (2.7)		1		
490	Martiniquians	Martinique	213							20 (9.4)		9 (4.2)				
180	Martiniquians (Negroid Lepers)		111							8 (7.2)		3 (2.7)				
27	West Indians	St. Vincent	748							65 (8.7)		20 (2.7)				
	West Indians	Dominica	664							63 (9.5)		10 (1.5)				
779	Caribs	Salibia Reserve Dominica	62			6 (9.7)				1 (1.6)						
	Black Caribs	Salibia Reserve Dominica	65			5 (7.7)			2	3 (7.7)						
	Others	Salibia Reserve Dominica	3			1										

REF.	POPULATION	PLACE	NUMBER TESTED	G6PD DEF.	SICKLE CELL	THALASSEMIA			HEMOGLOBIN TYPES							
						A_2	F	OSM. RES.	S	AS	SC	AC		AE	AN	
LESSER ANTILLES (CONT.)																
27	West Indians	Barbados	912							64 (7.0)		42 (4.6)				
	West Indians	St. Lucia	825							115 (14.0)		31 (3.8)				
TRINIDAD																
316	Negroes		204							19 (9.3)		6 (2.9)		1	1	
662	Negroes		175M	23 (13.1)												
	East Indians		153M	21 (13.7)												
CURACAO																
604	West Indians	District I	112M	5 (4.5)												
603	West Indians	District I	506						1	24 (5.1)	1	20 (4.2)				
604	West Indians	District II	238M	27 (11.3)												
603	West Indians	District II	660						3	56 (9.2)	2	40 (6.4)				
604	West Indians	District III	129M	17 (13.2)												

REF.	POPULATION	PLACE	NUMBER TESTED	G6PD DEF.	SICKLE CELL	THALASSEMIA			HEMOGLOBIN TYPES							
						A_2	F	OSM. RES.	S	AS	SC	AC				A
CURACAO (CONT.)																
603	West Indians	District III	336						1	18 (6.5)	3	27 (8.9)				
602	West Indians		2499		267 (10.7)											
66	West Indians		4746		206 (4.3)											
WEST INDIES																
677	West Indians	Panama	998		96 (9.6)											
129	West Indians	Providencia Island	42													42
COLOMBIA																
42	Tunebo	San Luis de Chuscal, Santander	100													100
265b	Ica	Sierra Nevada de Santa Marta	86													86
	Ica	Sierra Nevada de Santa Marta	74			0										
	Paez	Tierradentro Southwest Colombia	103													103
	Paez	Tierradentro Southwest Colombia	20			0										

REF.	POPULATION	PLACE	NUMBER TESTED	G6PD DEF.	SICKLE CELL	THALASSEMIA			HEMOGLOBIN TYPES							
						A_2	F	OSM. RES.		AS		AC		AD		A
COLOMBIA (CONT.)																
774	Katios	Cristiania Antioquia	193													193
	Katios	Dabeiba Antioquia	126													126
	Katios	Apartado Antioquia	19													19
	Chocos	San Juan River Valley	24													24
	Guahibos	San Pedro de Arimena, Mata	41													41
	Cunas	Caiman River	12													12
	Other Indians		16													16
476	Negroes and Mulattos	Puerto Tejada	489		46 (9.4)											
	Whites and Indians	Puerto Tejada	88		0											
572	Negroes	San Juan River Valley	95							14 (14.7)						
	Negroes	Quibdo, Choco	262			1	1			28 (10.7)		7 (2.7)		10 (3.8)		
	Mestizos	San Pedro de Arimena, Mata	69													69

REF.	POPULATION	PLACE	NUMBER TESTED	G6PD DEF.	SICKLE CELL	THALASSEMIA			HEMOGLOBIN TYPES							
						A_2	F	OSM. RES.	S	AS	SC	AC		AJ		A
COLOMBIA (CONT.)																
774	Colombians	Medellin	1000							11 (1.2)	1	1 (0.2)				
572	Colombians	Medellin	500			2 (0.4)										
	Colombians	Medellin	600			10			8	60	3			1		
66	Colombians		77		1 (1.3)											
VENEZUELA																
45	Pariri	Machiques, Zulia	71													71
	Shaparu	Los Angeles del Tukuko, Zulia	17													17
	Macoita	Sierra de Perija Zulia	138													138
	Irapa	Sierra de Perija Zulia	137													137
	Motilon	Sierra de Perija Zulia	71													71
148	Tukuko	Sierra de Perija Zulia	12		0											
	Yupa	Ayapaima, Sierra de Perija, Zulia	110		2 (1.8)											
517	Tukuko and Irapa	Sierra de Perija Zulia	85		0											

REF.	POPULATION	PLACE	NUMBER TESTED	G6PD DEF.	SICKLE CELL	THALASSEMIA			HEMOGLOBIN TYPES							
						A_2	F	OSM. RES.								A
VENEZUELA (CONT.)																
54	Motilones		112		2 (1.8)											
	Guajaribos		9		0											
45	Carina	Cachama, Mesa de Guanipa, Anzoategui	51													51
	Yaruro	Guachara, Apure	96													96
	Taurepane	Gran Sabana Bolivar	107													107
	Arecuna	Gran Sabana Bolivar	42													42
	Camaracoto	Gran Sabana Bolivar	81													81
	Makiritare	Alto de Continamo Amazonas	86													86
	Bare-Baniva	Puerto Ayacucho Amazonas	9													9
	Guahibo	Puerto Ayacucho Amazonas	167													167
	Piaroa	Puerto Ayacucho Amazonas	120													120
	Waica	Boca de Ocamo and Boca de Mavaca Amazonas	141													141
	Shirishana	Guaviare, Bolivar	46													46

REF.	POPULATION	PLACE	NUMBER TESTED	G6PD DEF.	SICKLE CELL	THALASSEMIA			HEMOGLOBIN TYPES							
						A_2	F	OSM. RES.		AS		AC		AD		A
VENEZUELA (CONT.)																
45	Panare	El Mantecal Bolivar	32													32
404	Warrau (Guayo)	Orinoco River Delta	81													81
	Warrau (Winikina)	Orinoco River Delta	72													72
403	Paraujano	Sinamaica Lagoon	120							1 (0.8)						
756	Paraujano	Sinamaica Lagoon	123	0												
286	Negroes	Paparo, Miranda	40		1 (2.5)											
43	Negroes	Curiepe	140							6 (4.3)		4 (2.9)		2 (1.4)		
	Negroes	Yaracuy	120							7 (5.8)		3 (2.5)		3 (2.5)		
756	Negroes	Tapipa	26M	3 (11.5)												
	Negroes	Tapipa	30F	4 (13.3)												
54	Negroes	Caracas	1163		76 (6.5)											
43	Mestizos	Pregonero	84									1 (1.2)				
	Mestizos	Fajardo	103							1 (1.0)						

REF.	POPULATION	PLACE	NUMBER TESTED	G6PD DEF.	SICKLE CELL	THALASSEMIA A_2	THALASSEMIA F	THALASSEMIA OSM. RES.	HEMOGLOBIN TYPES AS	AC	AD	AJ	AK
VENEZUELA (CONT.)													
209	Mestizos	Barquisimeto	213		9 (4.2)								
43	Mestizo Students	Caracas	168			1 (0.6)			1 (0.6)	1 (0.6)			
54	Mestizos	Caracas	3970		105 (2.6)								
	Whites	Caracas	1248		19 (1.5)								
516a	Venezuelans	Toas Island Zulia	133						11 (8.3)				
682	Venezuelans	Bolivar	233		22 (9.4)								
539a	Venezuelans	Bolivar	300			2 (0.7)			14 (4.7)	3 (1.0)		1	
295	Venezuelans	Trujillo Trujillo	300			2 (0.7)		14 (4.7)	5 (2.2)				
	Venezuelans	Valera Trujillo	300					33 (11.0)	1 (0.3)				
43	Venezuelans	Punto Fijo Falcon	210		11 (5.2)								
44	Venezuelans	Caracas	434			5 (1.2)			6 (1.4)				1
54	Venezuelans	Caracas	6381		198 (3.1)								

REF.	POPULATION	PLACE	NUMBER TESTED	G6PD DEF.	SICKLE CELL	THALASSEMIA A_2	THALASSEMIA F	THALASSEMIA OSM. RES.	HEMOGLOBIN TYPES	AS		AC		AD		A
VENEZUELA (CONT.)																
756	Venezuelans	Caracas	300	6 (2.0)												
296	Venezuelan Children	Caracas	315			3 (1.0)				3 (1.0)						
340	Venezuelan Children	Caracas	500					4 (0.8)		17 (3.4)		3 (0.6)		1		
66	Venezuelans		123		0											
GUYANA																
46	Wapishana	Aishalton	120													120
	Macushi	Lethem	118													118
	Acawai	Kamarang	87													87
44	Wapishana, Macushi, and Acawai		79			0										
SURINAM																
459a	Carib		40M	1 (2.5)												
	Carib		83F	3 (3.6)												
	Oyana		24M	4 (16.7)												

REF.	POPULATION	PLACE	NUMBER TESTED	G6PD DEF.	SICKLE CELL	THALASSEMIA			HEMOGLOBIN TYPES							
						A_2	F	OSM. RES.	S	AS	SC	AC				B_2
SURINAM (CONT.)																
459a	Oyana		15F	2 (13.3)												
364	"Red Indians"		?							(0.5)						
745	Bush Negroes	Village I	?		(17.0)											
	Bush Negroes	Village II	?		(25.0)											
425	Djukas (Bush Negroes)		343						4	46 (14.6)		9 (2.6)				
459a	Djukas (Bush Negroes)		63M	7 (11.1)												
	Djukas (Bush Negroes)		5F	0												
	Negroes	Moengo	110M	20 (18.2)												
	Negroes	Moengo	14F	0												
364	Djukas (Bush Negroes)	Kabel	519						1	87 (17.5)	3	27 (5.8)				
	Djukas (Bush Negroes)	Moengo	172						2	35 (22.1)	1	8 (5.2)				
	Djukas (Bush Negroes)	Stoelman's Island	275						1	31 (11.6)		9 (3.3)				
539	Djukas (Bush Negroes)	Upper Surinam River	311M	63 (20.3)		7 (2.3)				43 (13.8)		13 (4.2)				7 (2.3)

REF.	POPULATION	PLACE	NUMBER TESTED	G6PD DEF.	SICKLE CELL	THALASSEMIA A_2	THALASSEMIA F	THALASSEMIA OSM. RES.	HEMOGLOBIN TYPES		AS	SC	AC				A	B_2
SURINAM (CONT.)																		
539	Djukas (Bush Negroes)	Brokopondo Middle Surinam River	336M	65 (19.3)		3 (0.9)					60 (18.2)	1	14 (4.5)					7 (2.1)
	Djukas (Bush Negroes)	Tapanahony River	88M	14 (15.9)		1 (1.1)					19 (21.6)		2 (2.3)					
	Djukas (Bush Negroes)	North Surinam	115M	8 (7.0)		1 (0.9)					12 (10.4)		7 (6.1)					2 (1.7)
181	Creoles		789		88 (11.2)													
459a	Javanese		66M	2 (3.0)														
	Javanese		17F	1 (5.9)														
181	Hindus and Whites		231		0													
FRENCH GUIANA																		
140	Oyampi	Upper Oyapoc River	117			7 (23.9)	22										117	
	Oyana	Upper Maroni River	106			2 (13.2)	12										106	
	Emerillon	Camopi and Tampoc Rivers	33			3 (21.2)	4										33	
	Galibi	Maroni River Mouth	214			6 (3.3)	1				21 (9.8)		1 (0.5)					

REF.	POPULATION	PLACE	NUMBER TESTED	G6PD DEF.	SICKLE CELL	THALASSEMIA			HEMOGLOBIN TYPES							
						A_2	F	OSM. RES.		AS		AC				
FRENCH GUIANA (CONT.)																
140	Palikur	Oyapoc River Mouth	75			3	1 (5.3)			1 (1.3)						
144	Boni (Bush Negroes)	Maroni River	?							(17.9)		(6.8)				
721	Creoles	Cayenne	345							35 (10.1)		6 (1.7)				
256	Creoles	Cayenne	102		4 (3.9)											
	Europeans	Cayenne	36		0											
	Arabs	Cayenne	10		0											
	Syrians	Cayenne	3		0											
	Chinese	Cayenne	8		0											
BRAZIL																
628	Pariukur	Uaca and Urukua Amapa	98		0											
	Galiby	Curipy River Amapa	123		0											
	Caripuna	Curipy River Amapa	48		0											
	Indians (Mixed)	Curipy River Amapa	91		0											
368	Whites	Manaus, Amazonas	90		0											

REF.	POPULATION	PLACE	NUMBER TESTED	G6PD DEF.	SICKLE CELL	THALASSEMIA			HEMOGLOBIN TYPES							
						A_2	F	OSM. RES.	S	AS		AC				
BRAZIL (CONT.)																
594	Brazilians	Manaus, Amazonas	1642		57 (3.5)											
	Indians (Mixed)	Manaus, Amazonas	90		0											
	Brazilians	Codajas, Amazonas	672		25 (3.7)											
	Indians	Rio Andira Amazonas	100		0											
628	Canella	Barro do Corda Maranhao	299		0											
	Guajajara	Barro do Corda Maranhao	12		0											
368	Caraja	Bananal, Goyaz	86		0											
464a	Brazilians	Fortaleza, Ceara	179						2	6 (4.5)		2 (1.1)				
628	Brazilians	Aguas Bellas Pernambuco	166		3 (1.8)											
594	Brazilians	Paulo Afonso Bahia	200							9 (4.5)		1 (0.5)				
455	Whites	Salvador Bahia	249		0											
	Mulattos	Salvador Bahia	507		29 (4.9)											
	Negroes	Salvador Bahia	244		21 (8.6)											

REF.	POPULATION	PLACE	NUMBER TESTED	G6PD DEF.	SICKLE CELL	THALASSEMIA			HEMOGLOBIN TYPES							
						A_2	F	OSM. RES.		AS	SC	AC		AD	A?	
BRAZIL (CONT.)																
368	Mulattos	Itaparica Island Bahia	70		11 (15.7)											
502a	Whites	Northeast Brazil	660M	31 (4.7)												
	Light Mulattos	Northeast Brazil	127M	10 (7.9)												
	Dark Mulattos and Negroes	Northeast Brazil	996M	85 (8.5)												
491a	Brazilians	Northeast Brazil	2098							83 (4.0)		29 (1.4)				
594	Whites	Belo Horizonte Minas Gerais	72		0											
	Mulattos and Negroes	Belo Horizonte Minas Gerais	128		8 (6.2)											
	Whites	Belo Horizonte Minas Gerais	250							3 (1.2)				1		
	Mulattos	Belo Horizonte Minas Gerais	350							16 (4.6)		10 (2.9)		1	1	
	Negroes	Belo Horizonte Minas Gerais	400							46 (11.7)	1	12 (3.3)		2	1	
	Whites	Duque de Caxias Rio de Janeiro	105		0											
	Mulattos	Duque de Caxias Rio de Janeiro	120		4 (3.3)											

REF.	POPULATION	PLACE	NUMBER TESTED	G6PD DEF.	SICKLE CELL	THALASSEMIA			HEMOGLOBIN TYPES							
						A_2	F	OSM. RES.								
BRAZIL (CONT.)																
594	Negroes	Duque de Caxias Rio de Janeiro	720		37 (5.1)											
	Indians (Mixed)	Duque de Caxias Rio de Janeiro	17		0											
627	Negroes	Rio de Janeiro	890		93 (10.4)											
	Mulattos	Rio de Janeiro	140		11 (7.9)											
	Mixed Bloods	Rio de Janeiro	100		9 (9.0)											
	Whites	Rio de Janeiro	120		0											
	Mongoloids	Rio de Janeiro	30		0											
594	Negroes (Patients)	Rio de Janeiro	80		5 (6.2)											
	White Soldiers	Rio de Janeiro	1232		7 (0.6)											
	Mulatto Soldiers	Rio de Janeiro	454		19 (4.2)											
	Negro Soldiers	Rio de Janeiro	249		22 (8.8)											
368	Whites	Rio de Janeiro	86		0											
	Negroes	Rio de Janeiro	32		0											

REF.	POPULATION	PLACE	NUMBER TESTED	G6PD DEF.	SICKLE CELL	THALASSEMIA			HEMOGLOBIN TYPES							
						A_2	F	OSM. RES.	S	AS	SC	AC	C	AD	AG	
BRAZIL (CONT.)																
368	Mulattos	Rio de Janeiro	203		6 (3.0)											
101	Negroes	Santos, Sao Paulo	302		27 (8.9)											
	Mulattos	Santos, Sao Paulo	329		22 (6.7)											
	Negro Schoolchildren	Santos, Sao Paulo	117		3 (2.6)											
	Negro Asylum Inmates	Santos, Sao Paulo	55		2 (3.6)											
102	Whites	Santos, Sao Paulo	64		0											
594	Negroes	Sao Paulo Sao Paulo	330		16 (4.8)											
669a	Whites	Sao Paulo Sao Paulo	928			7 (0.8)			2	2 (0.4)		2 (0.4)	2	3	5	
	Mulattos	Sao Paulo Sao Paulo	110			2 (1.8)			1	6 (8.2)	2	1 (2.7)			1	
	Negroes	Sao Paulo Sao Paulo	330			10 (3.0)			3	23 (8.2)	1	2 (0.9)		2		
758	Whites	Sao Paulo Sao Paulo	234M	9 (3.8)												
	Whites (Lepers)	Sao Paulo Sao Paulo	323M	9 (2.8)												

REF.	POPULATION	PLACE	NUMBER TESTED	G6PD DEF.	SICKLE CELL	THALASSEMIA			HEMOGLOBIN TYPES							
						A_2	F	OSM. RES.								
BRAZIL (CONT.)																
758	Negroes (Lepers)	Sao Paulo City Sao Paulo	83M	8 (9.6)												
368	Japanese	Sao Paulo	89		0											
	Whites	Piracicaba Sao Paulo	87		0											
	Mulattos	Piracicaba Sao Paulo	41		1 (2.4)											
	Whites	Ilhabella Sao Sebastiao Island	77		0											
	Whites	Buzios and Vitoria Sao Sebastiao Island	73		1 (1.4)											
	Mulattos	Ilhabella Sao Sebastiao Island	43		2 (4.6)											
594	Whites	Curitiba Parana	123		0											
	Mulattos	Curitiba Parana	145		6 (4.1)											
	Negroes	Curitiba Parana	198		8 (4.0)											
628	Bororo	Northern Mato Grosso	121		0											

REF.	POPULATION	PLACE	NUMBER TESTED	G6PD DEF.	SICKLE CELL	THALASSEMIA			HEMOGLOBIN TYPES							
						A_2	F	OSM. RES.								A
BRAZIL (CONT.)																
628	Taunay and Lalima	Miranda District Mato Grosso	4		0											
	Mixed (White-Indian)	Miranda District Mato Grosso	1424		0											
	Tereno	Southern Mato Grosso	230		0											
	Cayua	Southern Mato Grosso	239		0											
	Cadueo	Southern Mato Grosso	17		0											
	Guarani	Southern Mato Grosso	8		0											
	Laiano	Southern Mato Grosso	10		0											
	Quinquinan	Southern Mato Grosso	3		0											
	Mixed Indians	Southern Mato Grosso	80		0											
510	Xavante	Sao Domingoes Mato Grosso	79	0												79
507a	Xavante	Simoes Lopes and Sao Marcos Mato Grosso	211	0												211

REF.	POPULATION	PLACE	NUMBER TESTED	G6PD DEF.	SICKLE CELL	THALASSEMIA			HEMOGLOBIN TYPES							
						A_2	F	OSM. RES.		AS		AC		AD		A
	BRAZIL (CONT.)															
594	Cayapo	South Para	96	0												96
368	Caingang	Palmas Parana	77		0											
263	Guarani	Nonoai Rio Grande do Sul	47		0											
	Guarani (Mixed)	Nonoai Rio Grande do Sul	5		0											
	Caingang	Rio Grande do Sul	334													334
	Caingang	Rio Grande do Sul	27		0											
	Caingang (Mixed)	Rio Grande do Sul	106													106
	Caingang (Mixed)	Rio Grande do Sul	22		0											
772	Whites	Porto Alegre Rio Grande do Sul	102M	4 (3.9)												
	Whites	Porto Alegre Rio Grande do Sul	141F	7 (5.0)												
	Mestizos	Porto Alegre Rio Grande do Sul	101M	11 (10.9)												
	Mestizos	Porto Alegre Rio Grande do Sul	257F	37 (14.4)												
679	Mestizos	Porto Alegre Rio Grande do Sul	320							9 (2.8)		2 (0.6)		2		

REF.	POPULATION	PLACE	NUMBER TESTED	G6PD DEF.	SICKLE CELL	THALASSEMIA A_2	THALASSEMIA F	THALASSEMIA OSM. RES.	HEMOGLOBIN TYPES	AS		AC				A
BRAZIL (CONT.)																
772	Mulattos	Porto Alegre Rio Grande do Sul	99M	15 (15.2)												
	Mulattos	Porto Alegre Rio Grande do Sul	225F	31 (13.8)												
679	Mulattos	Porto Alegre Rio Grande do Sul	357							21 (5.9)		6 (1.7)				
772	Negroes	Porto Alegre Rio Grande do Sul	116M	13 (11.2)												
	Negroes	Porto Alegre Rio Grande do Sul	197F	37 (18.8)												
679	Negroes	Porto Alegre Rio Grande do Sul	337							30 (8.9)		3 (0.9)				
CHILE																
298	Chileans	Santiago	9362		9 (0.1)											
299	Chileans	Santiago	1037	0												
298	Mapuche (Araucanians)	Temuco	450		0											
241	Mapuche (Araucanians)	Temuco	116	0												116
	Pehuenche (Araucanians)	Lonquimay	113	0												113
299	Alacaluf	Puerto Eden	45	0												

REF.	POPULATION	PLACE	NUMBER TESTED	G6PD DEF.	SICKLE CELL	THALASSEMIA A$_2$	THALASSEMIA F	THALASSEMIA OSM. RES.	HEMOGLOBIN TYPES							A
BOLIVIA																
779	Quechua	Altiplano	55			1 (1.8)										55
	Castellano	Altiplano	140			0										140
	Mestizos	Altiplano	235			5 (2.1)										235
	Fishermen	Altiplano	53			0										53
	Whites	Altiplano	30			1 (3.3)										30
	Negroes	Altiplano	2			0										2
	Indians	Altiplano	10			0										10
	Aymara	Altiplano	2017			33 (1.9)	5									2017
773	Aymara	Coroico and Caranavi Yungas and Anacoraimes Altiplano	521													521
	Tacana	Riberalta Beni	11													11
	Chama	Riberalta Beni	27													27
	Chacobo	Chacobo Beni	14													14

REF.	POPULATION	PLACE	NUMBER TESTED	G6PD DEF.	SICKLE CELL	THALASSEMIA			HEMOGLOBIN TYPES							
						A_2	F	OSM. RES.								A
BOLIVIA (CONT.)																
773	Itonama	San Ramon Beni	109													109
	More	MaMore Beni	67													67
	Siriono	San Pedro Beni	27													27
PERU																
469a'	Ticuna	Cushillococha Amazon River	122													122
	Yagua	Chimbote Amazon River	9													9
	Aguaruna	Santa Maria de Nieva Maranon and Nieva Rivers	151													151
	Piro	Bufeo Pozo Urubamba River	90													90
	Campa	Chicosa and El Encuentro Urubamba and Tambo Rivers	89													89
130	Isconahua	Eastern Peru	16													16
469a'	Isconahua	Calleria Ucayali River	14													14

REF.	POPULATION	PLACE	NUMBER TESTED	G6PD DEF.	SICKLE CELL	THALASSEMIA			HEMOGLOBIN TYPES							
						A_2	F	OSM. RES.								A
	PERU (CONT.)															
469a'	Shipibo	San Francisco Calleria and Panaillo Ucayali River	142													142
130	Shipibo	Eastern Peru	70													70
76	Lupaca (Aymara)	Jaillihuaya	58													58
75	Lupaca (Aymara)	Jaillihuaya	34M	0												
	Lupaca (Aymara)	Jaillihuaya	24F	0												
586a	Aymara		268	0												
469a'	Aymara	Puno	93													93
76	Colla (Quechua)	Paucarcolla	119													119
75	Colla (Quechua)	Paucarcolla	70M	0												
	Colla (Quechua)	Paucarcolla	50F	0												
586a	Quechua		66	0												
469a'	Quechua	Puno	181													181
75	Motilones	Tarapoto	50M	0												

REF.	POPULATION	PLACE	NUMBER TESTED	G6PD DEF.	SICKLE CELL	THALASSEMIA			HEMOGLOBIN TYPES							
						A_2	F	OSM. RES.		AS						A
PERU (CONT.)																
236	Peruvians	Cayalti	281							2 (0.7)						
586a	Whites		26	0												
	Metizos		44	0												
ECUADOR																
469a	Quechua	Andes Plateau	656													656
	Colorado	Santo Domingo de los Colorado	36													36
	Cayapa	Rio Cayapas	135													135
	Jivaro	Oriente Province	233													233
	Secoya	Cuyabeno Rio Aguarico	48													48

ADDENDA

Data contained in two recent studies add so significantly to our knowledge of the distributions of the abnormal hemoglobins that they are shown below; but no reference is made to them in the text.

REF.	POPULATION	PLACE	NUMBER TESTED	G6PD DEF.	SICKLE CELL	THALASSEMIA			HEMOGLOBIN TYPES							
						A_2	F	OSM. RES.	E	AE						
	BURMA															
	Burmese		414							[108] (26.1)						
	Mon		51							[12] (23.5)						
	Shan		99							[25] (25.3)						
	Karen		112							[6] (5.4)						
	Chin	North Burma	187							[2] (1.1)						

From: Flatz, G. (1967) Hemoglobin E: Distribution and population dynamics. Humangenetik, 3:189-234.

REF.	POPULATION	PLACE	NUMBER TESTED	G6PD DEF.	SICKLE CELL	THALASSEMIA			HEMOGLOBIN TYPES							
						A_2	F	OSM. RES.	S	AS	SD	AD	C		AJ	
ADDENDA (CONT.)																
IRAN																
	Iranians (Patients with no anemia)	Shiraz	200									2 (2.0)				
	Iranians (Patients with anemia)	Teheran	400			70 (17.5)			3	17 (5.3)	1		1		1	

From: Rahbar, S., Beale, D., Isaacs, W. A., and Lehmann, H. (1967) Abnormal haemoglobins in Iran. Observation of a new variant - Haemoglobin J Iran ($\alpha_2 \beta_2$77 His → Asp). British Medical Journal, 1:674-677.

Milton Keynes UK
Ingram Content Group UK Ltd.
UKHW020008071024
449327UK00031B/2704

9 780202 362649

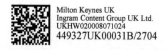